FESTSCHRIFT
The Institute of Nuclear Medicine
50 Years

University College NHS Foundation Trust
and
University College London

October 2011

Dedication:

The families of the Staff of the Institute of Nuclear Medicine

Acknowledgements

We are most grateful for the significant secretarial and editing support given by Mariam Cullum and Hansa Jadeja, and their many years of dedicated service to the Institute.

We wish to acknowledge all the present and past staff, who over many years, offered loyalty and commitment, with valuable contributions. We also acknowledge the meritorious contributions made by two past staff: Professor P H Jarritt and Dr. Durval Costa.

ISBN 978-3-642-24714-9 Springer-Verlag Berlin Heidelberg New York

Bibliographic information Deutsche Bibliothek
The Deutsche Bibliothek lists this publication in Deutsche Nationalbibliographie;
detailed bibliographic data is available in the internet at <http://dnb.ddb.de>.

Springer Medizin
Springer-Verlag GmbH
ein Unternehmen von Springer Science+Business
springer.de

© Springer-Verlag Berlin Heidelberg 2012

Cover Images represent:
- Treatment of paediatric cancer (whole body)
- Diagnosing abnormal focus of hyperinsulinism in the pancreas of 3 month infant (Section image)
- Localizing site of refractory Temporal Lobe Epilepsy in non lesional MR
- Pre-clinical iodine-125 labelled state-dependent sodium channel (VGSC) tracer in Balb/C mice with apparent uptake in brown adipose tissue.

Planning: Diana Kraplow, Heidelberg
Project management: Dr. Astrid Horlacher, Heidelberg
Typesetting and cover design: Fotosatz-Service Köhler GmbH – Reinhold Schöberl, Würzburg

SPIN 80114646   18/5141 – 5 4 3 2 1 0

Content

Part I: The first 25 Years
1961–1985

E.S. Williams and P.J. Ell

Part II: Growth and Progress 1986–2011

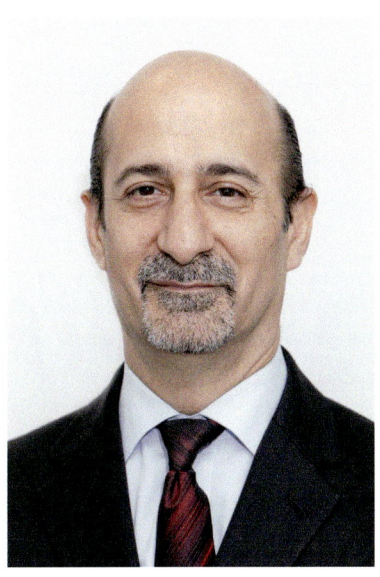

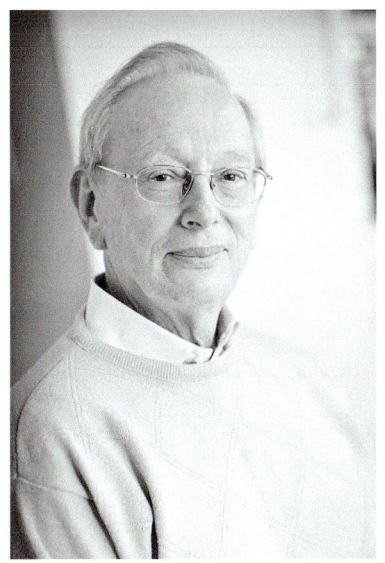

Dr. Jamshed Bomanji MD PhD FRCP FRCR
Head
Department of Nuclear Medicine

Professor Peter J. Ell FMedSci Dr. HC
Senior Investigator NIHR
Consultant Physician UCLH
Emeritus Professor UCL

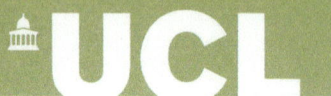

September 2011

How best to describe Peter Ell? An icon? A beacon? An inspirational leader? All are accurate but none completely captures the influence and inspiration that Peter has brought to the development of nuclear medicine. His reputation has been global and remarkable.

The 50th birthday of the Institute is therefore most worthy of celebration, and this book provides an important historical record. Peter has laid foundations which will bear the weight of much future development in this critically important area in which UCL and UCLH have so strong a combined interest.

University College London Gower Street London WC1E 6BT
Tel: +44 (0)20 7679 7234   Fax: +44 (0)20 7388 5412
www.ucl.ac.uk/provost   Email: provost@ucl.ac.uk

6

University College London Hospitals **NHS**

NHS Foundation Trust

Chief Executive's Office
Trust Headquarters
2nd Floor Central
250 Euston Road
London
NW1 2PG

It is a great privilege to celebrate the Golden Jubilee of the Institute of Nuclear Medicine with this impressive Festschrift. It is a historical document, narrating the creation of the Institute in 1961 by Sir Brian Windeyer, up to the present time. Already in 1985, Sir Brian Windeyer stated that the Institute had undoubtedly achieved an important place in modern medicine and it continues to flourish today.

UCL and UCLH have created an impressive powerhouse of biomedical research and clinical practice over recent years, built upon their historical strengths. The Institute of Nuclear Medicine has played an important part in this success and I would like to pay tribute to Professor Peter Ell for his visionary leadership of the Institute for much of its existence.

In all these years, the Institute has been at the forefront of the development of this medical speciality, based on the application of the radioactive tracer methodology. It is in this field that the vision "Atoms for Peace" finds its highest expression.

The Festschrift documents the relentless and admirably progress achieved, over these 50 years. Possibly much before the concept of translational medicine become a bye word for modern research endeavour, the Institute has put in practice this concept, in cancer, cardiovascular and neurodegeneration.

Nuclear Medicine is a technological demanding and resource intense activity. It is truly multidisciplinary and requires the dedicated expertise of many disciplines: health physics, radiation physics, computer modelling, statistical analysis, technical and nursing expertise, and last but not least, the dedication of medical staff.

The Institute has superbly met these challenges. The UCLH Trust Board, supported by the UCLH Charity Trustees are proud to continue to support the Institute – now housed in a brand new department, it clearly continues to lead, stimulate and engage. Current investment in the UK's first PET/MR in the new ground-breaking Cancer Centre is a taste of what's in store for the next 50 years.

On behalf of the Board, and our grateful patients, I wish the Institute every success for the future.

Sir Robert Naylor
Chief Executive
University College London

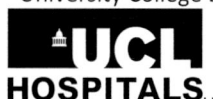

HOSPITALS UCL Hospitals is an NHS Foundation Trust comprising: The Eastman Dental Hospital, The Heart Hospital, Hospital for Tropical Diseases, National Hospital for Neurology & Neurosurgery, The Royal London Hospital for Integrated Medicine and University College Hospital (incorporating the former Middlesex Hospital and Elizabeth Garrett Hospitals

Comprehensive Biomedical Research Centre

Translational research for patient benefit   University College **NHS**
London Hospitals
NHS Foundation Trust

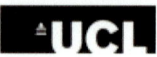

It is a great pleasure to acknowledge the international strength and superb leadership of the Institute for Nuclear Medicine. As a cutting edge discipline, the relevance of this area of expertise continues to increase.

One of the main planks of the current experimental medicine agenda is the ability to stratify patients based on complex characteristics. This is important in order to best target new therapies, or indeed, prevent unwanted side effects of interventions. There is no better example of a technology able to support such a programme as nuclear medicine. The ability to use probes for apoptosis, angiogenesis, cell proliferation and receptor status, to name a few, will become increasingly important in the ability of UCLH/UCL to deliver the best forms of stratified and experimental medicine. Placing this expertise together with the recent purchase of a PET/MR platform really places our institution in a good position.

I am delighted that the NIHR UCLH/UCL Comprehensive Biomedical Research Centre has been able to support some of the recent developments of the Institute, and, importantly, allow clinical academics the time to maximize the opportunity to exploit these technologies for key research initiatives.

On this occasion of the retirement of Peter Ell, I would like to pay tribute to his superb leadership, which not only has led to the current level of strength, but also will underpin the continual growth of the Institute in years to come.

Deenan Pillay

Deenan Pillay, Professor of Virology and Director NIHR UCLH/UCL CBRC
University College London, Cruciform Building, Gower Street, London WC1E 6BT

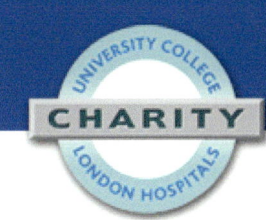

The Charity has a long history of involvement with and support of the Institute of Nuclear Medicine and its outstanding development program and clinical service.

Since early 1999, when the Institute began work with Positron Emission Tomography, the Charity has been a contributor both in early-stage development and in funding major initiatives such as the first PETCT scanner in the United Kingdom (the first patient investigated in January 2002 at UCLH). Today, the Charity continues this close association and interest, not least through having Professor Peter Ell as one of our seven Trustees.

This Festschrift is testament to the professional development of the Institute from the early days of growth to the remarkable resources and dedicated professionalism available today. Over these 50 years, frequent restructuring has occurred to meet advances in improvements in health services and patient care. It has been one of the great strengths of the Institute to be able to meet all these challenges whilst maintaining consistent and constant progress.

Over the years, the staff of the Institute have rightly achieved international recognition and are widely seen as proud ambassadors for Nuclear Medicine.

Today, on behalf of all the Charitable Trustees, I would like to say how delighted we are to renew our long-term association with and commitment to the Institute by funding the first fully integrated PETMR in the country. It is hoped that the integration of PET and MR information will bring new knowledge in many of the most significant areas in medicine, enhancing the understanding of disease mechanisms, refining the unique pathology signature for each patient, and enabling early recognition of disease modification and response.

With considerable past achievements, exciting future development plans and highly dedicated staff we congratulate the Institute for the last 50 years and look forward to further progress and success.

Yours sincerely,

Chairman
UCLH Charity

9

Senior Staff of the Institute of Nuclear Medicine

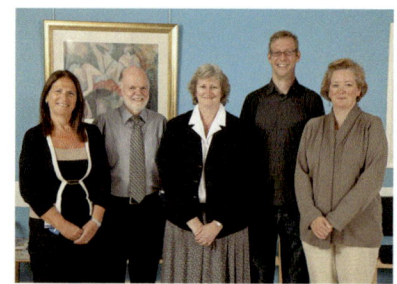

From Left:
Professor Simona Ben Haim, Professor Brian Hutton, Dr. Elizabeth Prvulovich,
Dr. Eric Arstad, Mrs. Wendy Waddington
Below: Dr. Ashley Groves and Dr. Irfan Kayani. Missing from this group are Dr. Ian Cullum
and Dr. Leon Menezes

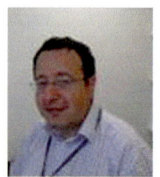

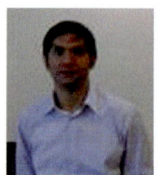

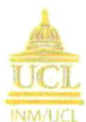

The Staff of the Institute of Nuclear Medicine

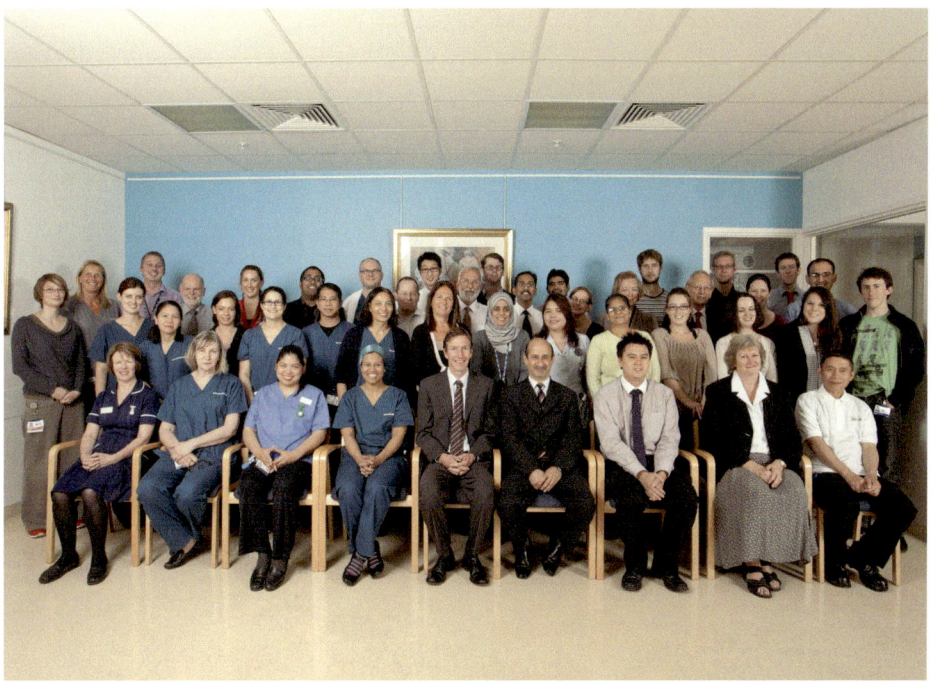

Part I: The first 25 Years
1961–1985

Institute of
Nuclear Medicine

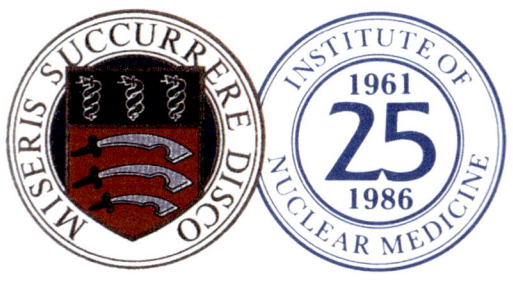

E.S. Williams

M.D., B.Sc., PhD., F.R.C.P., F.R.C.R.

and

P.J. Ell
M.D., M.Sc., P.D., M.R.C.P., F.R.C.R

Acknowledgments

This account could not have been prepared without the close co-operation of past and present members of the staff, and we warmly record, in particular, the help of Professor R.P. Ekins, Drs Britton, Keeling, Jarritt and Cullum as well as our appreciation of the dedication of Miss Joan Potter for patiently producing many drafts of the manuscript.
The Institute of Nuclear Medicine – the First 25 Years.
E.S. Williams and P.J. Ell, London, September 1986

Foreword

Progress during the past quarter of a century in the medical use and development of radiopharmaceuticals, and the benefit derived from their application, especially in diagnostic services, has been outstanding. The use of the term Nuclear Medicine to embrace all applications of radioactive materials in diagnosis or treatment or in medical research apparently emerged only in the early 1950s by which time the Middlesex Hospital and Medical School, as explained by Sir Brian Windeyer in his preface, had already established itself as a leader in the field and indeed had through the then Professor of Medical Physics – Sidney Russ – in 1921 led the world by setting up the first organisation concerned with X-ray and Radium protection. It was, however, thanks to the foresight of Brian Windeyer and Professor J.E. Roberts that the concept of an Institute of Nuclear Medicine emerged. This volume, as well as recognising the debt owed to these pioneers, succinctly sets forth the contributions made by the Institute and marks the 25th anniversary of its foundation. The authors, Edward Williams and Peter Ell are, of course, especially suited to produce this record because of their first hand experience, having been respectively past and present Directors of the Institute. In Bloomsbury and in the new University College and Middlesex School of Medicine we recognise the tremendous service and Academic contributions made by the staff of the Institute of Nuclear Medicine. This volume should provide inspiration and encouragement to all those associated with or interested in the still developing and expanding field of Nuclear Medicine.

Denys Fairweather M.D., F.R.C.O.G
Vice-Provost (Medicine), University College London
and Head (Elect) of the University College and
Middlesex School of Medicine, University College London

Foreword

This Medical School is very proud of the Institute of Nuclear Medicine which was founded here 25 years ago. The foresight of Sir Brian Windeyer together with the expertise of Dr. Edward Williams in its earlier years and later with Dr. Peter Ell, has assured the place of Nuclear Medicine as an important discipline in medical care and research. My sincere congratulations go to them for all that they have achieved. Now that we are forming a single School of Medicine with University College I am sure the Institute will continue to be of major national importance.

W.W. Slack M.A., M.CH., F.R.C.S.
Dean
The Middlesex Hospital Medical School

Preface

I am very pleased to have been invited to make some contribution to this 25th anniversary of the Institute of Nuclear Medicine as I am delighted that it has developed from two other organisations in which I had interest and association, the Department of Radiotherapy and the Department of Physics as Applied to Medicine.

I went to the Middlesex Hospital and Medical School in 1930 to be employed as a Radium Officer and was given an office in the Department of Physics in which Professor Sidney Russ held the chair. In 1921 he had started the British X-ray and Radium Protection Committee which was the first such organisation in the world. In 1930 X-ray treatments of patients were carried out by the radiologists who were using X-rays for diagnostic purposes as by far their main concern. Radium had been originally used mainly as a surface application but was used more and more by intracavity and interstitial applications into normal body cavities or by direct insertion into the tissues by surgeons and gynaecologists. The dermatologists continued with surface applications.

Radium supplies were kept in the Department of Physics and Professor Russ was involved with a certain amount of investigation into the effects obtained by its use. The Radium Officer's post was to keep records, supervise the proper retention and provision of the radium supplies and it was necessary to keep close contact with what was being done. Gradually the Radium Officers had more to do with the actual treatment of patients and it was becoming obvious that more patients had to be treated by both X-rays and radium. This led to the necessity to create, in place of the Radium Officers, some Radiotherapists who could take on both duties.

In 1937 a new Department of Radiotherapy had been created at the Middlesex with new X-ray therapy apparatus and facilities for dealing with the radium and it was to work here that I became a radiotherapist. It was obvious that it was important to continue close association with the Department of Physics as Applied to Medicine which continued to supply radium to the new department.

In 1946 Professor J.E. Roberts was appointed to take over the Physics Department and by 1948 had arranged more laboratory services in the upper part of the Barnato-Joel Laboratories. The activities during the war had made more radioactive substances available and I remember being greatly interested in the treatment of a thyroid condition by ^{131}I. A registrar and nursing sister were stationed there, having been supplied by the Radiotherapy Department and the work continued to increase and promote interest.

By 1961 Professor Roberts had need to extend his staff to cope with the considerable amount of work involved as I was then Dean as well as Professor in charge of the Radiotherapy Department I was able to agree with him that a larger organisation was necessary.

This new department "The Institute of Nuclear Medicine" was installed in a new building with a considerable grant made available for the purpose by an outside donor.

Dr. Edward Williams, then a registrar in the Radiotherapy Department and previous trained in Physics, was working in the new Institute and with Professor Roberts as Director he was appointed Deputy Director. Two years later Professor Roberts resigned to make way for Williams to become the new Director. Williams became the first Professor in Nuclear Medicine of the University of London. Recently, Dr. Peter Ell has become the new Director of the Institute, carrying it into the second quarter century since its institution.

As an academic subject, Nuclear Medicine continues to flourish, its influence being felt in other branches of medicine. As a diagnostic service, it is now firmly established in this country and elsewhere, as a means towards early detection of disease and the monitoring of organ function.

There is now in the United Kingdom one university-based post-graduation course leading to a Diploma in Nuclear Medicine and this is a "Mastership of Science (Nuclear Medicine) in the University of London". The Royal College of Radiologists also now requires candidates for its diploma to have studied and gained experience in Nuclear Medicine and one of the important duties of the Institute of Nuclear Medicine is to provide teaching in these matters.

This department of the Middlesex Hospital and Medical School which has pioneered so much of this work has undoubtedly achieved an important place in modern medicine.

Emeritus Professor Sir Brian Windeyer

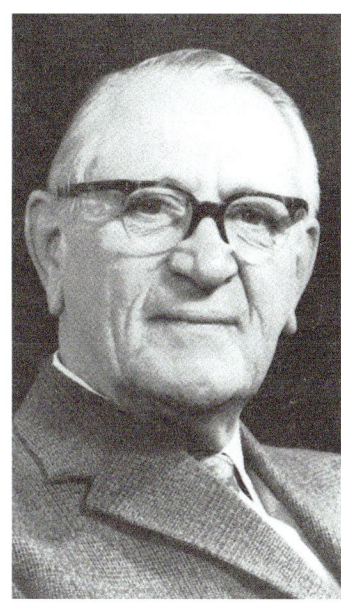

Fig. 1.
Sir Brian Windeyer, Dean of the Middlesex Hospital Medical School at the time of the Foundation of the Institute of Nuclear Medicine (1961)

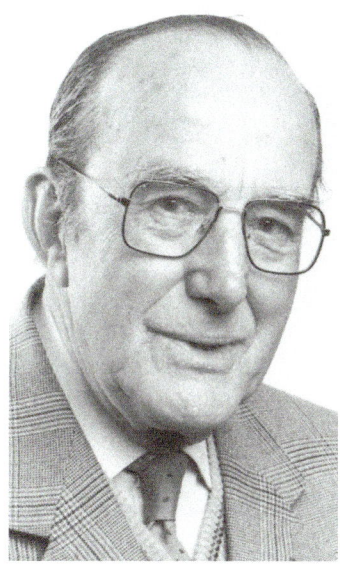

Fig. 2.
Professor J.E. Roberts, first Director of the Institute (1961-1963)

Introduction

This monograph has been prepared in order to give our generous sponsors, and to those who have collaborated with us, a brief account of the contribution made to the subject during the first quarter of the century of the existence of the Institute of Nuclear Medicine. It is also intended to represent a small recognition of our debt to Professor Sir Brian Windeyer and Professor J.E. Roberts, who, in the late 1950s, conceived the idea of such an Institute and also to all the present and past members of staff who, over so many years, have actively contributed with loyalty and dedication. We also hope that those new to the subject or establishing it elsewhere will derive encouragement from it.

E.S. WILLIAMS   P.J. ELL

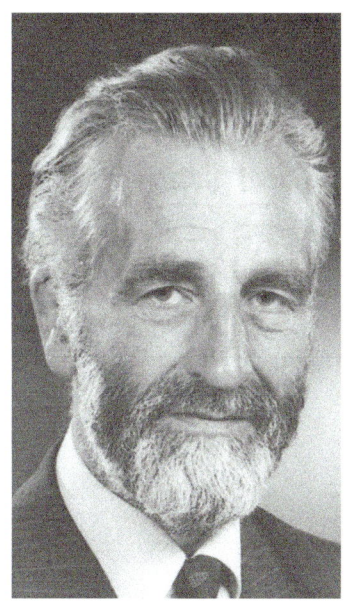

Fig. 3.
Professor E.S. Williams, Director of the Institute
(1963-1985)

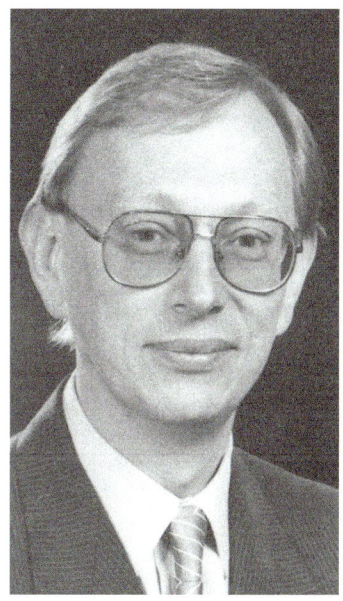

Fig. 4.
Dr. P.J. Ell, the present Director of the Institute
(1986-).

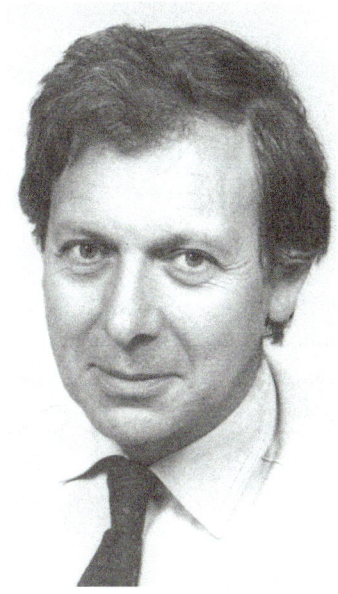

Fig. 5

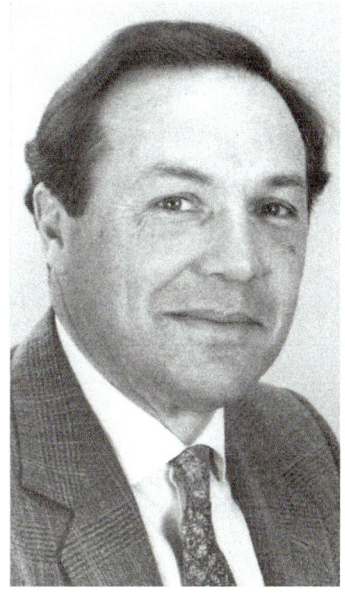

Fig. 6

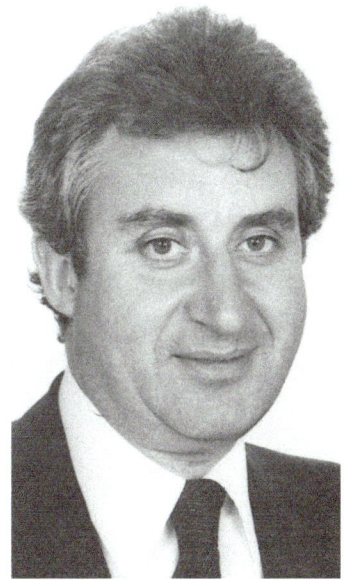

Fig. 7

Fig. 5
Professor R. P. Ekins, Deputy Director
Of the Institute (1968-1981)

Fig. 6
Dr. D.H. Keeling, first Physician in charge of
the Nuclear Medicine Clinic (1965-1973)

Fig. 7
Dr. K.E. Britton, Consultant Physician
In charge of the Nuclear Medicine
Clinic (1973-1976).

What is Nuclear Medicine?

The World Health Organisation has stated that "Nuclear Medicine" is taken to embrace all applications of radioactive materials in diagnosis or treatment or in medical research, with the exception of the use of sealed radiation sources in radiotherapy (1). A number of other definitions have been proposed in the recent literature, though when the term first became widely used its introduction was unaccompanied by precise definition.

How did the term come into use? In 1951 the editorial board of the American Journal of Roentgenology and Radium Therapy decided to express its special interest in the field by a change in the title of that journal. The words "and Nuclear Medicine" were added. A brief editorial on the subject can be read in its January 1952 issue, the fist to be graced with the extended title. This editorial is quite vague and avoids precisely defining the extended field of interest. Perhaps it is reasonable to allow a sort of literature "case law" to build up before attempting to formulate such a definition as that put forward by the WHO.

This branch of medicine is, in the United Kingdom, greatly influenced by the history of the use of radioactive materials here. During the Second World War British resources had been used in the collaborative development of nuclear fission so that in the late 1940s clinical work with radioactive traces had become possible in the larger hospitals. For example, there is a very complete record of a study being carried out in the Middlesex Hospital on a case of thyroid disease in 1948. Iodine 131 was used and the layout of the laboratory sheets suggests that this was but one of a series. A clinical diagnostic service had thus by then already become available and no doubt this was the case in some other centres in this country.

The pre-war establishment of radiotherapy and the progress made then in medical physics, and especially radiation physics as applied to medicine, made it natural that these two specialities should assume a large share of the responsibility for developing the clinical use of radioactive tracers. Thus, in some centres the medical physicists took the leading role, and by degrees, set up a routine radioisotope diagnostic service. In other centres the main interest was among the radiotherapists who, in due course, found themselves setting up a service, usually in close collaboration with physicists. In yet other centres general physicians played a leading role.

Many new techniques and new medical applications of techniques were of transatlantic origin but although nuclear medicine was not then recog-

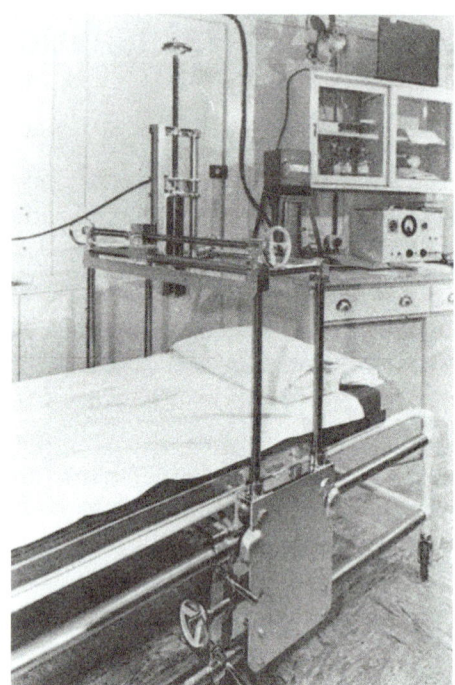

Fig. 8 One of the first clinical scanners, in operation in the Middlesex in the early 1950s

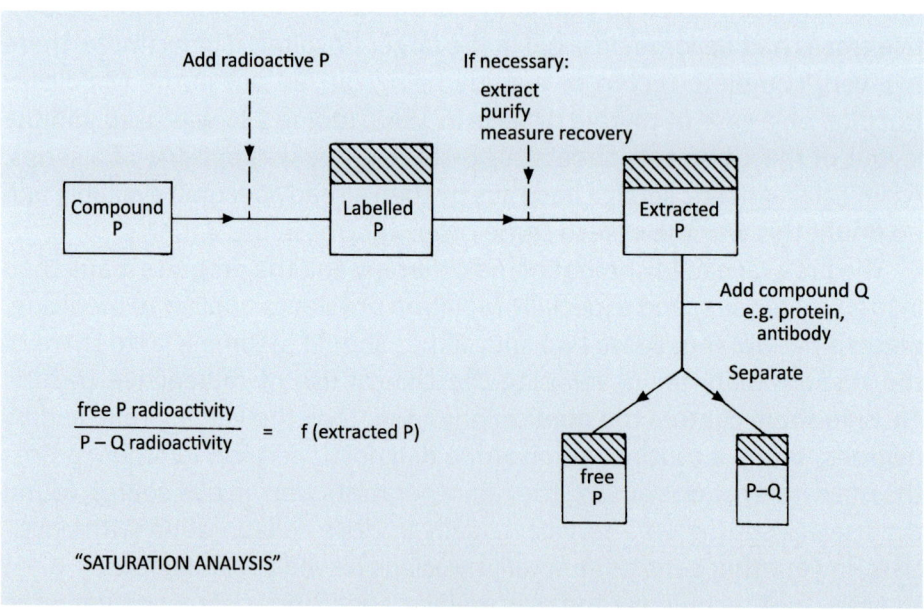

Fig. 9 Diagram of Ekins' original concept of saturation analysis

nised as a separate entity the work that others would designate by this term was rapidly developing here. The most widely applied photo-multiplier in medicine was for many years the British EMI tube. In these days of the dominance of imaging devices as a major clinical application of radioactive traces it is sobering to reflect that probably one of the first fully operational automatic clinical scanners was developed at the Institute of Cancer Research (2). Other centres in a number of countries worked on the development of such scanners and one was in use here in the middle 1950s, at first not automatic (3) but later automated and with colour display (Fig. 8).

Professor Tait and collaborators at the Middlesex showed that even with a simple application of radioactive tracers (4) fundamental biological discoveries could be made (5). Following his discovery of aldosterone (6), he and his staff developed the analytical tracer methods on which his continued endocrinological discoveries depended.

Perhaps one of the most important advances in tracer methodology was the discovery of saturation analysis. Professor Ekins had in the later 1950s been concentrating on the use of specific binding agents as a means of microanalysis using radioactive tracers. He published his first paper on this in January 1960 (7) (fig. 9).

These quoted examples are very selective, the intention being to give a picture of the sort of contribution which was made in the field in this country during the earlier years of nuclear medicine. Until about the late1960s there was no significant interest shown in the subject by diagnostic radiologists but with the advent of short-lived nuclides and more effective radiopharmaceuticals as imaging agents it was quickly recognised that certain nuclear medicine techniques were complementary to the use of X-rays. From that time, diagnostic radiologists have shown an increasing interest in the subject.

The medical use of radioactively labelled materials (radiopharmaceuticals) is still in a state of rapid evolution. Nuclear Medicine is listed as a specialty by the National Health Service and consultants in Nuclear Medicine have been appointed in large centres. At the same time there is no bar to others using nuclear medicine techniques, subject, of course, to the observance of the appropriate regulations relating to the use of ionizing radiations.

In view of the still-expanding diagnostic scope of nuclear medicine and the likelihood of new fields being opened up to useful functional studies it is apparent that many more consultants in nuclear medicine are likely to be needed during the next decade, but little provision has been made for training them or for financing the posts. In comparable member states of the European Economic Community there are more consultants trained in nuclear medicine per head of population than there are in this country and the same is true of the United States of America. Either a massive training effort must be quickly launched or the work will be in the hands of those inadequately trained to do it competently and safely, and also to be able rapidly to apply clinically the results of current research.

There are about 30 full-time practitioners in nuclear medicine in this country if one makes a reasonable extrapolation to account for the passage of time and of practitioners in Scotland since the report on manpower in England and Wales was published in 1984 (8). All major hospitals are now equipped with facilities for the provision of nuclear medicine service but often the clinician in charge has other responsibilities in addition to those of nuclear medicine. Extrapolating from the results of a survey of the Hospital Physicists Association it is probable that there are now of the order of 300 imaging devices in use in the United Kingdom. Most of these have a dedicated computer and are capable of being utilized for a wide variety of investigations.

Academic research in the field of nuclear medicine has been carried on in this country at least since before the end of the Second World War. At the present time it is probable that all medical schools as well as some universities and colleges not having a medical faculty are carrying out research either in some branch of nuclear medicine in its broadest sense or research using nuclear medicine instruments or techniques. Consonant with the growth of the subject in the applied, the hospital, context very little of this great amount of research effort is actually called "nuclear medicine" where those doing the research are consciously working with an aspect of nuclear medicine, as such, in mind they are likely to be doing it within, for example, an academic department of medical physics, of medicine, of radiotherapy, and so on.

Only one university-based postgraduate course leading to a diploma in nuclear medicine exists in the United Kingdom. This is the Master of Science (Nuclear Medicine) course of the University of London. Other examining bodies, notably the Royal College of Radiologists, require candidates for its examinations to have studied, and gained experience in, nuclear medicine. Additionally some nuclear medicine organisations headed by consultants in the subject have one or more junior doctors in training but these will, typically, not be following an academic course, but will be acquiring "in-service" training and experience. Many of these will be aiming to use this period for its utility in aiding their career in another specialty.

A British "learned society" for those interested in nuclear medicine was established in the early 1960s. From small beginnings it has grown to a current membership of about 320 and numbers among its members some who have made significant contributions to the subject. It is a society for people whose interest is mainly or wholly in nuclear medicine but it invites membership from a variety of disciplines and backgrounds. A number of these have been actively engaged in the field since the immediate post-war period. The British Nuclear Medicine Society aims to provide a forum for discussion, to hold meetings for the reporting of research results and of clinical experience and to act as a focal point to which those engaged in nuclear medicine can turn to make contact with others in the field. It is not a professional body: it does not conduct examinations; it is not concerned with remuneration or conditions of service.

A Possible Job Description of a Specialist in Nuclear Medicine

The scope of a specific appointment is likely to differ in detail from that of another, but otherwise similar, appointment elsewhere. The following description is intended to be typical but it is probable that some of the responsibilities mentioned may in some appointments not be part of the work of the nuclear medicine specialist. A nuclear medicine specialist, however, could be expected to be capable, if required, of assuming any of the responsibilities to which allusion is made.

The specialist is first a trained physician able to take clinical responsibility, while undergoing investigation, of all patients referred to him. He will have a sufficiently broad medical knowledge to be able to discuss clinical problems with his colleagues responsible for treatment and hence be able to give a reasonable opinion on the likely value of the alternative methods of investigation available.

The specialist will work from a department of which he will be in immediate charge. Such a department may or may not be administratively a part of a larger departmental organisation. For the purpose of the present description it is sufficient to state that the specialist will work from a suite of rooms in which nuclear medicine is practised and within that suite he will carry the ultimate responsibility. For simplicity this suite will be referred to as the Nuclear Medicine Department.

The Nuclear Medicine Department could deal with:

a) All aspects of in vivo investigation using radioactive tracers, including e.g. imaging, dynamic studies, whole body counting, absorption studies, etc.
b) In vitro studies incidental to in vivo investigation e.g. radioactive assay of labelled red cells sequentially obtained from a patient on whom successive external probe counting is being carried out
c) In vitro studies using radioactive tracers where no radiopharmaceutical has been administered to the patient This could include the microassay of hormones and other biologically important compounds by saturation analysis and its variants (radioimmunoassay, radioenzymaticassay, etc).
d) Radiation protection services restricted to unsealed source hazards.
e) The therapeutic use of unsealed sources of radiation included patient follow up.
f) Teaching of both medical and ancillary staff not only of "nuclear medicine" as a subject but also as an integral part of medical education in its widest sense.

If the Nuclear Medicine Department undertook all of this work for a large hospital then it would be a large department with the nuclear medicine specialist at the head of a large multidisciplinary team. In a given appointment one or more of the subjects listed would be likely to be the concern of another specialist and dealt with in another department, but the training and experience of the Nuclear Medicine specialist must be such that he could competently undertake responsibility for any combination (or all) of these subjects.

References

1. The Medical Uses of Ionizing Radiation and Isotopes. World Health Organisation Technical Reports Series No. 492: 1972.
2. An automatic method of studying the distribution of activity in a source of ionizing radiation. W.W. Maynford and S.P. Newberry, *British Journal of Radiology, 25*, 589-596, 1952.
3. An isoptope survey couch. B.R. Worsnop. *British Journal of Radiology, 28*, 116, 1955.
4. Assay of mixed radioisotopes, J.F. Tait and E.S. Williams, *Nucleonics, 10*, 47-50, 1952.
5. Further studies on the properties of a highly active mineralocorticoid. H.M. Grundy, S.A. Simpson, J.F. Tait, and W. Woodford. *Acta Endocrinologica, 11*, 199-220, 1952.
6. Isolierung Eines Neuen Kristallisierten Hormons aus Nebennieren mit Besonders Hoher Wirksamkeit auf den Minerealstoffwechsel. S.A. Simpson, J.F. Tait, W. Wettstein, R. Neher, J.W. Eaw, and T. Reichstein, *Experimentia, 9*, 333-339, 1953.
7. The estimation of thyroxine in human plasma by an electrophoretic technique. R.P. Ekins, *Clinical Chimica Acta, 5*, 453-459, 1960.
8. *Health Trends, 16*, 52, 1984.

Early Days

The Institute of Nuclear Medicine grew out of the success of the Department of Physics Applied to Medicine here. That department was from 1912 housed in the Barnato-Joel Laboratories and has Sidney Russ, a pioneer in medical applications of ionizing radiation, as its head. He became Joel Professor of Physics in 1920, being the first Professor of Medical Physics in the world. In 1946 Professor J.E. Roberts succeeded him and at once saw that the long tradition of specialization in radiation physics could be extended by exploiting for medical use the artificial radioactive isotopes of elements which were at that time beginning to be available as a by-product of fission in nuclear reactors.

A radioisotope laboratory was set up and instruments were designed and made so that specimens from patients could be measured for radioactive content and also the radiation emanating from specific organs could be measured. By 1948 a limited diagnostic service using a small range of radioactive materials was available to the Middlesex Hospital.

Over the next few years this service grew rapidly as regards the number of patients being examined as part of their routine "work-up", the scope of the useful tests available, and he number of studies being carried on as research projects. It was soon necessary for a medical man to take "on the spot" supervisory duties and also to allocate space in the laboratories to be modified and decorated in a suitable manner for patients to be investigated there. Soon the whole of the top floor of the Barnato-Joel Laboratories was in use for this purpose.

A registrar and a nursing sister were seconded from the Radiotherapy Department and physicists became more and more involved full-time with the diagnostic isotope service so that by the later 1950s a significant proportion of the commitments of the physics department was devoted to this work as well as to research projects which, while truly academic, would, if successful, lead to an improvement of, or extension of, the Isotope Diagnostic Service. By this time Professor Roberts found it necessary to extend his staff to include radiochemical expertise, so by degrees the problems being tackled were chemical or physico-chemical rather physical. Yet medical physics in its own right was extending its frontiers and deserved the full attention of a Professor with a staff of physicists.

So the idea evolved for the creation of a new department, the sole work of which would be the provision of an isotope service in the broadest sense but which would also be an academic department of the Medical School responsible for teaching the subject, carrying out research, and generally establishing in this country a centre of excellence in what by then had begun to be called nuclear medicine. Professor Roberts put forward the idea of such a separate department and he was enthusiastically supported by the then Dean, Professor Sir Brian Windeyer.

The Institute of Nuclear Medicine was established in June 1961 as this new separate department. The Nuffield Foundation showed a particular interest in the project and provided a substantial grant for the Institute to be installed in a purpose-built building. Naturally this took some years to design and erect, especially as the site was already occupied by buildings in one of which the Institute was rapidly expanding its activities. The new accommodation incorporated a number of special features which required the close cooperation of the director and architect over a prolonged period. This highly satisfactory "home" provided by our benefactors was formally opened on the 24th February 1969 by the Rt. Hon. Lord Todd, F.R.S., but by that date it had for some time been fully occupied for providing a nuclear medicine service to the Middlesex Hospital, for teaching, and research.

Initially Professor Roberts acted as Director of the new Institute as well as continuing as Head of the Physics Department. Dr. E.S. Williams was then on secondment from the Radiotherapy Department to the Isotope Unit and he was invited to become Deputy Director of the Institute of Nuclear Medicine. From the outset he was given almost complete autonomy and when, in 1963, Professor Roberts took a one year sabbatical leave, Dr. Williams became Acting Director. He was, on Professor Roberts' return, asked to accept ultimate responsibility as Director.

From the outset the Institute had a staff of varied interests and the research projects being tackled were wide. Some staff was seconded from the Physics Department and some from radiotherapy while others were supported by grants from the Medical Research Council and some from the British Empire Cancer Campaign (now the Cancer Research Campaign – CRC).

The policy at the time of the establishment of the Institute is best set out by reproducing an extract of a document from the time.

The primary purpose of the Institute is to provide for the consultant staff of the hospital the best possible diagnostic service using techniques based on radioactive isotopes. This in turn involves the development of new and improved techniques and collaboration in clinical research programmes initiated normally by members of the consultant staff. Apart from the spe-

cialised work of the British Empire Cancer Campaign and Medical Research Council groups, no research work is carried out nor planned in the Institute which does not have clinical application either immediately or at one short remove.

It should be emphasized that the large majority of the investigations require laboratory tests, not involving the continuous presence of the patient. At the same time it is important that the Medical Officers attached to the Institute should be in close consultation with the hospital staff in order that the maximum amount of information should be obtained from the interpretations of the tests. From this point of view the Institute should be considered on much the same lines as the Bland Sutton Institute or the routine laboratories of the Courtauld Insitute where thousands of investigations for clinical purposes are carried out without any suggestion of elaborate facilities for patients.

True, it would be an advantage to have a form of small metabolic ward for the observation of a proportion of patients undergoing isotope tests, but this idea has been abandoned for the time being.

Routine tests which are offered to and widely used by the consultant staff, include the following:

1) Thyroid uptake of ^{131}I
2) Excretion rate of ^{131}I
3) Assay of protein bound ^{131}I in plasma
4) Topographical distribution of ^{131}I in thyroid
5) Assay of exchangeable sodium
6) Assay of exchangeable potassium
7) Determination of total blood volume using ^{51}Cr
8) Determination of mean erythrocyte life and sites of their destruction using 51Cr
9) Assay of iron absorption using 59Fe
10) Determination of extra-cellular fluid space, using 82Br
11) Determination of vitamin B12m absorption, using 58Co labelled B12
12) Assessment of fat absorption using 131I labelled triolein
13) Assessment of serum/cerebrospinal fluid bromide ratio, using 82Br

In addition the Institute provides a dispensing and measuring service for the administration of therapeutic doses of radioactive materials.

Development and research projects, with direct clinical applications, include the following:
1) Assay of circulating thyroxine in plasma. This technique is fully worked out and tested and will be offered as a routine service as soon as equip-

ment not being constructed in the Physics Department is completed. It is the first major step in the study of thyroid function, which avoids the administration of radioactive material to the patient.

2) Hamolsky labelled tri-iodothyronine red cell uptake test for thyroid function. This is already on a semi-routine basis and over 100 cases have been tested.

3) Determination of circulating Vitamin B_{12} in plasma. This test, recently developed in the Institute, is of extremely high sensitivity and may prove to be of great clinical importance. If staff are available it is hoped to offer it as a routine test on a limited basis in the fairly near future.

4) Assay of circulating insulin in plasma. This test is under intensive development and should be ready for clinical trials later this year. There seems no reason why it should not eventually be offered as a routine test.

5) Assay of fat fractions in blood. This is an extension of the routine excretion test for fat absorption. It has been fully developed using ^{131}I triolein and is offered as a routine test on a limited basis. A programme of development is in hand to extend the test to a variety of saturated and unsaturated fats. There is a longer tem prospect for routine use.

6) In vivo localisation of liver metastases, using ^{198}Au. This is a limited study based on equipment at present available and can be expanded when equipment which is on order comes into use.

7) Determination of body bromide space. This is a clinical research project in collaboration with the surgical unit.

8) Investigations of the penetration of the epidermis by soaps.

Projects proposed mainly by clinical departments of the hospital which will be undertaken as staff and facilities become available, include the following:

1) Liver function tests using in vivo counting methods.

2) Renal function tests using in vivo counting methods.

3) Determination of C.S.F. volume.

4) Determination of C.S.F. globulins in disseminated sclerosis.

5) In vivo scanning of central nervous system and localization of brain tumours.

6) Determination of carbon dioxide space of "the metabolically active core" of the body.

7) Haematology:

a) In vivo determination of the limits of functioning bone marrow.

b) Study of the distribution of iron and the dynamics of iron turnover.

c) Labelling of platelets and determination of platelet life.

d) Study of haemodynamic problems.

By the standards of the time, this is a reasonably comprehensive list of diagnostic tests available but the changing pattern of tests can be assessed from the summary of current indications for tests offered on a routine basis (see 1976-1986 section). Some of these are similar to those offered 25 years ago but are now much more precise, usually offer more specific information, and are much more reliable. Some tests are no longer offered and this is because they have been superseded by diagnostic tests using chemical methods, or by imaging not using ionizing radiation (e.g. ultrasound). In general the radiation received by the patient to obtain clinically useful information is a fraction of what it was 25 years ago and radiation safety measures are much more strict. In addition the on-site manipulation of radiopharmaceuticals is now carried out in the most up to date sterile conditions in contrast to 25 years ago when preparation were made on an open bench.

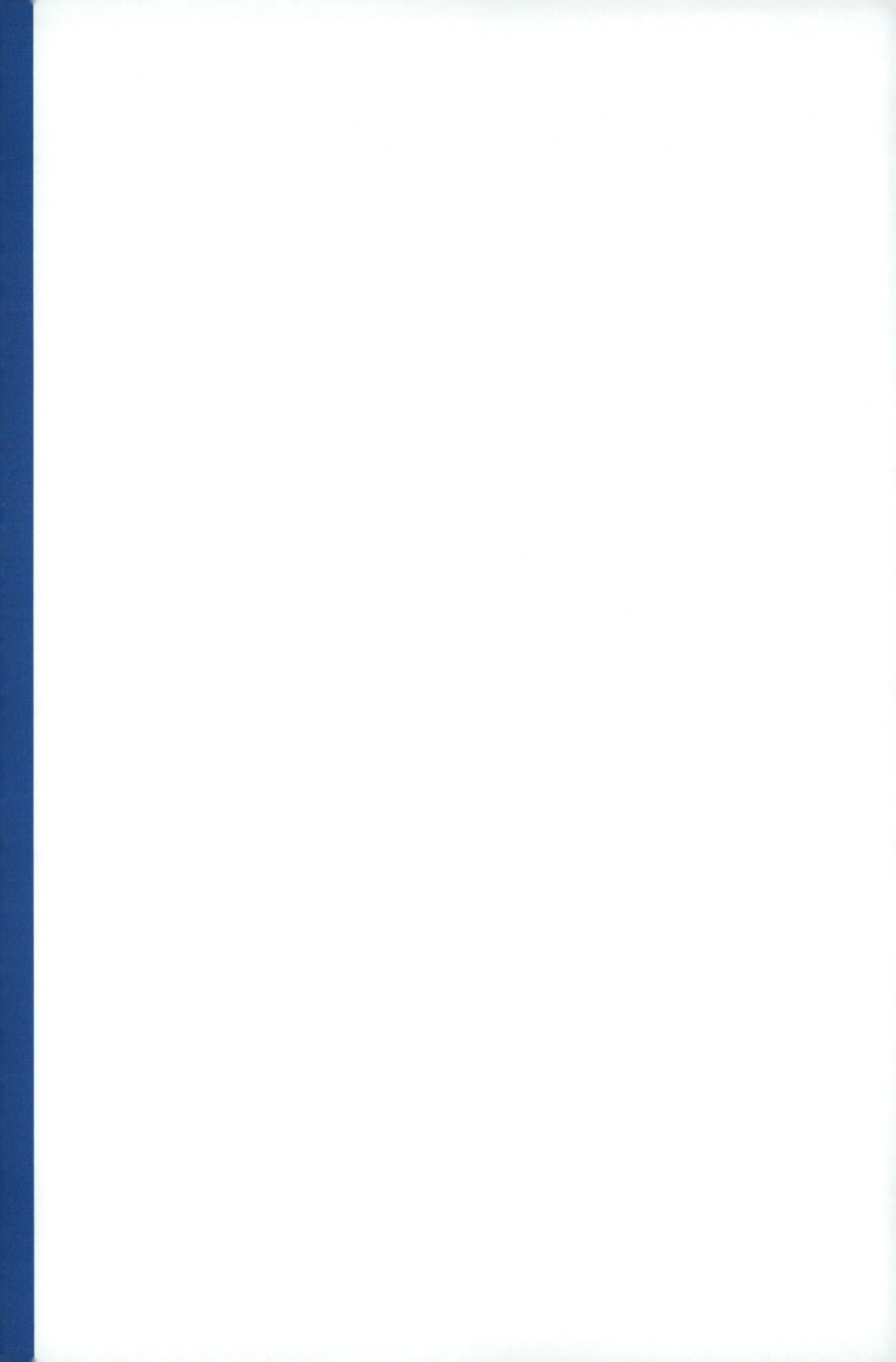

In Vitro Research and Development

From the outset the work of the Institute was divided into that where a specimen from a patient (blood, urine CSF, et.) was the basic material for study and that where investigations were carried out on a patient in person: "in vivo" studies. In routine diagnostic tests both were often required. For example in thyroid function testing, not only was the thyroid uptake of an administered dose of radioactive iodine measured but also a blood sample was obtained and the radioactive iodine bound to the blood proteins measured using an end-window Geiger-Muller(GM) counter. However, the research projects fell reasonably into one or other group.

R.P. Ekins (later Professor) was, from the beginning, in charge of the in vitro section. Early in his career as a member of the staff of the Department of Physics he had displayed interest in the use of radioisotopes in endocrinology. This arose from his association with the research activities of J.F. Tait, who, together with S.A. Simpson of the Courtauld Institute of Biochemistry, was engaged in studies on adrenal control of electrolyte balance while R.P. Ekin was developing a repertoire of radioisotope tests of thyroid function for routine diagnostic use. A problem encountered in each of these areas was the difficulty of measuring hormone levels in body fluids, knowledge of which was frequently required in the interpretation of experimental data.

A highly sensitive microanalytical technique for assay of steroid and thyroid hormones was developed by J.F Tait and J.K. Whitehead relying on the technique of "double-isotope derivative analysis". This technique relies on the formation of an isotopically labelled derivative of the hormone of interest using a hormone-reactive reagent (typically acetic anhydride) labelled at known specific activity with a radionuclide such as ^{3}H, ^{14}C or, more occasionally, one of the radioisotopes of iodine or sulphur. A tracer quantity of the hormone itself or of the hormone derivative – labelled with a second radionuclide – is added at a suitable point in the procedure to monitor recovery of the labelled, derivatised, hormone through the extensive purification steps which are typically required to isolate a highly purified sample. Measurement of the ratio of the two radioisotopes in this sample enables the amount of hormone initially present to be calculated.

This technique was of crucial importance in research on the physiological role and metabolism of a number of steroid hormones in the late 1950s and early 1960s (particularly aldosterone, testosterone, progesterone, etc.); nevertheless it is technically demanding and tedious, largely in consequence of the complexity of the purification procedure involved. Meanwhile in 1954 R.P. Ekins conceived and suggested a general analytical approach for the measurement of substances of biological importance which he termed "saturation analysis"; this essentially relied on reacting the substance to be measured (the "analyte") with a small "saturable" amount of highly specific "binding" protein (such as a specific serum hormone binding protein, specific antibody or a specific cell "receptor") so that, following reaction, part of the analyte would be protein bound and part would be "residual", or "free", Ekins calculated that, under appropriate conditions, the ratio of these two fractions would provide a sensitive measurement of the total amount of analyte present. In order to observe the analyte "distribution ratio", Ekins visualised the initially addition of a small quantity of "tracer" analyte – labelled with a radioisotope or other marker – to the reaction mixture.

Ekins had specifically identified the measurement of serum tyroxine (T4) as an important objective which might be achieved using this approach. The specific serum protein, thyroxine binding globulin(TBG) appeared to possess the physico-chemical properties required and radiolabelled T4 was commercially available. Nevertheless the lack of funding required to purchase the latter prevented Ekins proceeding, until, in 1957, his monitoring of a patient given large doses of ^{131}I for the treatment of metastatic deposits of a primary thyroid carcinoma, fortuitously provided him with small samples of serum containing ^{131}I-labelled T4. Using simple "home-made" electrophoretic equipment and a basic end-window GM counter, Ekins relied, throughout 1957, on blood occasionally taken from this patient to develop a saturation assay for serum T4. During this year, Ekins also worked with a Finnish visit (A. Harjanna) on the development of a microdiffusion method for the radioiodination of proteins to high specific activity as a prelude to the development of antibody-based saturation assay methods for protein hormones (1). This iodination technique subsequently permitted Ekins to continue with work on the assay for T4 until he was able to purchase commercial supplies of radiolabelled T4.

This research was successful, enabling Ekins to submit a description of the technique for publication in 1959 (2). At a meeting of the Middlesex Hospital Research Society in January 1960, Ekins described the general method of "saturation analysis", discussing its possible application, using specific binding proteins or antibodies, for the measurement of protein hormones, vitamins and haptens. Nevertheless, it was not considered appropriate to publish the approach as a general methodology until it had been applied to other substances. Together with R. Barakat, a visitor from Iran, Ekins developed a method for the measurement of vitamin B12 (3). Meanwhile Drs. Berson and Yallow had described (1960) the "radioimmunoassay" of serum insulin, a method conforming to the principles enunciated by Ekins.

Considerable controversy subsequently erupted between Berson and Yallow and Ekins regarding the fundamental theory of "saturation assay" design, a controversy which culminated in major confrontations at meetings in Boston (1967) and Liege (1968). Central to this controversy was the differing perceptions of the concepts of "sensitivity" and "precision" held by the two groups, Ekins insisting on the fundamental importance of statistical components in the definitions of these terms (4). Differences in the concepts of sensitivity and precision inevitably led to differing theories of "assay design" (i.e. the choice of reagent concentrations and characteristics for the attainment of optimum assay performance). The concepts advanced by Ekins are now accepted as correct, and the approach to assay design proposed by him (relying for example, on the evaluation of the "precision profile" of the assay system) is now being increasingly adopted notwithstanding the influence on the field, which is still exerted by the ideas of Berson and Yallow.

At an early stage of development of the thyroxine (T4) assay blood was accepted from patients where the result would be likely to influence clinical management and within a few years a routine assay service was set up which rapidly expanded to include a range of hormones, then of other substances of medical importance. Initially the routine T4 assay reports were examined and certified by the Medical Registrar in the Institute of Nuclear Medicine because this assay replaced the traditional in vivo methods of determination of thyroid functional status. After some time it became clear that there was a frequency distribution of the results in the euthyroid, hyperthyroid and hypothyroid range. Occasionally this frequency distribution from one assay would appear inappropriate and this form of medical quality control was able to identify systematic errors in some assays. The analysis of 1500 request forms by Drs. Britton and their results led to the development of a cost-effective strategy for thyroid function tests (5). This was based on the concept of a Decision Aiding Range rather than a normal range, for the latter always gives false positive and false negative results if, as is usual, biological variation causes overlapping distributions of results in those with a normal thyroid as compared with those whose thyroid is abnormal.

A decision aiding range is one where, if the result was normal there was a high probability (greater than 99.9%) that the patient was normal, and if the result was abnormal then there was a high probability that the patient was abnormal, either hyperthyroid or hypothyroid. Owing to the overlap of the distributions of the conventional normal range with the conventional abnormal range a new range was defined, the borderline range, in which there was uncertainty as to whether a result indicated a normal or abnormal patient and this was then used to define the progress to the next, more specific, test. Thus five categories of results were obtained: definitely high, borderline high, normal, borderline low and definitely low.

The strategy for thyroid function tests was based on using T4 with the free thyroxine index as a first line, tri-iodothyronine (T3) if the T4 result was borderline hyperthyroid and thyroid stimulating hormone (TSH) if the T4 result was borderline hypothyroid. The laboratory automatically followed on with the second line test if the T4 fell into one of these borderline categories. A number of clinical and therapeutic modifications on the strategy helped to cope with the request for all studies, for example, in pituitary based thyroid disorders. This approach was shown to reduce the number of unnecessary T3 and TSH assays done at that time and led to the concept of decision aiding ranges rather than normal ranges. Applying the strategy showed that clinical uncertainty occurred in 48% of the requests and uncertainty after the T4 was reduced to 22% and after applying T3 to the borderline high and TSH to the borderline low, the uncertainty was reduced to less than 2%, to which a thyrotrophine releasing hormone (TRH) test would then be applied (4). This approach has now to some extent been superseded by the development of supersensitive TSH assays and measurements of the free hormones.

More recently, Ekins' major contributions in the analytical field have centred on the development of immunoassays for "free" hormones in blood (i.e. the non protein-bound moiety, widely regarded as the physiologically active fraction) and the development of new "ultra-sensitive" immunoassays relying on lanthanide-chelate flurophors and "time resolution" fluorescence measurement techniques.

The measurement of free hormones by immunoassay has emerged as an area of great importance in the past five years, largely because of the application of such methodology to the routine diagnosis of thyroid disease. Ekins and his colleagues played a pioneering role in this area, which involves entirely novel immunoassay principles (6,7). Considerable controversy has nevertheless centred on it, largely in consequence of its commercial importance and the unjustified claims made by certain manufacturers. Ekins has played a significant part in resolving this controversy, and in identifying scientifically sound material from the claims and counter claims advanced by different manufacturers.

The development of ultra-sensitive, non-isotopic, immunoassay techniques has also assumed major importance in the past few years. Ekins' work in this field commenced in the mid-1970s at which time considerable doubts existed regarding the possibility of developing assay techniques significantly superior in sensitivity to conventional RIA (8). Following detailed mathematical analysis of he physico-chemical reactions underlying various forms of immunoassay design, Ekins concluded that sensitivities several orders of magnitude higher than those yielded by RIA were potentially achievable using one particular design, provided labels could be identified displaying specific activities significantly greater than radioisotopes. These ideas led to the establishment of a collaborative project with E. Soini, Research Director of LKB/Wallace, centred on the use of lanthanide-chelate compounds as antibody-labelling agents. These compounds possess unique fluorescence decay" properties which make them particularly suitable in the context of pulsed light, time-resolution, fluorescence measurement techniques (9). These techniques enable the fluorescence of the labelled substance to be rapidly distinguished from "background" fluorescence, and implicitly enable very high detection sensitivities to be achieved. One of the Ekins'group, S. Dakubu, developed a new method enabling these properties to be exploited in the context of immunoassay, and it is this method which forms the basis of the DELFIA immunoassay kits now being marketed by LKB/Walllac. This is the most sensitive commercially available immunoassay methodology in the world today.

In view of the success of his work and of his ability to attract financial help from grant-giving bodies this section of the Institute was given the status of a sub-department of the Medical School. The University of London awarded Dr. Ekins the title of Professor and in 1982 his sub-department became a full Department of the Medical School with him as its head. The recognition, almost 25 years before, that the medical use of radioactive materials merited the separation of the work from the Physics Department and the formation of a new department, had now, in effect, been repeated by a similar recognition that radioactive tracer-based microassay work was now so far reaching in research and in routine diagnosis that it in turn should continue as a department separate from mainstream, nuclear medicine.

References

1. A simple microdiffusion technique for the radioiodination of proteins. R.N. Bannerjee, and R.P. Ekins, *Nature, 192, 746-747,* 1967.
2. The estimation of thyroxine in human plasma by an electrophoretic technique. R.P. Ekins, *Clinica Chimica Acta, 5, 453-459,* 1960.
3. The assay of vitamin B12 in blood: a sample method. R.M. Barkat, and R.P. Ekins. *Lancet, II, 25-26,* 1961.
4. The fundamental principles governing the attainment of high sensitivity and precision in radioimmunoassay techniques and their exemplification in a method for the assay of serum insulin. J. Albano, and R.P. Ekins. *Acta Endorcrinologica Supplement 138, 61,* 1969.
5. A strategy for thyroid function tests. K.E. Britton, V. Quinn, B.L. Brown and R.P. Ekins. *British Medical Journal, iii, 350-352,* 1975.
6. The radioimmunoassay of serum free tri-iodothyroxine and thyroxine in *Radioimmunoassay in Clinical Biochemistry, (ed. C.A. Pasternak), 187-194,* 1975.
7. The radioimmunoassay of free thyroid hormones in serum. R.P. Ekins, and S.M. Ellis in *Thyroid Research, (eds. J. Robbins and L.E. Braverman), 597-600,* 1976.
8. More sensitive immunoassays. R.P. Ekins. *Nature, 14-15,* 1980.
9. Pulsed-light, time-resolved fluoroimmunoassay. N.J. Marshall, S. Dakubu T. Jackson, and R.P. Ekins. In *Monoclonal antibodies and developments in immunoassay, (eds. A. Albertini and R.P.Ekins), 101-108,* 1981.

In Vivo Research and Development up to 1976

In the early ears, much attention was paid to the distribution of radioactive materials in the whole body, the changes of this with time, the rate of excretion and so on. A whole body counter using large sodium iodide detectors in a low background (chalk) room was constructed in the basement of the old building. The system was extended and developed and led eventually to a relatively novel slit shield scanning whole body counter which was designed and built in the Institute, and was one of the prototypes for a whole generation of similar systems. Part of the design was performed by computer simulation also a relatively novel approach for the period.

The Institute became interested in gamma cameras at an early time having received one of the first to be used in the U.K. as a result of a gift from Eco-electronics: it had an enormous five inch (!) field of view. This led to experiments to see if a conventional radiological image intensifier could potentially be used for imaging by addition of an appropriate scintillator at its front surface. Limited success was achieved.

The use of computers in nuclear medicine was pioneered at the Institute, both for imaging, and in renography. After a long battle to obtain funds, a paper tape punch was attached to one of the rectilinear scanners, and used for many years as the source for data for (limited) image processing. One of the original problems tackled was that of detection of abnormal parathyroid nodules by dual isotope subtraction.

As a result of the interest in such image processing, it was decided to interface a minicomputer to a gamma camera. No such systems were available commercially at that time and the system eventually installed by Dr. Todd-Pokropek was one of the very early computers to be used dedicated to a gamma camera. The first such system had a total memory of only 4 k, half being used for the software, and the other half for data. This was a very early virtual memory system and it was eventually expanded to 8 k, and used to develop much of the early nuclear software in Assembler, since compilers for languages such as Fortran were not then available. This system, and others like it, generated considerable commercial interest (indeed some of the programs then written are still in use) and most current gamma camera software was developed along the lines suggested by such systems.

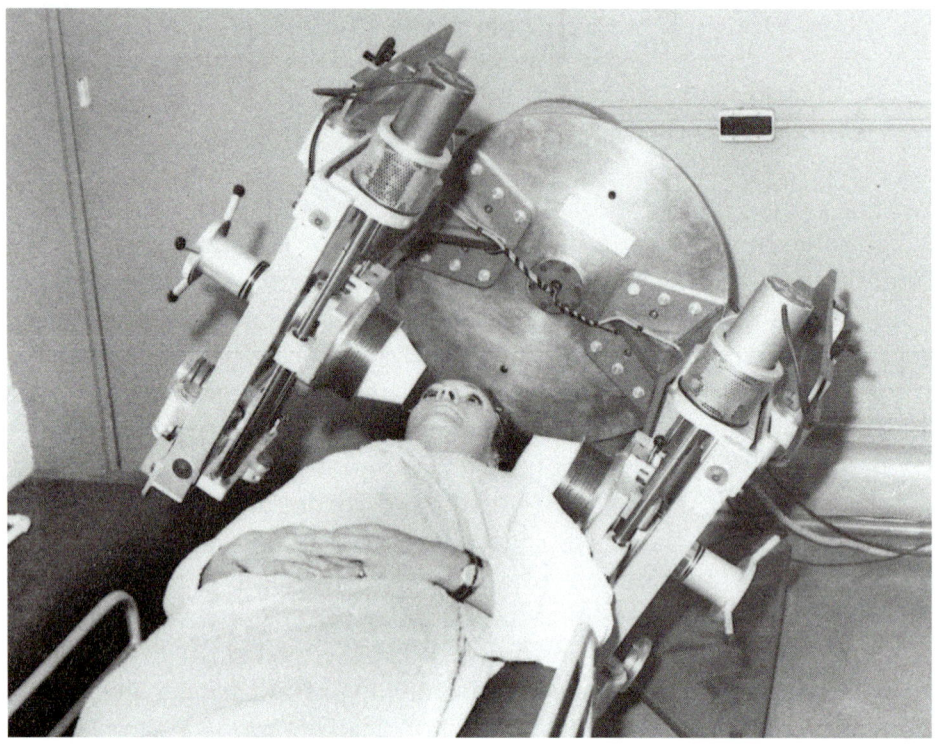

Fig. 10 Keeling and Todd-Pokropeks' single photon emission tomographic (SPET) scanner, the first section scanner in Europe, built in 1969

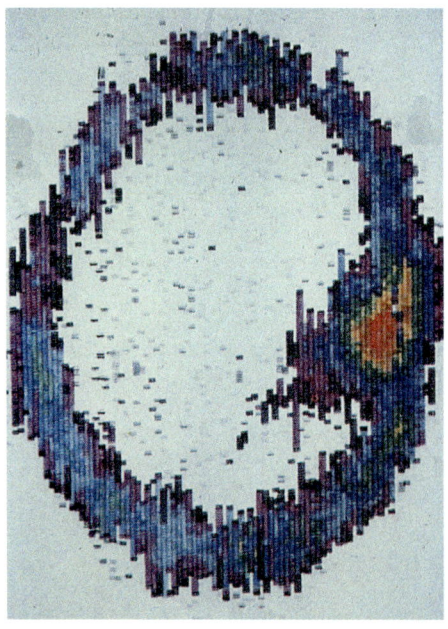

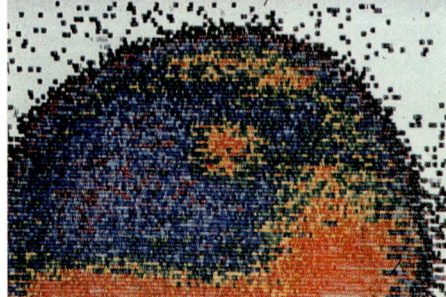

Fig. 11 Initial clinical work with the brain section scanner. A planar and transaxial section san of the brain is shown with a peripheral lying tumour in the fronto-parietal lobe. A study recorded in 1971

In 1968 Keeling and Todd-Pokropek had the idea of developing a section scanner to perform tomography. After obtaining a grant of £6,000 they built, in 1969, with the aid of J & P Engineering, the first tomographic system in the U.K. (and probably in Europe). The system was based on two rectilinear scanning frames which could be used to perform conventional scanning, or to produce a single slice tomogram. This entailed developing a tomographic reconstruction package on the minicomputer, and initial results were reasonably successful. (Figs 10 and 11). The prototype system was never widely used as a result of being rather unreliable clinically. However, published results predate those from the EMI-CT scanner by a number of years (1,2).

Much of this research was carried out using the Institute's own mechanical and electronic workshop facilities which were outstanding for the time. This infrastructure has throughout these 25 years been unique in its versatility to build and modify equipment in response to in-house design. Amongst a number of smaller devices, a whole body counting system, a thyroid uptake probe system, special purpose lead and tungsten collimators, and Perspex phantoms were all made available.

Keeling and Todd-Pokropek built and operated (occasionally with useful clinical results) a very early radionuclide subtraction unit for pancreas

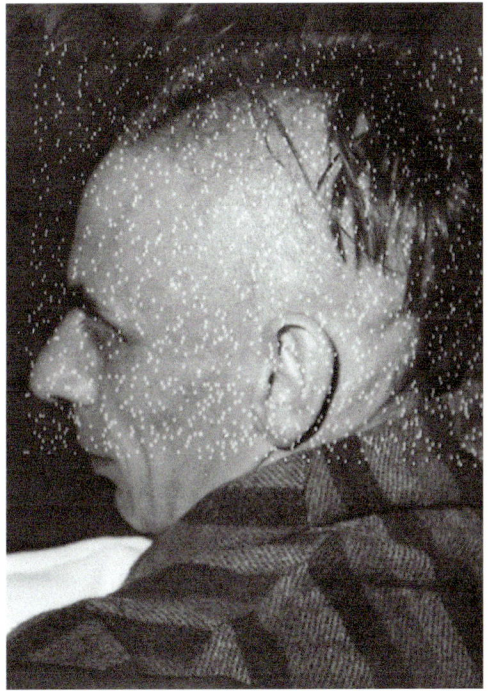

Fig. 12 A ^{197}Hg-chlormerodrine brain scan recorded in November 1963, with the Mecaserto scanner. Image interpretation as a fine art!

49

scanning at the beginning of the 1960s (3) ^{99}Tc^m was already used, labelling antimony sulphide colloid, and of course ^{75}Se-selenomethionine. With Magdi Yacoub, Keeling undertook early work on red cell survival on patients with both mechanical and pig heart valve replacements (4,5). At the beginning of 1965, the then Mecaserto Scanner was upgraded at the Institute from its original thimble size crystal, to a magnificent three-inch size detector! Brain scanning with arsenic and mercury compounds and ^{131}I radioiodinated human serum albumin became much more feasible (Fig. 12) and a variety of clinical studies were undertaken (Fig. 13) (6).

In 1968, much time was spent looking at new Indium-113m generators and pharmaceuticals, the Institute receiving the second Indium generator for medical use in the U.K. (FIG. 14). Keeling reported on this work (these materials were not yet in use in Europe) to a joint Scandinavian meeting in September 1969 (7). In 1970, Keeling investigated Gallium-67 in a series of

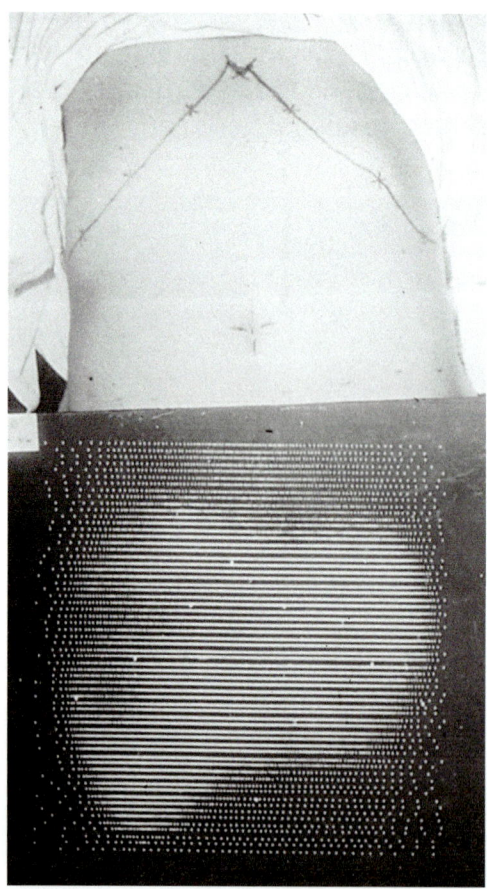

Fig. 13 One of the first ^{99}Tc^m antimony sulphide liver scans performed at the Institute in 1966, demonstrating liver metastases

patients with tumour. These were the first human subjects investigated with this radionuclide this side of the Atlantic. Almost 20 years hence, Gallium-67 citrate scanning is still being used, albeit in a more defined set of clinical indications.

Among the early clinical applications of the computer/gamma camera system referred to was to improve the then relatively poor quality of brain images. Qualitative techniques were developed by Britton and Brown including the production of realistic brain images using an unsharp masking technique which came to be known as the Canterbury filter. This process demonstrates the true base of the brain, the pituitary and posterior fossae clearly but it was soon appreciated that image enhancement by itself could be misleading with "noise blobs" able to mimic tumours. The key to the computation of brain scans was the realisation that every suspect lesion

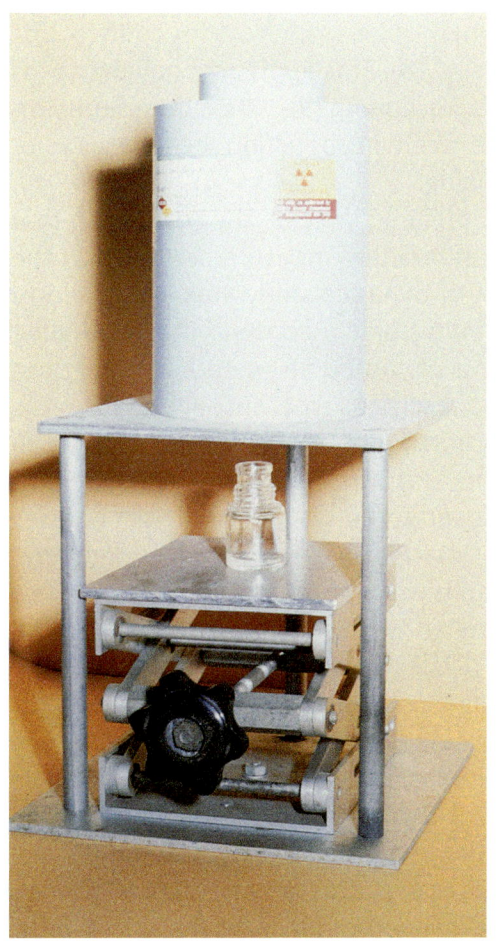

Fig. 14 An example of an early $^{113}In^m$ Indium generator in use at the Institute in 1968

thrown up by an optimised qualitative display had to be tested quantitatively for its significance. Thus, maps of the variation in normal uptake in the views of the processed brain scan had to be developed. These were obtained by showing a series of computer displays of brain images to doctors studying here for the degree of MSc in Nuclear Medicine telling them that all brain images were abnormal, whereas in fact all but four were normal. By manipulating the images to look as normal as possible they were then forced to say where they thought the abnormality was. Since these were in fact noise blobs, the range of variation was discovered. In practice once suspected areas were identified, regions of interest were set up and the image had then to be returned to the unprocessed state for the quantification to be applied, since only in the unprocessed state was the statistical approach valid because the pixel contents were independent of each other. It was shown that qualitative plus quantitative computer analysis improved the detectability over conventional transparent film. A 10% change was significant in the hemisphere whereas for a film a 30% changes was necessary for detectability (8). This approach, however, was swamped by the developed of X-ray CT scanning (9), which then supplanted radionuclide brain studies until the recent introduction of the new radiopharmaceuticals for grey matter imaging.

In parallel with the development of static imaging the realisation that nuclear medicine was primarily about function measurements led to the rapid development of various forms of dynamic study. Initially, the form of recording was graphical, using multi-point recorders. Brain scanning gave way to attempted measurements of carotid and cerebral blood flow. Dramatic experiments were carried out with buckets suspended from the ceiling and plastic tubes representing aortic and carotid arteries over which detectors were placed. There were measuring cylinders to collect the outflow, by-passes to induce turbulence and three-way taps to inject boluses of radioactivity. This work led to the description of disturbances of carotid flow, when it was turbulent and when it was non-turbulent. Based on this approach, special collimators for settling over the patient's aorta and the internal carotids viewed through the orbits were designed and applied, and carotigraphy was developed (10). Significant carotid stenosis, that is sufficient to alter volume flow, affected the activity-time curve dramatically on one side as compared with the other. Determination of the spectrum of transit times showed differences in sub-critical stenoses and were related to turbulent flow which was thought to be embologenic (11).

While the development of apparatus for carotigraphy was continuing, renography was developing. The crudely anatomical approach to interpreting the curves as the vascular spike, secretory phase and excretory phase, were shown to be nonsense in physiological terms, the vascular spike not representing blood flow to the kidney, the secretory phase not representing tubular secretion and the excretory phase representing the amount left behind in the kidney, not the amount coming out. A physiological approach to the interpretation of the renogram was developed by Britton and Brown which showed that most of the indices previously used bore little relationship to the function of the kidneys because of the considerable contribution of non-renal background activity to the recorded curve. In order to correct for this, a method of computer assisted blood background subtraction renography was developed known by the acronym of CABBS at a time when acronyms were just becoming fashionable (12). This approach allowed the contribution of one kidney to total function to be measured accurately (13).

It led to the analysis of the truly representative kidney curves by deconvolution. Much effort was put into deconvolution analysis since the linear system approach clearly modelled the anatomy and physiology of the kidney, which is made of up of tubes (the nephrons) in a much more realistic (isomorphic) way than the compartmental model. A requirement of a compartmental model, that there is rapid mixing in each compartment compared with the rate of exchange between compartments, was clearly a non-contender for stimulating events in the nephrons of the kidneys. This approach led to the measurement of the spectrum of renal transit time and to the demonstration that in normal kidneys the transit time distribution was bimodal (14). Studies in rabbits and pigs jointly with Wilkinson at King's College Hospital comparing this approach with microsphere distribution confirmed that the first mode represented the transit of cortical nephrons which, having short loops of Henle, takes a short time and the second mode represented the transit of juxta-medullary nephrons which, having long loops of Henle, took a longer time (15). This was the first rigorous approach to the measurement of intra-renal blood flow distribution in man, which has now been developed into a technique for the gamma camera using [123]I Hippuran.

In order to put these theories into practice, in co-operation with Nuclear Enterprises Ltd., a new system of renography was designed and built by Britton and Brown, known as the renograpy couch (16). This Rolls-Royce for renography appeared externally to look like a hospital couch, (Fig. 15), but unfolded to reveal three detectors and all the electronics and included an automatic analogue CABBS system (Fig. 16). The couch could be lowered or elevated and one could be seen strolling through the hospital to do kidney

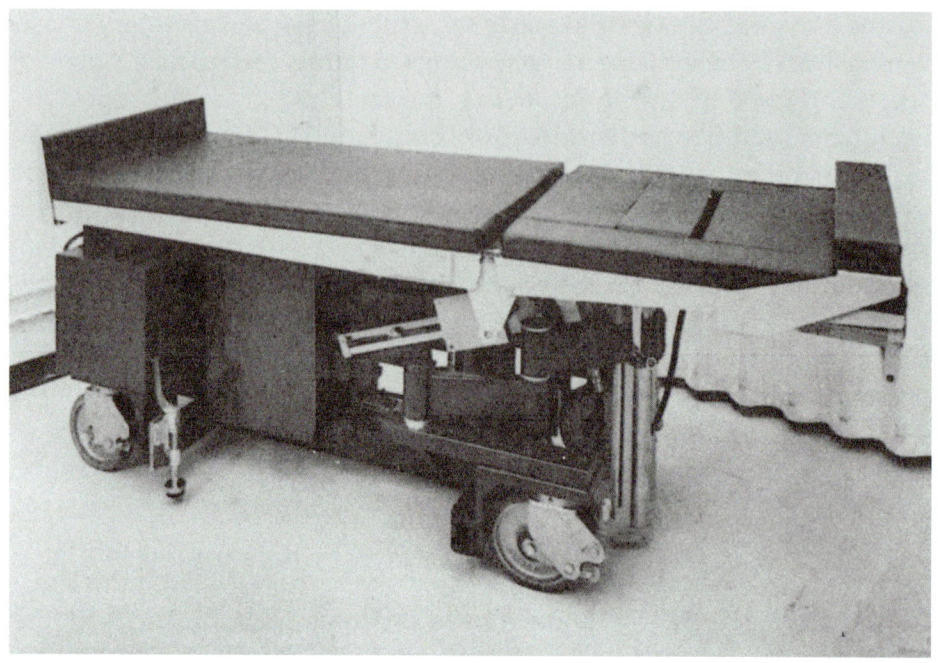

Fig. 15 Mobile renography couch packed. Designed by Britton and Brown

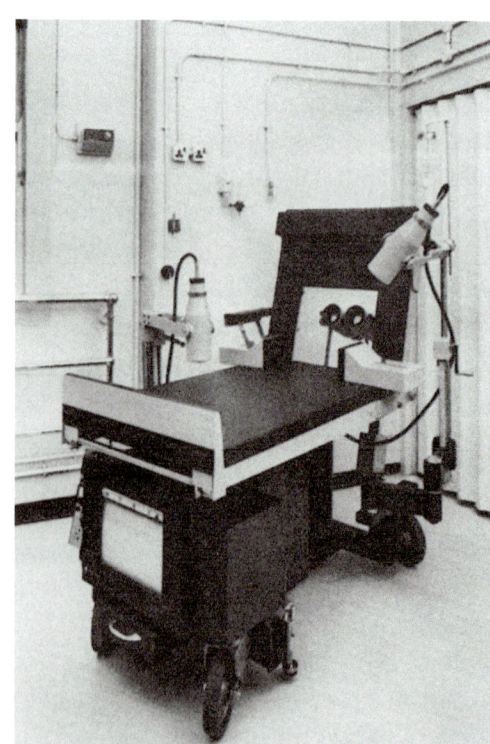

Fig. 16 The mobile renography couch unpacked, showing the back support raised and the detector. On the left of the multi-point recorder, the analog computer assisted blood background substraction (CABBS) unit can just be seen

function studies in patients in the equivalent of the intensive care unit, raising the couch to the level of the hospital bed, sliding the patient over and then unfolding the equipment to carry out the study. It showed, for example, that a burglar who had fallen out of a fourth floor building window suffering internal haemorrhage had not in fact damaged his kidneys. Six of these machines were built and distributed by the Department of Health, but unfortunately they were not a commercial success because of their high expense compared with a simple static three-probe system.

However, "Tomorrows World" somehow heard of this strange machine and insisted that it was taken to their studio in White City so that a genuine renogram was performed in front of the television cameras. The prototype machine was parked among the Grecian columns of the set of "Up Pompeii", looking slightly incongruous. Then, in rehearsal, the machine was duly set up with Brown as the patient, Britton as the doctor, and a genuine injection of radioactive Hippuran was given and the recordings made. When it came to the live performance the "patient" was duly set up and the detectors placed over the back and an injection given under the television cameras, which were to return 20 minutes later at the end of the programme to see the completed results. Unfortunately, the ticking of the multi-point recorder could be heard during the other presentations and the floor manager insisted that the machine be turned off. Furthermore, one of the probes, so carefully set up, started to fall away from the back of the patient, due to a mechanical fault, the size of the patient fortunately concealing this from the cameras. During this interval, the doctor could be seen mending the probe with an allen key and re-playing the previously recorded normal renogram, adjusting the analog computer so that the second result overlaid the first result, just in time to come up on cue to state how well the patient's kidneys were working!

This work on the kidney led to the writing of a monograph entitled *"Clinical Renography"* (14). While it outlined the physiological basis of renal function tests using radioactive compounds, reading between the lines it was really about how a medical doctor and a medical physicist learn each other's language and how to work together. The opening paragraph of the preface summarised this problem:

> "The disciplines of medicine and physics are like oil and vinegar – often shaken together often appetising but not easily miscible. This monograph is an attempt to blend the soothing oil of medicine with the acid reality of physics in a study of one area of common interest: how a kidney works. The result may be criticised for having insufficient clinical salt by masters of the art of medicine and for insufficient scientific pepper by professors of the practice of physics,

but we hope this mixture will be to the taste of the general physician and surgeon who find a need for a test of the function of each kidney without the danger or discomfort to the patient, whether he be well or seriously ill."

It became clear that an understanding of the new physiological basis of the interpretation of the renogram required a new look at renal physiology. The data on the handling of compounds such as insulin and para-amino hippurate (PAH) summarised in Homer Smith's book on the kidney, were determined after injecting many grams of the appropriate compound, whereas for radionuclide renography fractions of milligrams were injected. Thus; for example, owing to weak protein binding ortho iodo hippurate used for renography is only filtered to the extent of 6%, not 20% as for PAH. Developing the bolus hypothesis of renography led to considering how far the kidney's physiological functions relevant to renography could be considered to work purely on a mechanical basis, dependent on the physical properties of a series of tubes made of living cells and the effects of filtration, pressure gradients, diffusion, osmosis and active transport.

Work with Peter Cage, a computer engineer, led to the development of the Bootstrap model of urinary concentration. The problem with the conventional counter current hypothesis was that the single effect of active transport of sodium is limited to the cells of the thick ascending limb of the loop of Henle, yet the conventional theory required active sodium transport to be present also in the thin descending limb. The engineering approach based on the alternate diffusions of sodium and urea down concentration gradients and their interaction at different levels in the renal medulla demonstrated that a thermodynamically sound system could be developed without postulating active transport in the thin ascending limb (17).

In the cortex, the Thurau loop system of renin-dependent renal autoregulation was developed by resolving its conflict with American work in this field and published as a hypothesis in *The Lancet* (18). One of the problems of the loop hypothesis had always been that experimentally different arteriolar tone could be shown in some circumstances to increase within a few seconds of a rise in perfusion pressure yet it takes 30-40 seconds for filtered salt to reach he juxta-glomerular apparatus. In the best "Eureka" tradition of a bath provided the answer. When turning on the shower and finding that the water is too hot, one turns on the cold tap. The force of the shower immediately increases but it takes several seconds for the cold water to find its way along the hose and cool the hot water. Thus, in the nephron, a change of pressure at the juxta-glomerular apparatus, increases the passive component of salt reabsorption. The increased salt delivery comes along 3-40 seconds alter. Both effects increase afferent arteriolar tone through local salt-dependent renin release.

During this time a close association developed between the Atomic Energy Research Establishment at Harwell and the Institute of Nuclear Medicine leading to the first use of their cyclotron-produced radioisotopes in patients. In particular they were able to produce ^{123}I free of ^{124}I using their 55 MeV cyclotron. The first studies of thyroid uptake of pure ^{123}I were undertaken and after many difficulties ^{123}I-labelled BSP (bromosulphthalen) was produced. The problems encountered included the alkalinity of the ^{123}I, the low molar concentration, the low amount of carrier iodine and the heterogeneity of BSP itself. A technique was developed were added potassium iodide was found to be necessary and liver, gall bladder and biliary images were obtained long before the development of HIDA compounds. The high count rate allowed good mathematical analysis of the data and it was shown that the traditional compartmental model of hepatic clearance was at fault, taking no account of the 10-18 minute delay between hepatic uptake and biliary excretion of BSP, a matter confirmed by T-tube sampling after biliary surgery (19). Thus, a linear model of the liver was found to be more appropriate and deconvolution analysis was undertaken in the hope that the effect of one pint of beer on the liver could be demonstrated. The tri-modal transit time distribution was difficult to explain and thought to be due to different time relationships of gluconated, sulphated and free BSP. Studies with Di BSP which was not so conjugated however, show the same tri-model transit time distribution. It remains unexplained.

References

1. A new approach to brain scBanning. Keeling, D.H. *Proceedings of the Second Congress of the European Association of Radiology,* Amsterdam, Excerpta Medica, Amsterdam, June 1971.
2. Tomographic reconstruction. Todd-Pokropek, A.E. *Proceedings of the Second Congress of the European Association of Radiology,* Amsterdam, Excerpta Medica, Amsterdam, June 1971.
3. Problems in the visualisation of the pancreas. Keeling, D.H. and Williams, E.S. Abstract: *Brit. J. Radiol.* 40, 798, 1967.
4. Chronic haemolysis following the insertion of ball valve prostheses. Keeling, D.H. and Yacoub, M.H. *Brit. Heart J.* 30, 676, 1978.
5. Red cell survival after homograft replacement of the aortic valve. Yacoub, M.H., Keeling, D.H., Kothari, M., Patterson, M and Ross, D.N. *Thorax,* 24, 283, 1969.
6. The preparation of Technetium-99m for clinical use. Keeling, D.H. and Bryant, T.H.E. *Radioactive Isotope in Klinik und Forschung,* Band. VIII. Urban and Schwarzenberg. 1967.
7. Some experience with Indium generators and compounds. Keeling, D.H., *Brit. J. Radiol.* 42, 236, 1969.

8. Clinical use of quantitative brain imaging. Britton, K.E. Cruz, F.B., Brown, N.J.G. In *Proc. 13th Int. Con. of Int. Medicine* Helsinki 1976.

9. EMI and radioisostope brain imaging. Britton, K.E., Williams, E.S. *Lancet* 2,pp.477 and 660, 1976.

10. A feasibility study of a screening test for abnormalities of carotid blood flow using technetium 99m. Britton, K.E. *J. Neurol. Neurosurg. Psych.* 33, 379-382, 1969.

11. MSc Disseration, University of London. The determination of abnormalities of blood flow using external counting techniques with special reference to carotid blood flow, 1971.

12. Clincal use of computer assisted blood background subtraction (CABBS) renography. Sub-title: Investigation of the "Non-functioning kidney" and renal artery stenosis by the use of I-131 Hippuran renography modified by computer assisted blood background subtraction (CABBS). Britton, K.E. and Brown, N.J.G. *Brit. J. Radiol.* 41, 57-579, 1968.

13. The theory of renography and analysis of results. Brown, N.J.G. and Britton, K.E. *Radionuclides in Nephrology.* Ed. Blaufox, M.D. and Funck-Bretano, J.L. pp 315-324, Grune and Stratton, New York.

14. *Clinical Renography,* Britton, K.E. and Brown, N.J.G. Lloyd-Luke Ltd., London, 1971.

15. Validation of "transit renography" for the determination of the intrarenal distribution of plasma flow: comparison with the microsphere method in the anaesthetized rabbit and pig. S.P. Wilkinson, M. Vernardi, P.C. Pearce, K.E. Britton, N.J.G. Brown, L. Poston, M. Clarke, R. Jenner and Roger Williams. *Clin. Sci. and Mol. Med.* 55, 277-283, 1978.

16. Mobile CABBS renography. Britton, K.E. and Brown, N.J.G. *Computers in Radiology,* S.A. Karger, Basel, 454-458, 1970.

17. A "Bootstrap" model of the renal medulla. Britton, K.E., Cage, P.E. and Carson, E.R. *Postgrad. Med. J.* 52, 279, 1979.

18. Renin and renal autoregulation. Britton, K.E. *Lancet* 2, 329-333, 1968.

19. Computer assisted blood background subtraction (CABBS) hepatography with ^{131}I and ^{123}I bromosulphthalein. Britton, K.E., Suwanik, R., Tuntawiroon, C., Premoydin, M., Reuben, A., Narasimha, K., Myers, M., Wood, T.P. and Brown, N.J.G. In *Dynamic Studies with Radioisotopes in Clinical Medicine and Research,* International Atomic Energy Agency 9SM 185) Vienna, pp. 157-171, 1974.

In Vivo Research and Development: 1976–1986

As from 1976, a major re-equipment programme was initiated at the Institute by Ell, the present director. With the passage of time, some of the existing apparatus had become obsolete, no modern Anger gamma camera or data processing equipment was available and whole body imaging facilities were rather limited (Figs. 17,18,19,20). Despite the increasing difficulties in attracting NHS funds for the provision of a clinical service, the next 5 years saw a substantial fund-raising programme being launched. This permitted the Institute to meet the challenge posed by a very rapidly changing specialty and the emerging clinical applications of single photon emission tomography (SPET) and nuclear cardiology. The Special Trustees of the Middlesex Hospital and the Sir Jules Thorn Charitable Trust supported a number of important research projects: within 5 years, a new large field Anger gamma camera and associated computer system, a second small field of view gamma camera, a dedicated SPET unit for tomography of the brain, and a dedicated SPET unit for tomographic studies of the whole body, were acquired. This represented fund raising (Figs 20,21) equivalent to a grant of over £300,000.

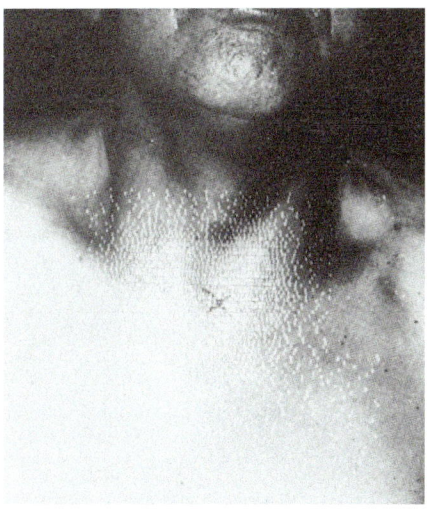

Fig. 17 Scanning in the mid-1960s, with [131]I. A patient with retrosternal goitre

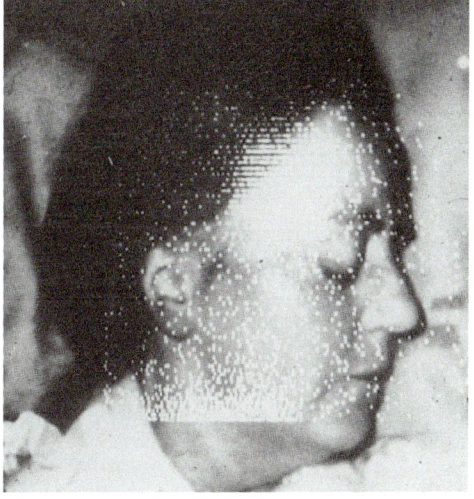

Fig. 18 Scanning in the mid-1960s, with [131]I. A patient with carcinoma of the the thyroid and a skull deposit

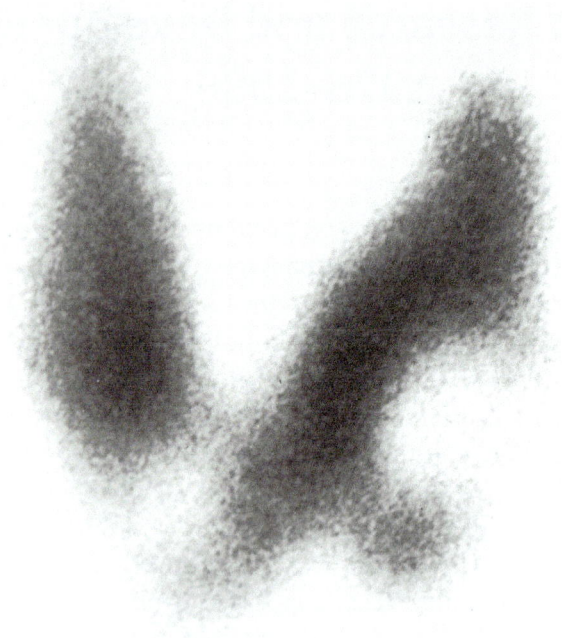

Fig. 19 For reference, a modern Anger gamma camera image of a patient with multi-nodular thyroid goitre

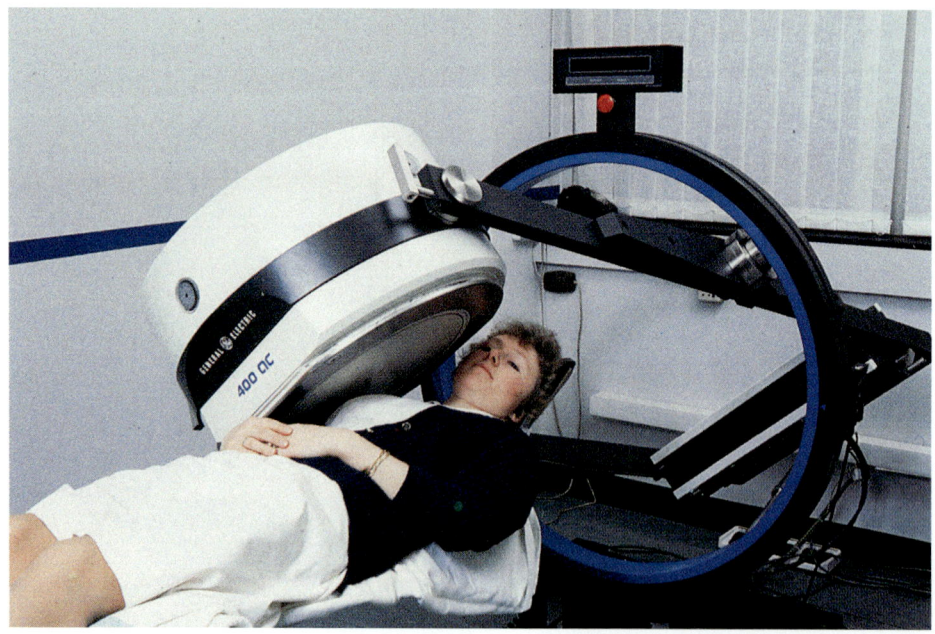

Fig. 20 A 1986 single photon emission tomography rotating Anger gamma camera

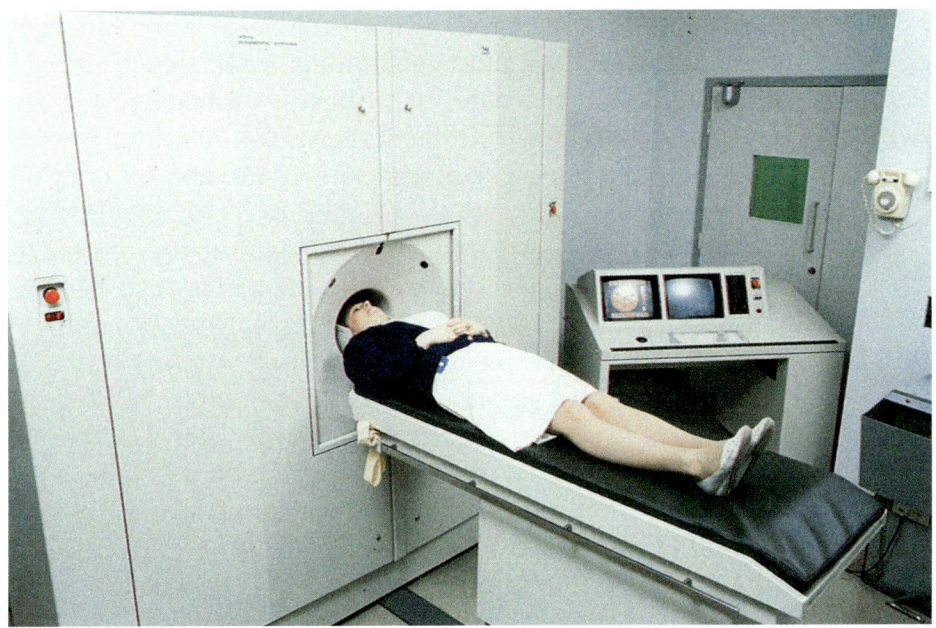

Fig. 21 A modern dedicated single photon emission tomography unit for imaging the brain

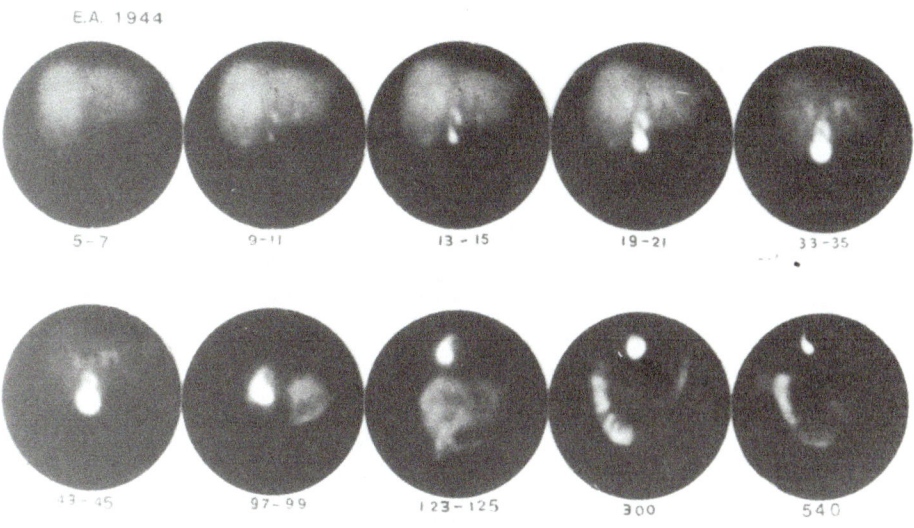

Fig. 22 A normal hepatobiliary study recorded with $^{99}Tc^m$ HIDA. The frame time is shown in minutes, a fatty meal given at 45 minutes after intravenous trace administration

By the beginning of the 1980s, the Institute was again in the forefront of its field of interest, being the most modern equipped Department of Nuclear Medicine in the U.K., on a par with the best institutions worldwide. With these developments on the instrumentation side, the Institute made significant inroads into the clinical field, with a new generation of radioactively labelled compounds.

[99]Tc[m] Imidodiphosphonate was formulated, labelled and first applied to man, by Ell et al., in 1977 here. This opened the clinical area of acute myocardial infarct imaging, with the Institute and the Department of Cardiology reporting on the efficacy of this diagnostic approach in a large series of patients. Transmural myocardial infarction and subendocardial necrosis could be detected with sensitivity of 95 and 75%, respectively (1a,1b).

[99]Tc[m] Plasmin was introduced as a non-invasive counting technique for the exclusion of deep venous thrombosis (DVT); in comparison with X-ray phlebography, useful data emerged, the technique allowing for the reliable exclusion of DVT. [99]Tc[m] Plasmin permits early, rapid, safe and economic screeing of DVT 15 minutes after intravenous administration (2).

A [99]Tc[m] labelled ethylhydroxyiminodiacetic acid derivative was the first [99]Tc[m]-labelled tracer used in man for investigation of bile flow. The work was carried out at the Institute in 1977 and the initial experience was reported

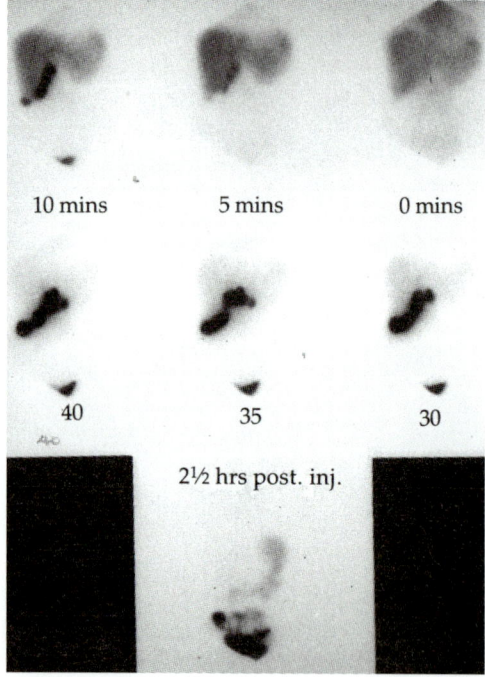

10 mins   5 mins   0 mins

40   35   30

2½ hrs post. inj.

Fig. 23 A typical hepatobiliary study of a patient post-gastric surgery with biliary reflux into the stomach

in 1978 (3). Radionuclide hepatobiliary studies are now routinely performed in the majority of nuclear medicine departments, mainly as the first port of call in the diagnosis of acute cholecistytis, but perhaps more significantly in the demonstration of biliary reflux and/or leakage (Figs. 22, 23). The sensitivity of the nuclear medicine method, couple with data processing capability, provides quantitative information on the transit of bile. This is of particular interest in patients with biliary dyskinesis (4) and there is recent interest in this methodology in the evaluation of liver transplantation.

[123]I-labelled amines and diamines (isopropylamphetamine-IMP and propanediamine-HIPDM) were first used in the UK y Ell (1981 and 1982) as radionuclide markers for regional cerebral blood flow in man (rCBF) (5). Tomographic maps of rCBF were recorded in a variety of clinical entities, and the phenomena of luxury perfusion, cross-cerebellar diaschisis and rCBF positive, but X-ray CT negative, stroke were clearly demonstrated (Figs. 24,25). There has been a significant worldwide interest in SPET and rCBF, particularly in view of the almost specific pattern which has been demonstrated in rCBF loss in the senile dementias of the Alzheimer type.

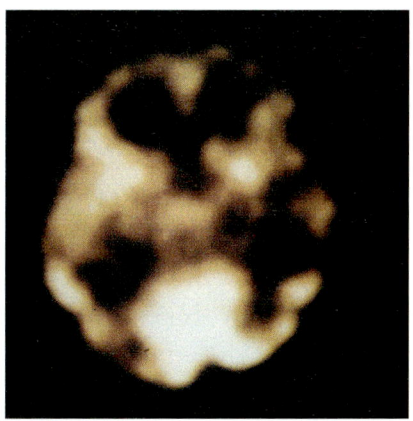

Fig. 24 One of the first ^{123}I-isopropylamphet-amine studies recorded in the Institute at the beginning of 1982, it shows the transaxial distribution of regional cerebral blood flow in a normal brain

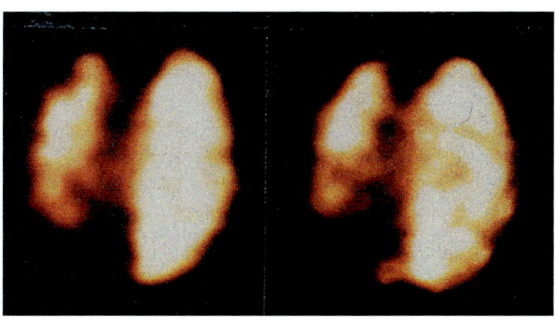

Fig. 25 An ^{123}I-HIPDM study of cerebral blood flow in a patient with established multiple stroke

The application of these techniques to man led to the U.K. Amersham Award for Radiopharmacy conferred by the British Nuclear Medicine Society being awarded to Mr Lui, a member of the Institute's staff.

Recently (1984) Dr. Ell and co-workers, in collaboration with Amersham International, have evaluated a range of entirely new compounds, leading to the first worldwide studies of rCBF in man with a ^{99}Tc^m-labelled tracer. These studies carried out from August 1984 onwards, received the accolade of Image of the Year, during the 1985 Annual Meeting of the Society of Nuclear Medicine (USA) (Figs. 26, 27).

A number of publications underline the importance of this discovery (6), and a programme of joint research has been initiated with the Stroke Unit at Charing Cross Hospital. Significant funds have already been identified and it is hoped that SPET and the new tracers will bring new insights into the management and treatment of this condition.

From the clinical application aspect, this period of the Institute's activity centred around two major areas of development: 1) the application of radioactive tracers to the study of cardiac function and disease – nuclear cardiology; b) the development of single photon emission computed tomography aimed at the 3 dimensional investigation of a radioactive tracer distribution in man and the measurement of absolute amounts of tracer (in vivo autoradiography).

The first programme, nuclear cardiology, has been uniquely successful. With an initial setting up grant in 1979 (£120,000, the Sir Jules Thorn Charitable Trust) a subsequent grant of £80,000 from the same Charity for two Fellowships in nuclear cardiology in 1982, the research programme into the

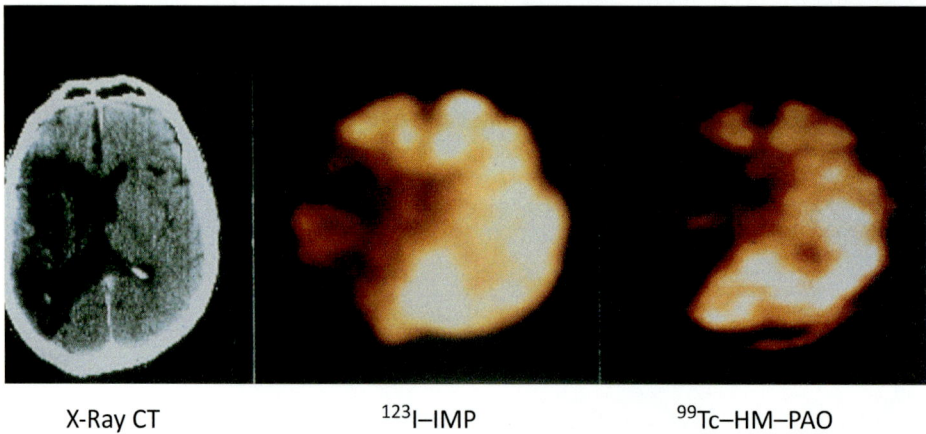

X-Ray CT ^{123}I–IMP ^{99}Tc–HM–PAO

Fig. 26 The first study made with the new ^{99}Tc^m-labelled agent aimed at depicting cerebral blood flow in man is shown in comparison with X-ray CT and ^{123}I-IMP studies

(a)

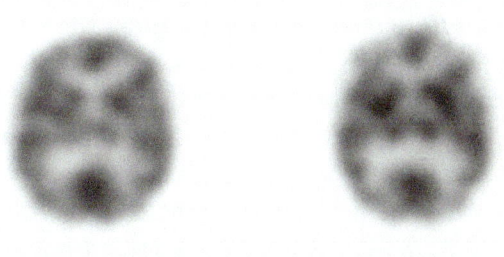

(b)

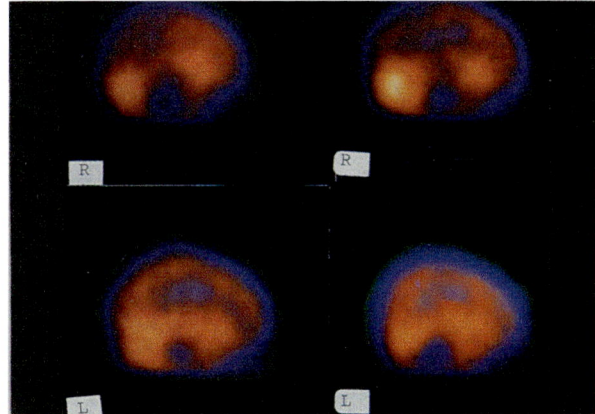

(c)

Fig. 27 (a) The normal distribution of $^{99}Tc^{m}$-labelled HMPAO in man. Note excellent detail, with clear visualisation of basal ganglia.
(b) A regional cerebral blood flow study in a patient with hemiplegic migraine. Sagittal section scans show extensive blood flow abnormality in the left frontal lobe and right parietal lobe.
(c) The high resolution X-ray CT scan is normal

broad area of coronary artery disease, its detection and monitoring, led to an environment where in 1986 20-25% of all routine investigations at the Institute are being carried out in patients with cardiac disease.

With Brown and Jarritt, we were first in the U.K. to apply the Fourier Transform to: the analysis of left ventricular time activity curves and the derivation of parametric images of amplitude and phase, time of end systole (TES) and the time of end diastole (TED), the evaluation of patterns of ventricular contraction in patients with conduction abnormality and the determination of left ventricular volume and ejection fraction by radionuclide tomographic techniques (7,8,9). Gated pool emission tomography was described as a new technique for the investigation of cardiac structure and function, and nuclear cardiology were successfully applied to the preoperative assessment of patients undergoing surgery. There is now an established place for the application of nuclear cardiology and the monitoring of cardiac disease and its treatment (diagnosis and follow-up of ventricular aneurysm, shunting, valvular regurgitation, pre-therapy assessment of cardiotoxic drugs often used in oncology), the radionuclide techniques replacing some of the more invasive investigations in the assessment of patients with coronary artery disease (Figs. 28,29,30). In a recent survey (1986), one-third of all routine nuclear cardiological studies were person-

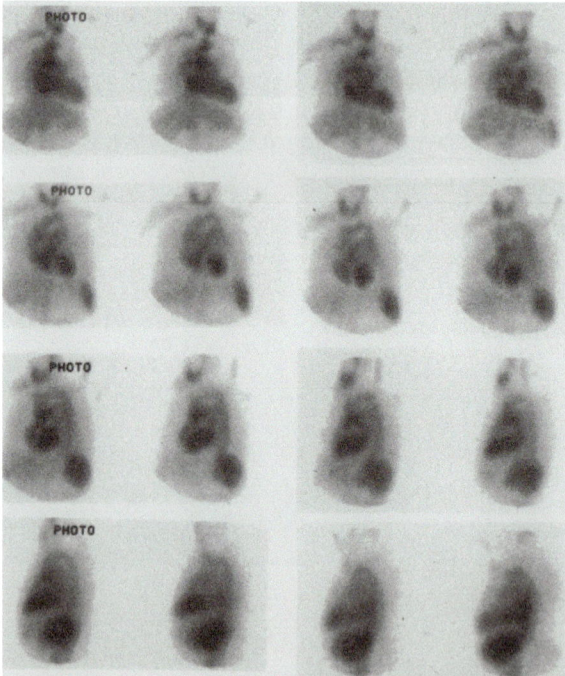

Fig. 28 A study of the heart undertaken with ^{99}Tc^m-labelled red cells and multiple planar projections recorded over 360 degrees. The blood pool within the thyroid, heart, right and left ventricles, liver and spleen, is clearly visualised

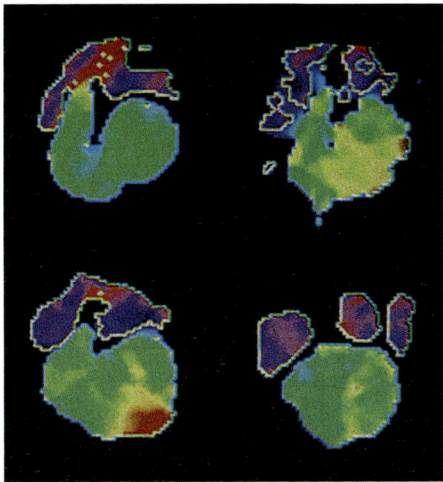

Fig. 29 Images of cardiac phase depicting the timing of ventricular contraction. On the top left, the colours green and light blue depict normal and simultaneous contraction of both ventricles. On the top right, the yellow colour depicts asynchronous contraction of the left ventricle in a patient with ischaemic heart disease. Bottom left demonstrates dyskinetic contraction of the left ventricle in a patient with a typical aneurysm. Bottom right, the same patient after surgical removal of the left ventricular aneurysm

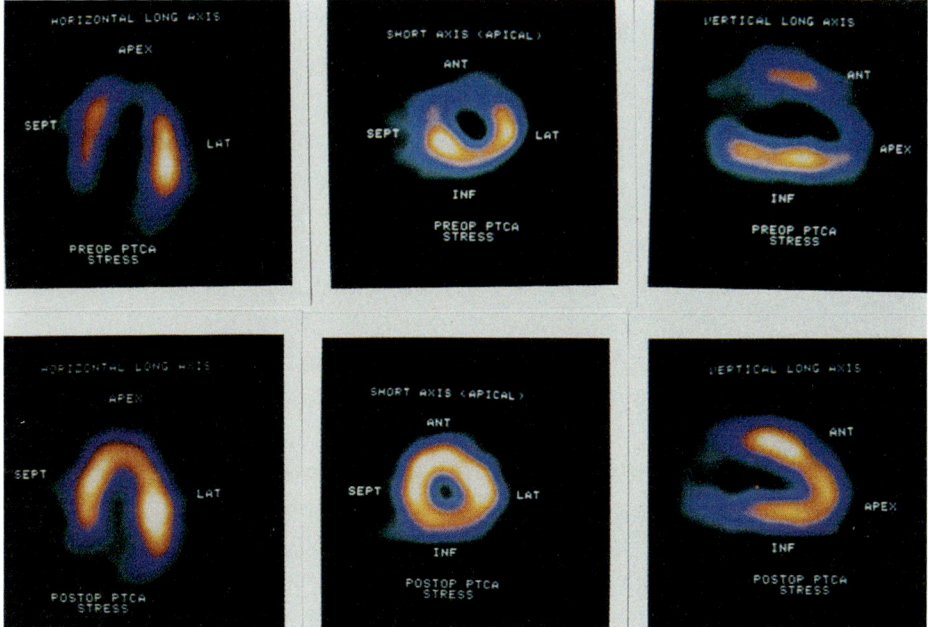

Fig. 30 A typical tomographic study recorded with ^{201}Tl, depicting the perfusion of the myocardium at rest and after PTCA (percutaneous transluminal coronary artery) dilatation. Significant perfusion deficits demonstrated pre-operatively have resolved after successful intervention

ally classified by the consultant physician as having contributed to the surgical management of the patient, and in a further 7% of these studies, invasive and more costly catheter procedures could be avoided.

Although the tomographic scanner designed here was not developed beyond the prototype stage, the initial clinical data pointed to the advantages of emission tomography with improved image contrast and lesion detection, and this was at a time when transmission computed tomography (X-ray CT sanning) had yet to be developed. Single photon emission tomography (SPET) late became a major research project in the Institute, since the initial setting up grant by the Special Trustees (£80,000) and Union Carbide USA (£80,000) in 1978.

This time, the BBC and "Tomorrow's World", came to the Institute. A programme was seen on TV in April 1979, where a first prototype of new tomographic brain scanner began clinical activity. This apparatus is still in operation, due to the dedication and expertise of the physics staff here.

SPET research was aimed at the investigation of clinical utility in Oncology (detection of primary and secondary tumours, and secondary tumours in the brain and the liver) and the quantitative assessment of tracer distribution in man (measurement of phosphate uptake in bone in pg/ml, assessment of cardiac ventricular volume in ml, and cerebral blood flow in ml/min/g). Particular emphasis was placed on the development and application of SPET in the assessment of patients with neurological and psychiatric disease with the newly developed ^{123}I and ^{99}Tc^{m} lipophylic tracers and in the 3 dimensional investigation of myocardial perfusion in man, using ^{201}Tl chloride, or one of its possible substitutes.

Data relevant to diagnostic oncology led to the publication by Ell et al. of the first worldwide large clinical series on brain and liver deposits (10,11). Evidence was made available, demonstrating the feasibility, utility and sensitivity of SPET, as a routine diagnostic tool. With the introduction of SPET all brain, heart perfusion and liver colloid studied became routine in the Institute, replacing conventional planar investigations. The sensitivity of SPET in the detection of brain and liver deposits compared very favourably with other imaging techniques, such as XOray computed tomography and grey-sale ultrasound. This method is still in use, almost 10 years later, for the routine investigation of oncology referrals.

A special purpose methodology was developed, tested and clinically utilised, as far as SPET of the skeleton (skull) was concerned. Data was measured in pg of methylene diphosphonate taken up per ml of skull bone. Normal ranges were established and applied to the investigation of metabolic bone disease, and metastases in the skeleton. Clear differences in tracer uptake were measured between normals, patients with Paget's disease, hyperparathyroidism and osteomalacia. It was demonstrated that monostotic Paget's may influence skeletal turnover as a whole, that the effect of vitamin D on osteomalacia could be monitored in terms of whole body skeletal turnover (sampling the skull as a segment of the skeleton largely independent from gravity and perfusion), and that peripheral skeletal deposits from carcinoma of the breast and prostate could lead to more widespread involvement of skeletal metabolism (12).

The Institute became a test bed for dedicated and general purpose SPET instrumentation. From 1976 to 1986, 5 major SPET apparatus were installed, tested, modified and put through clinical utilisation. The commercial value of these instruments approached £1,000,000. We became a source of reliable information concerning the performance of SPET units, providing worldwide guidance as to the state of the art of this technology, R & D trends, and possible clinical utilisation. In collaboration with Cambridge University, maximum entropy algorithms were tested and applied to image reconstruction, and Monte Carlo techniques were used for the investigation of collimator design and performance of single slice tomographic scanners.

The research carried out with SPET led to upwards of 30 scientific publications in refereed journals, and to the first (worldwide) publication of 3 atlases on the clinical application of single photon emission tomography. Over 1,000 clinical cases have now been studied with radionuclide tomography and a significant degree of know-how has been accumulated. The experience gained here, improvement in the radiation detectors, and the new lipophilic radiopharmaceuticals, have all significantly contributed to the establishment of SPET as a routine nuclear medicine tool in many hospital institutions, even non-university based, worldwide. Most new Anger gamma cameras installed in nuclear medicine departments offer tomographic capability, and it is predicted that SPET studied of the brain and heart will dominate the next decade of nuclear medicine activity.

The Current Clinical Role of Nuclear Medicine

A survey of routine clinical work at the Institute of Nuclear Medicine shows a doubling of the number of tests performed over the last 10 years. Emphasis on the detection of primary and secondary neoplasms (present in the mid 70s) has however been largely replaced by the evaluation of organ function (in the first half of the 80s). The single most notable change within this context occurred with the emergence of X-ray radionuclide brain scanning, X-ray CT becoming first port of call for most conditions leading to imaging studies of the brain. Recently however, radionuclide brain scanning is emerging with a new role, namely that of the investigation of cerebral blood volume and flow, and the demonstration of the distribution of some of the neuroreceptors (the dopamine and opiate receptors are the focus of most of the present attention). The routine radionuclide investigation of the cardiac patient, practically absent in the mid 70s, has shown an important growth, now accounting for 25% of all routine investigations. Despite the arrival of digital subtraction angiography, ventilation/perfusion lung scanning is well established as the first port of call investigation of a patient suspected of embolic disease. Diuresis renography plays an essential role in the assessment of the urological patient, and the radionuclide studies of the thyroid and the skeleton remain the bread and butter of the nuclear medicine clinic.

There has been a significant expansion in the clinical utilisation of radio-labelled cell products: red cells in the demonstration of haemorrhage, white cells in the detection of infection (Figs. 31,32) and platelets in the visualisation of clot. Non-specific tracers, such as ^{67}Ga-citrate, still have clinical value in the monitoring of patients with sarcoid, many centres applying this approach to the investigation of conditions such as lung cancer restaging of lymphomas, and AIDS. Tracers with specific uptake mechanisms such metaiodobenzylguanidine (Fig. 33) have found a clinical role in the investigation of tumours of neurocrest origin, whilst a number

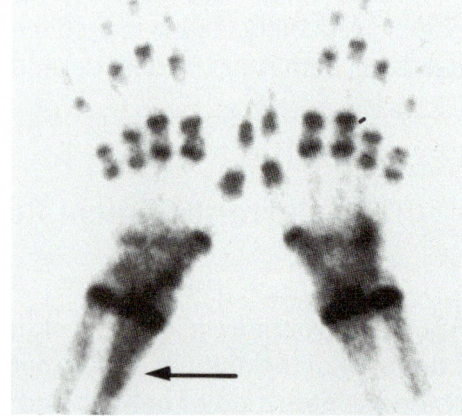

Fig. 31 A bone scan of the forearm and hand of a 7 year old child, demonstrating acute osteomyelitis of the distal component of the radius (arrow)

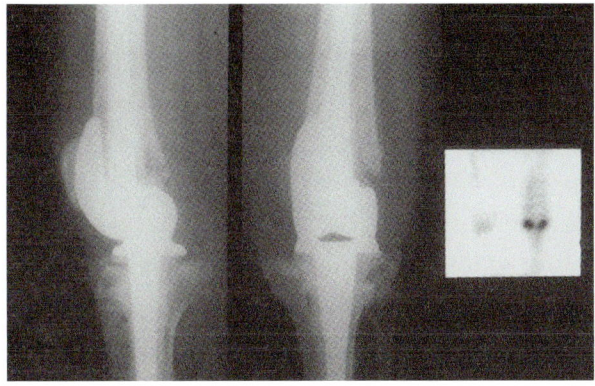

Fig. 32 A study recorded with ^{111}In-labelled leuco-cytes demonstrating the site of infection in a patient with a prosthesis of the knee

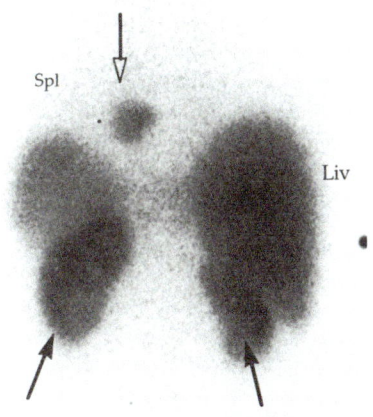

Fig. 33 A patient with metastatic malignant phaeochromocytoma. The nuclear medicine study undertaken with compounds which concentrate in the liver and spleen (colloid), in the kidneys (DMSA) (closed arrows) and in the malignant deposit (mIBG) (open arrows)

of new tracers (^{99}Tc^m pentavalent DMSA, ^{123}I MIBG, ^{201}T-chloride) have led to successful visualisation of deposits from medullary carcinoma of the thyroid. In gastroenterology, there is a growing awareness of the unique role of radionuclide tracer methodology in the assessment of oesophageal motility and gastric emptying, in the detection of biliary leakage and reflux, and the demonstration and detection of small and large bowel disease.

Costing of nuclear medicine has demonstrated the relative economy which can be achieved in an efficiently organised environment. On average, nuclear medicine costs are equivalent to those of conventional fluoroscopy (13), being significantly cheaper than CT, DSA or contrast angiography, and only slightly dearer than conventional diagnostic ultrasound (see page 66).

71

There follows a brief outline of clinical indications:

Brain
- As a filter to X-ray CT or NMR imaging in oncology.
- Regional cerebral blood flow studies in stroke, sub-arachnoid haemorrhage and transient ischaemia
- Differential diagnosis of dementia
- As the localising technique for activation (e.g. temporal lobe epilepsy).
- As a monitor of CSF flow (hydrocephalus, shunt patency).

Eye Studies
- As a monitor of flow and obstruction to flow.

Salivary Gland Studies
- As a monitoring technique of impaired tracer uptake, obstruction or impaired flow.

Thyroid
- Thyroid function testing
- Nodule assessment
- Thyroiditis assessment
- Differentiation of Grave's disease, Plummer's disease, adenoma.
- Assessment of optimal treatment in thyrotoxicosis.
- Monitoring of carcinoma and metastases (Fig. 34)
- Treatment of carcinoma and metastases.

Lungs
- Ventilation and perfusion studies in embolic lung disease (diagnosis and treatment monitoring) (Fig. 35)
- Sarcoid – assessment of involvement; activity versus treatment.
- Carcinoma of the bronchus: pre-operative assessment.
- Chronic obstructive pulmonary disease: baseline and follow-up studies
- Extravascular lung water.
- Leaky lungs.

Heart
- Detection of ischaemic heart disease.
- Heart disease monitoring: pre and post operative CABG procedures.
- Acute myocardial infarction: assessment and prognosis.
- Function assessment: ejection fractions, ventricular volumes, ejection rates.
- Detection of aneurysms and pseudoaneurysms.
- Monitoring of therapy.

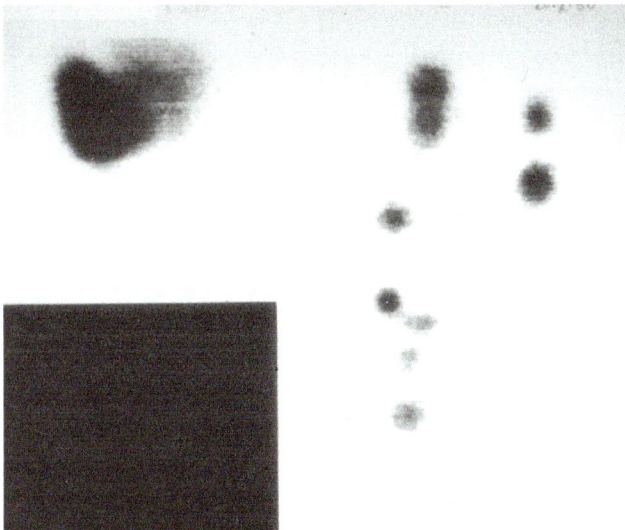

Fig. 34 A patient with follicular carcinoma of the thyroid sown on the left, and on the right the ^{131}I neck and mediastinal survey post surgical removal of the thyroid demonstrating iodine avid metastases in neck and mediastinum

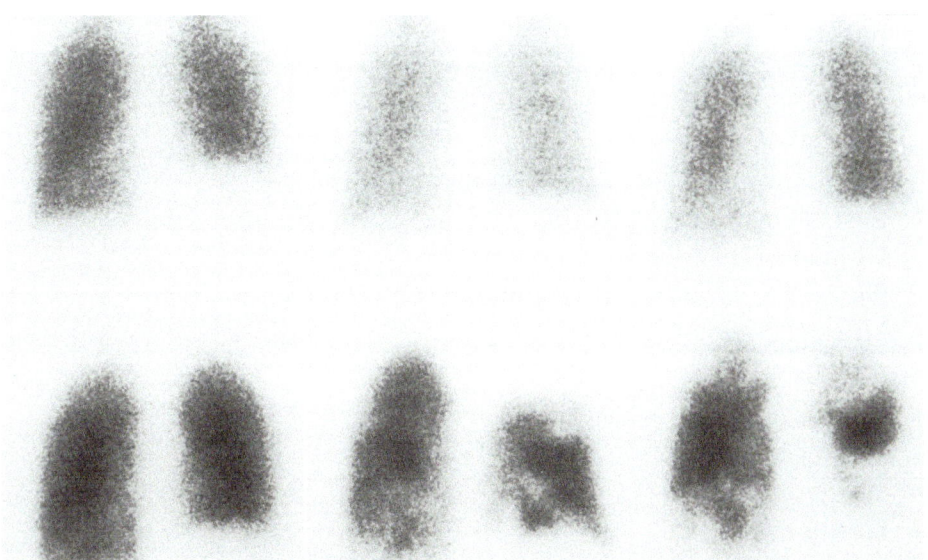

Fig. 35 Ventilation studies (top row) and perfusion studies (bottom row) shown in a patient with recurrent pulmonary emboli. Three studies (posterior projection) shown from the same patient over a period of 6 months, demonstrating progressive deterioration of perfusion due to recurrent embolic phenomena

- Valvular regurgitation assessment.
- Pre-operative assessment of patients in general surgery.
- Cardiotoxic drug therapy monitoring.
- Assessment of conduction disease and pacing.

Gastrointestinal Tract
- Oesophagus:
  Transit time study, study of motility.
  Reflux identification.
  Barrett's syndrome.
- Stomach:
  Gastric emptying for solids and liquids.
  (dumping, pre- and post-operative studies.
  Pre- and post-medication studies.
- Small bowel:
  Detection and activity assessment in Crohn's disease.
- Large bowel:
  Detection and activity assessment in Ulcerative Colitis.
- Spleen and liver:
  Space occupying lesion detection (in many circumstances, first port of call).
  Hepatobiliary flow studies.
  Acute cholecystitis diagnosis (first port of call).
  Biliary reflux detection and measurement.
- Meckel's diverticulum
- Gastrointestinal bleeding detection.
- Gastrointestinal absorption and excretion studies: Schilling test – Vitamin B12.
- Bile acids – malabsorption studies.

Haematology
- Red cell mass.
- Red cell life.
- Plasma volume.
- Splenic uptake.
- Splenic mass.
- Iron kinetics.
- Bone marrow imaging.

Kidneys
- Measurement of GFR, ERPF, and individual renal function.
- Diuresis renography and hydronephrosis/obstruction – diagnosis and monitoring (Fig. 36).

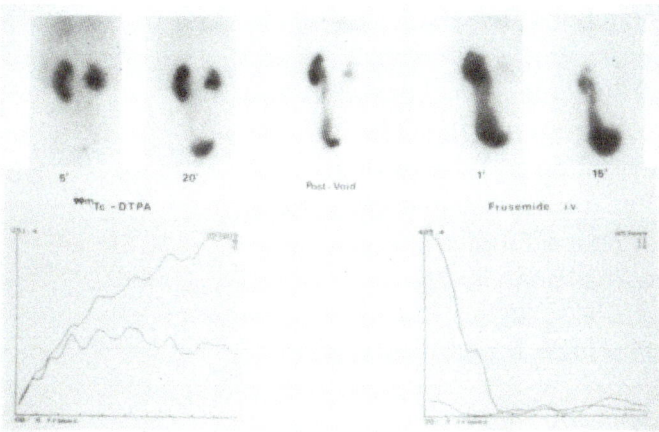

Fig. 36 Typical renographic study with [99]Tc[m]-labelled DTPA. Images demonstrate the functional information available from radionuclide renography in a patient with unilateral obstruction responsive to frusemide, and with significant reflux

- Demonstration of scarring and reflux.
- Acute tubular necrosis/rejection monitoring.

Oncology:
- Detection and monitoring of neoplasia in brain, thyroid, liver and bone.
- Detection of neoplasia of the parathyroid and adrenal glands and tumours of neurocrest origin.
- Sarcoid detection and monitoring.

Whole Body Imaging
- Soft tissue:
  Pyrexia of unknown origin work up.
  Non-Hodgkins and Hodgkins lymphoma work up and monitoring.
- Whole body bone:
  Deposit detection, mainly of Ca. breast, lung, stomach and colon.
  Individual osteoporosis and osteomalacia assessment and follow up.
- Whole body bone marrow:
  To demonstrate sites of active marrow, marrow expansion,
  marrow deposits.
- Lmphoma scintigraphy
  As an adjuvant for radiotherapy field planning.
  As a technique for lymph drainage monitoring.
  As a technique for monitoring oedema.

Orthopaedics and Benign Bone Disease.
- Osteoid osteoma: localisation
- Rod implant monitoring: detection of pseudoarthrosis.
- Femoral head necrosis: diagnosis (fig. 37)
- Caisson disease: localisation and monitoring.
- Prosthesis monitoring: loosening/infection.
- Infection (diagnosis and monitoring.
- Diagnosis of fissure/small bone fractre.
- Localisation of Paget's (Figs. 38,39).
- Detection of metabolic bone disease and HPOA.

Deep Vein Thrombosis
- As a technique to reduce X-ray phlebography and monitoring of DVT versus treatment.

Therapy
- Thyroid:
  Hyperthyroidism
  Carcinoma (mainly follicular, papillary or mixed histology)
- Malignant effusions: pleural and peritoneal.
- Chronic effusions: knees
- Neuroblastoma
- Phaeochromocytoma.
- Intractable skeletal pain in malignancy

In Summary
From what has been outlined so far, it is apparent that nuclear medicine is an important general tool in medical diagnosis, individual monitoring and, in some circumstances, treatment. These techniques are economic. A simplified outline of the costs of nuclear medicine in vivo tests is given in order to substantiate this statement and differentiate the nature of costing.

Average Costing of Test (in vivo) Middlesex Hospital Medical School

Salaries	Radiopharmaceuticals	Display & Sundries	Other
£25	£12.50	£5	£7.50

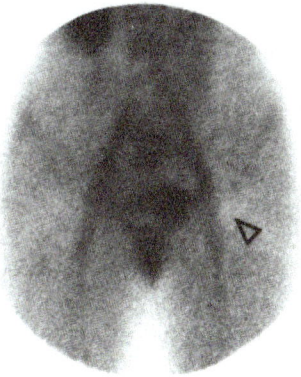
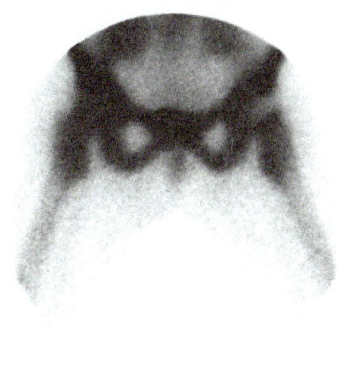

Fig. 37 Bone scan (left perfusion phase and right metabolic phase of patient with avascular necrosis of the head of the femur. The arrow points to the perfusion deficit

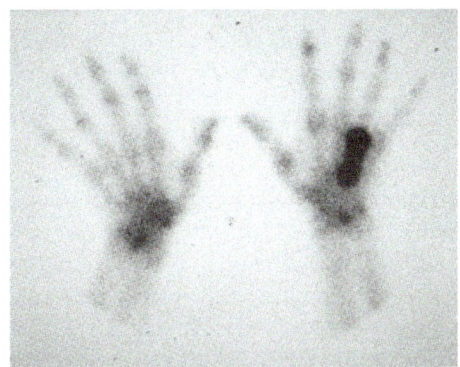

Fig. 38 A patient with monostotic Paget's disease of the third metacarpal bone

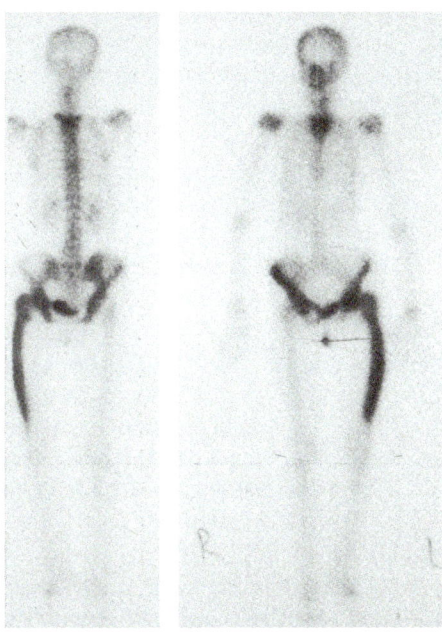

Fig. 39 A typical bone scan of a patient with advanced Paget's disease of bone

References

1a. $^{99}Tc^m$ Imidodiphosphonate. A superior radiopharmaceutical for in vivo positive myocardial infarct imaging. I. Experimental Data. P.J. Ell, R. Langford, P. Pearce, D. Lui, A.T.
Elliott, N. Woolf and E.S. Williams. *British Heart Journal* XL, 3, 226-233, 1978.

1b. $^{99}Tc^m$ Imidodiphosphonate. A superior radiopharmaceutical for in vivo positive
myocardial infarct imaging. II. Clinical Data. S. Joseph, P.J. Ell, P. Ross, R. Donaldson,
A.T. Elliott, N.J.G. Brown, W. Somerville and E.S. Williams. *British Heart Journal* XL,
3, 234-241, 1978.

2. 99m-Tc-Plasmin: A new test for the detection of deep vein thrombosis. J.M. Deacon,
P.J. Ell, A. Anderson and O. Khan. *British Journal of Radiology*, 53, 673-677, 1980.

3. Experimentelle und Klinische Ergebnisse der Gallenwegsszintigraphie mit 99-m-Tc-
Diethyl-IDA. H Deckart, P.J. Ell, K.F. Pfitzmann, A. Blottner, J. Brunhober, R. Janiszewski
und J. Welland. *Radiologie und Radiotherapie, 1,* 122-123, 1979.

4. A quantitative study of biliary dyskinesia using 99m-Tc-EHIDA. P.H. Jarritt, E. Pagtakhan
and P.J. Ell. *Nuclear Medicine Communications, 7,* 280, 1986.

5. Cerebral Blood Flow with Iodine-123 labelled amines. P.J. Ell, M.J.G. Harrison, D. Lui,
Lancet, II 1348-1352, 1983.

6. Regional cerebral blood flow mapping with a new Tc-99m-labelled compound. P.J. Ell,
I.D. Cullum, D.C. Costa et al. *The Lancet, II,* 5-51, 1985.

7. Patterns if Vnetricular Contraction in patients with conductive abnormality studied by
radionuclide angiocardiography. S.R. Underwood, S. Walton, P.J. Laming, P.J. Ell, R.W.
Emanuel, R.H. Swanton. *British Heart Journal,* 51, 568-575, 1984.

8. Left ventricular volume and ejection fraction determined by gated blood pool emission tomography. S.R. Underwood, S. Walton, P.J. Laming, P.H. Jarritt, P.J. Ell, R.W.
Emanuel, R.H. Swanton. *British Heart Journal,* 53, 216-222, 1985.

9. Gated blood pool emission tomography: a new technique for the investigation of
cardiac structure and function. S.R. Underwood, S. Walton, P.J. Ell, P.H. Jarritt, R.W.
Emanuel, R.H. Swanton. *European Journal of Nuclear Medicine,* 10, 332-338, 1985.

10. Emission and transmission brain tomography. P.J. Ell, J.M. Deacon, D. Ducassou and
A. Brendel. *British Medical Journal,* 280, 438-440, 1980.

11. A comparison between emission and transmission computed tomography of the liver.
O. Khan, P.J. Ell, P.H. Jarritt, I.D. Cullum and E.S. Williams. *British Medical Journal,*
283, 1212-1214, 1981.

12. The skull uptake test. A new investigative and perhaps diagnostic tool. P.J. Ell, I.D.
Cullum, P.H. Jarritt and D. Lui. *Nuclear Medicine Communications,* 5, 215-216, 1984.

13. Costs of nuclear medicine procedures. P.M. Bretland. *Nuclear Medicine Communications,* 7, 310-311, 1986.

Physiological Research

Nuclear Medicine is largely a diagnostic specialty but it differs from others (e.g. radiology) in that the data obtained depend upon the functional state of the system being investigated. Often information is obtained in a time-related form (so-called dynamic studies) and is presented graphically with relevant functional parameters plotted against time. Images of the distribution of radioactivity in the body are functional images and only incidentally demonstrate anatomy. Some images are merely a convenient way of displaying for rapid assimilation massive amounts of computer-processed data. These are "parametric" images, such as, for example, the phase image of myocardial contraction.

Studies to establish "what is normal" can make a significant contribution to human physiology and such contributions have been made by the Institute, particularly in the field of nephrology and of endocrinology. However, in one field physiological research was carried out as a special interest not elated to the development of diagnostic techniques and for this reason it is explained here at some length.

As a life-long mountaineer, Professor Williams at an early stage decided to carry out research on the effect on man of the adverse environment encountered mountaineering. His first two studies were carried out while he was still a medical student, the first being an investigation of what level of "field" work was feasible under the arduous conditions typical of this "pastime". This took place during a Himalaya-training traverse of the Bernese Oberland in 1955 and although exploratory in nature, results were obtained which were integrated into a later publication (1).

In 1956 he took charge of all aspects, financial, protocols, etc., of the scientific work of a small-scale climbing expedition to the Karakoram, a range of very high mountains just to the north-west of the Himalayas (K2, the second highest mountain in the world is here, as also is the largest single concentration of the world's highest summits).

At that time it was thought that the "stress" of oxygen lack, of extreme exercise, and of cold, would lead to maximising adrenal cortical function and it had been theorized (2) that such abnormal unremitting stress could lead to a degree of adrenal cortical failure, which might be a major factor in the slow "deterioration", and inevitable death, of those staying at high altitudes (say, above 20,000 ft/6,00 m) for protracted periods of time.

In the early 1950s attention had been focused on the sodium and potassium content of saliva as an indirect, but convenient, means of studying adrenal cortical function in patients (this was before it was appreciated that the three cellular "zones" of the adrenal cortex each had specific functions and that changes in sodium and potassium excretion from the body, as mirrored by the salivary content of these electrolytes, were not necessarily a reflection of overall adrenal function). This was the method used for studying abnormal function during this expedition.

This was only one of a series of projects all of which were completed and the results published, but it is the one that led to work which was only possible by the use of radioactive tracers – in the application of nuclear medicine to this field. Nuclear medicine research directed at elucidating pathophysiology was, by Williams, repeatedly applied to further studies of human response to an adverse environment, particularly oxygen lack. This was not primarily high altitude research for its own sake: going very high produced in healthy people a condition simulating that common to a number of pathological conditions where oxygen exchange between the alveoli of the lungs, and the blood, is impaired.

In the light of the pre-suppositions of the mid-1950s the salivary electrolyte results were totally unexpected. Instead of a stimulation of "adrenal function: gross depression was demonstrated when the mountaineers under study were no higher than 10,000 ft (3000 m) altitude.

A functional index used at the time was the sodium-potassium ratio and in one person this rose to heights recorded previously only in Addison's disease. Yet to all outward appearances he and his expedition colleagues were not only healthy but exceptionally fit. As this unexpected and (then) inexplicable data had been obtained and "worked up" by a student it was not published but in 1959 Williams (now medically qualified) organized a similar study, though at lower altitude, on the Mont Blanc Massif. Similar results were obtained and the earlier results were then published (3). In the light of this confirmation, funds were raised to set up (in 1960) a major study involving a number of weeks stay near the summit of Mont Blanc. Now, for the first time, nuclear medicine techniques were used. Aldosterone had already been extensively studied and an analytical method using radioactive tracers for its assay in urine was available in the Middlesex Hospital Medical School.

Once again the work relating to the theme of this chapter was only one of the studies carried out but nuclear medicine had no impact on the development of the other undertakings (e.g. complex psychological testing; the arduous task of documenting eosinophilia in an environmental temperature almost always sub-zero, etc.). The implication of the salivary elec-trolyte results was that aldosterone secretion had been "switched off" on ascent to a moderate altitude but, in 1960, only urinary content of this hormone and that in 24 hour samples, could be measured. It was felt how-ever that a direct measure of the *excretion* of this hormone would be one step nearer to elucidating this curious homeostatic puzzle.

The urine had to be kept frozen which presented no problem as the 2 litre plastic bottles had merely to be left outside. But they also had to be transported to the laboratories here without thawing. Insulated boxes were designed by Williams and made here and a helicopter lift at roughly week-ly intervals was arranged, the samples being delivered within minutes to a waiting lorry in the valley and whisked to Geneva airport (arrangements having previously been made with the French and Swiss Customs authori-ties). A colleague here was telephoned by the lorry driver so that speci-mens could be collected at Heathrow from the plane, prior arrangements had also been made with the airport authorities. The next stage was a dash by road to deep-frozen storage. In this complicated logistical operation no single 24 hour specimen was lost or damaged nor did any thaw. The (then) laborious aldosterone assay results confirmed that the early sample of urine contained no detectable amount of the metabolite of aldosterone production. Later samples showed a slow return of the urinary aldosterone metabolite levels towards (but by no means reaching) each individual's pre-expedition concentration (5,6).

This use of the in vitro nuclear medicine technique of "derivative analysis" confirmed the inferences drawn from the previous indirect salivary electro-lyte findings. During the next few years nuclear medicine techniques applied to endocrinology rapidly advanced and Williams wished to apply these to prove that the reduction aldosterone metabolite concentration in the urine from those at high altitude reflected reduced secretion of this hormone form the adrenal glands. The urinary results alone, of course, could have been accounted for by postulating, for example, that oxygen lack had resulted in aldosterone being metabolized in such a way that it produced metabolites ignored by the assay procedures which had been employed.

A colleague, Dr. J.D.H. Slater, a physician with a special interest in the kidney, and in the renin-angiotensin-aldosterone system, had supervised successful research in this field using radioactive hydrogen (tritium) and had worked on a method of measuring the secretion rate from the adrenal glands of aldosterone and cortisol. He and his colleagues were therefore in a position to make a direct measurement of the secretion rate of aldoster-one in subjects at high altitude.

Dr. Slater readily agreed to collaborate and became a very active member of the expedition team. Rates of aldosterone and cortisol secretion were measured in all member of the high altitude team over a 24-hour period on days 3-4, 8-9, and 13-14, at about 11,500 ft (3,500 m). The 24-hour urinary excretion of the metabolite of aldosterone measured on the earlier expedition was also measured in two subjects on a series of days through-out the stay at high altitude.

Even with the mild degree of oxygen lack the aldosterone secretion rate fell by an average of 65% of the measured rate in the same subjects before the expedition and the earlier urinary excretion results were confirmed. It was interesting that the cortisol secretion rate rose on ascent and fell again on descent, a result in accordance with the expectations as regards response to "stress" which it had been hoped to document in the studies en years before (6,7).

Dr. Slater continued his interest in the relationship of oxygen-lack to the subjects of his special clinical interest and in 1969 he collaborated in an experiment on four subjects carried out in the decompression chamber of the Institute of Aviation Medicine at Farnborough. Changes of serum renin activity, heart rare, blood pressure, renal sodium, potassium and metadren-aline excretion, as well as alveolar gas tensions were recorded during 2-3 hour exposures at an atmospheric pressure equivalent to an altitude of 14,000 ft (4,300 m) (8).

Williams' many periods spent in the mountains had impressed on him the common occurrence of oedema both at high and low altitudes. Although by the middle 1960s the occurrences of, and dangerous nature of, both pulmonary and cerebral oedema as important features of the (sometimes fatal) condition known as "mountain sickness" was becoming well docu-mented, no reference seems to have been made to peripheral oedema until Williams did so in summarising his work thus far before a meeting of the Royal Society (5). Anecdotal evidence had also suggested a correlation between exercise and acute mountain sickness so with this in mind the occurrence of oedema after extreme exercise as well as the above apparent correlation it was decided to turn attention to this new field. The decision was to some extent influenced by the fact that human physiologists in the U.S.A. with a full-time commitment to the subject had taken up the work described above and were intending to extend it rapidly. In particular the Mount Logan permanent research station at about 17,000 ft (5,200 m) with its great resources, was beginning to build on this pioneering work.

Preliminary work was carried out in British mountains with such success in 1976 that a full-scale field study followed in 1977 (9). It was found that exercise in the form of hill walking caused a retention of sodium and of water, and a reduction in packed cell volume. These findings were interpreted as indicating a movement of water from the intracellular to the extracellular space and also an expansion of the plasma volume. The response seemed to be related to changes in the handling of electrolytes rather than of water, because the concentration of arginine vasopressin did not change throughout the study, but the urinary sodium/potassium excretion ration increased on stopping exercise, suggesting a change in the secretion of aldosterone by the adrenal glands.

In order to verify and extend these findings a further study was carried out in British hills in 1979 (10). This second study confirmed that water was significantly retained during the days of exercise as compared with the 'control' days and repeated careful measurements on the lower leg demonstrated an increased lower leg volume during exercise whether or not signs of leg oedema could be demonstrated. During the exercise period plasma aldosterone concentration and plasma renin activity rose and there was a highly significant correlation between these values and sodium retention.

It was now felt that sufficient knowledge of the relevant effects of mountaineering exercise without oxygen lack had been established to arrange a similar exercise study under mildly hypoxic conditions. The army had shown considerable interest in this work and in 1980, with supports from its resources, an appropriate study was arranged in the European Alps at about 10,000 ft (3,000 m) altitude (11). The design of the experiment was similar to those on British hills; controlled diet throughout; a period of study without stress; the stress period (daily mountaineering); and finally a recovery period without stress. In the Alpine study the first four and the last four days of the experimental period were spent semisedentary at 2,900 feet (900 m) altitude and the middle five days were spent mountaineering at between 8,900 ft and 11,900 ft (2,700 m and 3,600 m, respectively).

A retention of both sodium and water was demonstrated during the period of exercise and the plasma volume increased but there was no change in the plasma sodium concentration so that a significant expansion of the extracellular space was inferred. The detailed results were similar to those resulting from comparable exercise at sea level and opposite to the effect of altitude previously demonstrated (and by now confirmed by others) on resting subjects.

In 1981 the evolution of these studies was interrupted as Williams was invited to be a member of the British Mount Kongur Expedition to China.

There were two main objectives: to make the first ascent of then highest unclimbed summit in the world, and to carry out further physiological studies at very high altitudes (12). Later in the same year these studies were extended to higher altitudes by United States scientists on Everest.

Soon afterwards a protocol was arranged to expand the exercise-at-altitude studies already briefly described. Cooperation of the United States Army was obtained and a month's use of its laboratory on the summit of Pikes Peak, in Colorado, was agreed (14,110 ft/4,300 m). This was the first British party to stay on the peak for physiological research since the famous studies carried out there in the early years of this century.

Any reader interested in the detailed results of this research which has extended as a part-time interest over so many years is referred to the literature, some references to which have been made in this chapter. The inclusion of this topic here serves to emphasise how the use of radioactive tracers has had an impact on almost all branches of medical research in addition to giving rise to the clinical medical specialty of nuclear medicine.

References

1. Effect of altitude on basal palmar sweating: P.C.P. MacKinnon, I.L. MacKinnon, and E.S. Wiliams. *British Medical Journal, I,* 199-201, 1959.
2. L.G.C.E. Pugh – private communication.
3. Salivary electrolyte composition at high altitude. E.S.Williams *Clinical Science, 21,* 37-42, 1961.
4. Aldosterone excretion and potassium retention in subjects living at high altitude, P.J. Ayres, r.c. Hurter, E.S. Williams and J, Rundo. *Nature, 191,* 78-80, 1961.
5. Electrolyte regulation during the adaptation of humans to life at high altitudes. E.S. Williams. *Proceedings of the Royal Society,* B, *165,* 266-280, 1966.
6. Potassium retention during the respiratory alkalosis of mild hypoxia in man: its relationship aldosterone secretion and other metabolic changers. J.D.H. Slater, E.S. Williams, R.H.T. Edwards, R.P. Ekins, P.H. Sonksen, C.H. Beresford and M. McLauglin. *Clinical Science, 37,* 311-326, 1969.
7. Control of aldosterone secretion during acclimatization to hypoxia in man. J.D.H. Slater, R.E. Tuffley, E.S. Williams, C.H. Beresford, P.H. Sonksen, R.H.T. Edwards, R.P. Ekins and M. McLaughlin. Clinical Science,37,327-341,1969
8. Serum renin activity during exposure to hypoxia. R.E. Tuffley, D. Rubenstein, J.D.H. Slater and E.S. Williams. *Journal of Endocrinology, 48,* 497-510, 1970.
9. Effect of exercise of seven consecutive days hill-walking on fluid homeostasis. E.S. Williams, M.P. Ward, J.S. Milledge, W.R. Withey, M.W.J. Older and M.L. Forsling. *Clinical Science, 56,* 305-316, 1979.
10. Sodium balance, fluid homeostasis and the renin-aldosterone system during the prolonged exercise of hill walking. J.S. Milledge, E.I. Bryson, D.M. Catley, R. Hesp, N. Luff, B.D. Minty, M.W.J. Older, N.N. Payne, M.P. Ward and W.R. Withey. *Clinical Science, 62,* 595-604, 1982.

11. Fluid and electrolyte homeostasis during prolonged exercise at altitude. W.R. Withey, J.S. Milledge, E.S. Williams, B.D. Minty, E.I. Bryson, N.P. Luff, M.W.J. Oldere and J.M. Beeley. *Journal of Applied Physiology 55,* 409-412, 1983.
12. Cardiorespiratory response to exercise in man repeatedly exposed to extreme altitude. J.S. Milledge, M.P. Ward, E.S. Williams and C.R.A. Clarke. *Journal of Applied Physiology, 55,* 1379-1385, 1983.

Teaching

From the outset teaching has been a main commitment of the Institute. At first most of this was on an ad hoc basis, visitors being accepted to gain experience in nuclear medicine not only from an academic point of view but also in order that they could return to their own hospital to set up a diagnostic service.

Such visitors were medical doctors, scientists, radiographers, and technicians. The period of stay varied from a few weeks to two or three years and in many cases the visitors contributed materially to the research of the Institute and higher degrees were obtained. At an early stage the token staff was increased by appointing a registrar and this enabled a doctor to obtain the "in depth" experience now recognised as an essential to anyone proposing to make a career in nuclear medicine. All of the holders of this post 9except the most recent who are still in a medical training grade) are now consultants although not all have made their career in nuclear medicine. Young doctors have recognised that a registrarship in nuclear medicine gives invaluable experience in investigating a wide variety of diseases and also an insight into the advantages and limitations of the tracer method for research in their chosen field of medicine, whether this be endocrinology, neurology, cardiology, etc.

Co-operation between nuclear medicine and diagnostic radiology makes it desirable that some trainee radiologists should spend preferably a registrarship in nuclear medicine but if this is not possible nuclear medicine should be included in the rotation programme of such trainees. This is a feature of the teaching of the Institute but from time to time a doctor aiming to make a career in radiology has occupied the registrar post in the Institute.

During the first few years it became evident that those coming here for training in nuclear medicine techniques or to gain experience in the provision of a routine diagnostic service wished to obtain a certificate of evidence that they had received training in the subject. The Director wished to set up a course leading to a Diploma in Nuclear Medicine, the training being of a practical nature and aiming to equip the trainee to return to his own hospital and be able to set up a basic nuclear medicine service and, as time passed, to develop this according to local needs.

At that time the University of London was averse to instituting new Diploma courses and after much negotiation a course was instituted to conform in pattern to the then relatively new series of medical MSc's. The MSc course in Nuclear Medicine was arranged in collaboration with the Royal Postgraduate Medical School and the Institute of Cancer Research, so from the first it was an intercollegiate course. A particular student was attached for his day by day training to one of the collaborating Schools of the University but he attended a single course of lectures, practicals and demonstrations and in addition he was strongly advised to attend seminars which were from time to time arranged here and elsewhere in London and also to attend the nuclear medicine symposia of the British Nuclear Medicine Society, the British Institute of Radiology and (later) of the London Nuclear Medicine Club.

The course became popular especially with visitors from abroad, and other Schools of the University applied to be recognized as Collaborating Schools in this intercollegiate course; there are now (in 1986) eleven such recognized Schools. In spite of the vastly increased fees resulting from the Government's policy of requiring all such courses to be financially self-supporting the numbers applying for the course have tended to remain steady. It is necessary to be selective in accepting would-be students byt of the order of 20 students take the course each year.

The MSc (Nuc.Med.) has come to be recognized worldwide as providing a sound introductory training in the subject and although it was conceived as being no more than that – introductory to a further 2-3 years of full time in-service training – it has, in some countries, been treated very much as an "exit" qualification, and is accepted as evidence that the professor of the degree is qualified to take charge of a nuclear medicine diagnostic service.

Master of Science in Nuclear Medicine (Faculty of Medicine)
The course aims to provide a training for medical practitioners wishing to gain a qualification in Nuclear Medicine and to follow careers either in Nuclear Medicine as one of the diagnostic services within the Health Service, in general medicine where the individual aims to make considerable use of radioactive materials, or in such branches of medical research as require an adequate knowledge of the techniques of using these materials. The course is intended for medically qualified persons of adequate clinical experience.

Practitioners of Nuclear Medicine must have a thorough scientific training particularly in such parts of physics and chemistry as are essential to an understanding of the application of radionuclides in medicine. The course will emphasise this requirement within the context of their clinical use and because the course itself is essentially scientific it will lead to the degree of Master of Science in the Faculty of Medicine.

Course of Study
The course for the Degree is open to:
a) Graduates in Medicine of this or another university whose previous training has, in the opinion of the University, fitted them to profit by the course.
b) Other candidates who qualify for admission to Master's Degree course under Section 2 of the General Regulations for Postgraduate Student proceeding to a higher degree and whose experience fits them in the opinion of the School concerned to profit from the course.
The duration of the course will be twelve months full-time, or two years part-time.

Systematic Instruction
This shall be composed of lectures extending over at least two terms of the course.
The subjects of the course shall be:-
a) The principles of physics as applied to nuclear medicine, including radio-activity, properties of nuclear radiations, radiation dosimetry and instruments for radiation detection and measurement.
b) Basic radiochemistry including the manipulation of radioactive materials and the preparation of radiopharmaceuticals.
c) Radiation safety with special reference to the se of unsealed sources of ionizing radiation.
d) The application of radionculides and radiopharmaceuticals in medical diagnosis and investigation including visual presentation of radionuclide distribution, organ function studies, investigation of body composition, absorption studies, in vitro techniques and the comparison of results obtained with those derived from the use of other methods of investigation.

Clinical and Practical Instruction
During the period of the course the student must be attached to an approved institution or institutions where he/she will receive instruction in a wide range of clinical applications of radioactive materials and associated laboratory procedures and where he/she will obtain experience in the routine diagnostic and investigative use of radionuclides and radiopharmaceuticals. In the case of a student attending the course for 12 months, this attendance must be full-time.

Details of Examination

The examination will consist of two three-hour written papers and an oral examination. The written examination will commence on the fourth Monday in June of the year in which the student completes the course, and will normally cover, respectively, the scientific principles and the clinical applications of nuclear medicine. In addition a report on a topic approved by the candidate's teachers must be submitted not later than 31 August. The marking of the reports will be completed during September and the oral examination will commence on the fourth Monday in September. The report need not include original work, but should provide evidence of a thorough knowledge of the subject matter of the report. It should be related to the experience gained during the period of attachment to an approved institution mentioned above. The report should be of not more than 10,000 words.

Every student entering for the examination must apply to the Academic Registrar for an entry form, which must be returned completed together with the certificate of course of study thereon attested in accordance with the General Regulations for Approved Courses of Study. This completed form and the proper fee must be received not later than 1 February.

It will be evident from the first chapter of this book that nuclear medicine is heavily dependent upon collaboration with scientists, particularly physicists. In addition to the training of medical qualified men and women the staff of the Institute has contributed to physics courses, both undergraduate and post-graduate, lecturing on the physics of ionizing radiation and of the ever more complex apparatus used in detection, measurement, recording and data processing of this radiation as applied in nuclear medicine. Over the years our physics staff has taken an increasing lecturing and demonstrating commitment to such courses and currently our two physicists, Drs Jarritt and Cullum, have a significant lecturing role, e.g. in the MSc in Radiation Physics organised jointly by the Middlesex Hospital Medical School and the Medical College of St Bartholomew's Hospital.

The Institute has also been closely associated with the training of radiographers and from the first, radiotherapy radiographers rotated in pairs for two periods of two weeks for part of their training which related to the use of unsealed sources of radiation. In due course the College of Radiographers evolved the specification of a course which would lead to the Diploma in Nuclear Medicine of that College. The Middlesex Hospital's Schools of Radiography at once set up a course leading to that Diploma and the Director of the Institute became a Joint Director of our Schools of Radiography, a number of his staff lecturing on the course as well as pupils spending time in the Institute to gain advanced practical experience.

As nuclear medicine expanded its scope beyond that which could reasonably be expected to be part of the profession of radiographer the title of the Diploma was changed to "Diploma in Nuclear Imaging" so that most of the functional studies and in vitro work was excluded from the course, this being more appropriate to the specialist training of laboratory technicians.

The teaching commitment of the staff of the Institute extended to being invited to lecture at many centres throughout the country and this activity has continued unabated right up to the present. In the earlier years the Director was from time to time invited to visit provincial cities to advise Health Authorities on the setting up of a nuclear medicine service and a number of now well-established and well-known nuclear medicine departments developed from such a visit.

Teaching was also established beyond the confined of the Institute by didactic publications. After the first few years a small handbook was written with the object of describing briefly the tests available for routine diagnostic use. The intention was to make clear the limitations of a test, the medical problems in which it could be helpful and, briefly, how it was carried out so that appropriate preparation of the patient could be arranged. The booklet soon spread far beyond our own colleagues and requests for copes were received from far and wide. It was obvious that it was being widely used as a read reference handbook and a second revised edition was produced.

Then a monograph on probe renography had a great teaching impact as well as for some years also being a widely used "bench" reference book. With the rapid dissemination of nuclear medicine methods throughout most branches of medicine a need was felt for an elementary textbook to supplement the huge multi-author tomes which had appeared in the early 1970s. Such a short textbook was published in 1980.

With the rapid growth of new methods of study, new instrumentation and new radiopharmaceuticals it was decided to produce a series of brief monographs to enable those new to a particular advance, which was rapidly gaining acceptance to have at hand an up to date reference manual. This included the first ever published atlases of nuclear cardiology and single photon emission tomography (in 1980 and 1982).

The following is a list of the books, booklets and monographs produced from the Institute.

BOOKS AND MONGRAPHS

Williams, E.S.
Nuclear Medicine Handbook, pp 40, 1962
Second Edition 1966 (Institute publication).

Britton, K.E. and Brown, N.J.G.
Clinical Renography, pp. 298 (Lloyd Luke), 1971

Ell, P.J., Jarritt, P.H. and Deacon, J.M.
Atlas of Computerized Emission Tomography, pp. 255
(Churchill Livingstone), 1980.

Ell, P.J. and Williams, E.S.
Nuclear Medicine: an Introductory Text, pp. 208 (Blackwell) 1981.

Ell, P.J., Khan, O. and Jarritt, P.H.
Radionuclide Section Scanning, pp. 282 (Chapman & Hall), 1982.

Ell, P.J., Walton, S. and Jarritt, P.H.
Radionuclide Ventricular Function Studies, pp. 171
(Martinus Nijhoff), 1982.

Walton, S. and Ell, P.J.
An introduction to Nuclear Cardiology, pp. 58 (Current Medical Literature
Ltd), 1983.

Jarritt, P.H. and Ell, P.J.
*Gamma Camera Emission Tomography. Quality Control and Clinical Appli-
cations.* pp. 190 (Current Medical Literature Ltd) 1984.

The Future

University College and Middlesex School of Medicine

The creation of a new, single school of medicine, resulting from the unification of the two existing medical schools, the UCL School of Medicine and the Middlesex Hospital Medical School, formally commencing activity in 1987, will influence the future of the academic life in the Institute, at a time when it is in its 27th year of existence. The Institute, as the only academic organization entirely dedicated to nuclear medicine in the U.K., is looking forward to its contribution to the new School of Medicine. Staffed by a Professor, a Reader, a Senior Lecturer and Lecturer, it represents a small but efficient academic unit, its research activity leads to the publication of some 10-20 publications per annum in refereed journals, with a teaching commitment of the order of 400 hours per annum, and a history of considerable fund-raising. Grants received within the last 10 years, are listed below:

1978
Special Trustees, the Middlesex Hospital, £80,000 for the clinical evaluation of an emission tomographic brain scanner.
　　Union Carbide (USA): £80,000 for the evaluation of a new emission tomographic brain scanner.

1979
Sir Jules Thorn Charitable Trust: £120,000 for the clinical application of computerised emission body tomography and nuclear cardiology.

1980
Sir Jules Thorn Charitable Trust: £20,000 to employ a Senior Technician for 3 years for the application of emission tomography.

1982
Sir Jules Thorn Charitable Trust: £80,000 for two fellowships in nuclear cardiology over 4 years, in collaboration with the Department of Cardiology.

1984
International General Electric: $40,000 for the evaluation of area detector technology in DSPET and the clinical study of rCBF tomography.

Special Trustees, the Middlesex Hospital: £30,000 for the investigation of rCBF in patients post CABG: in collaboration with the Department of Surgery and the Department of Neurology.

Special Trustees, the Middlesex Hospital:£24,000 for studies in quantification of tracer distribution with SPET.

1985

Amersham International: £9,500 to employ a Research Assistant for a period of two years, for research into rCBF.

Amersham International: £3,000 for research into collimator design for brain SPET studies.

1986

Centocor: £86,000 for two fellowships in radioimmunoscintigraphy and the evaluation of labelled monoclonal antibodies for imaging purposes (2 years).

Bloomsbury

Recently (1985/86), the Institute has been asked to take on a district-wide role for the provision of a nuclear medicine service. This should result in a more rational utilisation of resources, higher efficiency, improved medical cover and financial savings. Despite the financial constraints imposed on the district, this new role is seen by the Institute as a positive challenger, which needs to re-define its activity, improve the utilisation of the considerable facilities available to the district in terms of nuclear medicine and an opportunity to concentrate its main activity in those areas where the district has considerable strengths: Oncology, Cardiology, Nephrology and Orthopaedics. The geographical spread of the service needs within Bloomsbury and the considerable reshaping which the district will go through over the next few years, underline even more the need for the Institute to adapt and respond adequately to the new requirements. Coordination of effort, radiopharmaceutical production, data processing and resources, all will help to improve the level of activity and the efficiency of the service. There is significant physics expertise and pharmacy know-how across the district, and a commitment to a first rate service. As a whole, the nuclear medicine activity in Bloomsbury represents the second largest patient care commitment in this specialty in the U.K.

Research

As the impact of the radionuclide tracer approach (mainly positron emission tomography – PET) grows in the neurosciences in general and their clinical

94

counterpart (neurology and psychiatry) so the application of more manageable nuclear medicine techniques in neurological and psychiatric disease in particular will expand. Amongst the most hopeful indicators of clinical progress, the combined measurements of cerebral blood volume and flow seem to point the way towards a greater pathophysiological understanding of cerebrovascular disease processes, leading to new information relevant to patient management in conditions such as acute stroke, transient ischaemia and sub-arachnoid haemorrhage. Tissue at risk can be demonstrated and a cohort of patients with stroke divided into groups at higher, medium and smaller probability of further involvement. Similarly there is significant interest in the evaluation of flow patterns in dementia, particularly in the differential diagnosis of senile dementias from the Alzheimer type and progress has been achieved in the evaluation of patients with schizophrenia.

Studies at rest and during intervention are progressively entering the clinical field. There is considerable progress in the area of neuroreceptor imaging and in the demonstration of neuroreceptor deficiencies in a variety of neurological conditions. Whilst PET has made a very significant contribution, the importance of PET findings requires translation into clinical practice, with techniques which can be applied in a day to day routine diagnostic service. The Institute will pursue research within this context, with a view to making available by means of SPET the potential clinical gain to be expected with the PET approach to medicine. Within this context the labelling of new radiopharmaceuticals with conventional non-positron emitting radionuclides is paramount, $^{99}Tc^m$-labelled red cells as a marker for regional cerebral bood volume, $^{99}Tc^m$-labelled hexamethylpropyleneamineeoxime (HM-PAO) as a marker for regional cerebral blood flow, ^{123}I-labelled amines as markers for cerebral blood flow, and more recently ^{123}I-D1+D2 dopamine receptor analogues have become available for clinical work. SPET techniques may therefore offer to a wider patient population what PET technology has been developing over the last 15 years in a highly sophisticated university and teaching environment.

The direct labelling of compounds with positron emitting nuclides of oxygen, carbon or nitrogen, allows for almost a limitless range of substrates to be made available to radionuclide tracer methodology. The constraints of PET imaging is in this context the ultimate specific activity which may be required for localisation studies in man. Non-imaging PET technology may therefore have a significant potential, the nuclear medicine probe of Normal Veall returning to the foray of nuclear medicine activity. Economy, portability and sensitivity are considerable attractions of this approach to PET studies (neurochemistry and related drug research representing an interesting field of application).

Radioimmunoscintigraphy is an expanding field in nuclear medicine which the Institute is about to address. Clot visualisation in general and the detection of secondary soft tissue spread in carcinomas of the breast and ovary will represent initial areas of further research. Fab'2 monoclonal antibodies will be investigated, first tagged onto "In and anti-fibrin and anti-platelet monoclonals used in the detection of clot.

Progress will be made in the general area of quantification of organ function, the radionuclide tracer being particularly suited for the investigation of a patient at rest and during a particular task. Less emphasis will be placed on conventional morphology-related studies for the localisation of disease, and more emphasis will be placed on the development protocols of the individual patient at time of presentation.

There is increasing emphasis in the stratification of patient data into different levels of risk assessment and outcome (prognosis). This is relevant to a number of areas in medicine, including the post-operative assessment of patient undergoing coronary artery bypass grafting. In this common clinical condition, the radionuclide tracer method appears particularly promising as a post-operative screen and predictor of myocardium at risk.

In the recent past, useful clinical information has been derived from the utilisation of rather non-specifically acting radiopharmaceuticals. This will be progressively replaced by more specifically acting tracers, which will be distributed in the body according to a previously determind model. A few can be named at this stage: ^{131}I or ^{123}I metaiodobenzylguanidine (MIBG) for the detection and eventual treatment of primary and secondary phaeochromocytoma and neuroblastoma; ^{111}In monocloncal anti-platelet antibody in the detection of clot; ^{123}I-labelled D1 and D2 receptor analogues for the detection and follow up of dopamine receptor concentration in the brain.

Finally, there is renewed interest in the application of nuclear medicine techniques to therapy. In terms of energy delivery per gram of tissue in man a target specific radiopharmaceutical will be significantly more efficient than any form of beam therapy. This explains the success of ^{131}I in the treatment of thyroid disease and supports the existing small-scale practice of the treatment of neurocrest tumours with ^{131}I and the treatment of intractable bone pain in patients with widely spread bony metastases with bone-localising radionuclides. Preliminary steps have been taken to utilise radioactively labelled and specifically acting monocloncal antibodies for the treatment of carcinoma and its metastases.

Contributions to Medical and Scientific Literature

Inevitably there are omissions from the list, especially of papers published in the earlier years. For ease of reference the list is divided into sections:-

Books and Monographs
Cardiology
Central Nervous System
Computer Applications
Endocrinology
General Topics
Nephrology
Oncology
Physiology
Radiation Protection
Radioimmunoassay and Related Topics
Technical Applications

Books and Monographs

1. Williams, E.S. Nuclear Medicine Handbook, pp40, 1962. Second Edition 1966, (Institute publication).
2. Britton, K.E. and Brown, N.J.G. Clinical Renography, pp298 (Lloyd Luke), 1971
3. Ell, P.J., Jarritt, P.H. and Deacon, M.J. Atlas of Computerized Emission Tomography, pp225 (Churchill Livingstone), 1980.
4. Ell, P.J. and Williams, E.S. Nuclear Medicine: an Introductory Text, pp 208 (Blackwell) 1981.
5. Ell, P.J., Khan O and Jarritt, P.H. Radionuclide Section Scanning, pp282 (Chapman & Hall), 1982.
6. Ell, P.J., Walton S. and Jarritt, P.H. Radionuclide Ventricular Function Studies, pp171 (Martinus Nijhoff), 1982.
7. Walton, S. and Ell, P.J. An introduction to Nuclear Cardiology, pp 58 (Current Medical Literature), 1983.
8. Jarritt, P.H and Ell, P.J. Gamma Camera Emission Tomography Quality Control and Clinical Applications. pp190, (Current Medial Literature), 1984.

Cardiology

9. Omar Y.T., Reith W.S. and Williams E.S. The Lancet 1963, I, 1025. The 131i-Triolein Fat Absorption Test in Coronary Artery Disease.
10. Ell P.J. "Scan analysis in Myocardial Infarction" Nuklearmedizin, XV, 157-159, 1976.
11. Ell P.J., Elliott, A.T., and Marcomichaelaidis I. "Myocardial Perfusion Imaging". The Lancet, I, 304, 1977.
12. Ell P.J. "A Cintigrafia do miocardio". Revista de Terapeutica e Clinica Medica, 3, 127-134, 1977.
13. Joseph S., Ell P.J., Langford, R.M., Pearce, P.C., and Woolf N. Tc99m Imidodiphospho-nate: a new radiopharmaceutical for positive myocardial infarction imaging. British Heart Journal, 39, 924, 1977.
14. Rocha A.F.G., Dohmann H.J.F., Ell P.J. and Murad-Netto S. In Conceitos actuais em cardiologia, 177-192. Dohmann and Rocha, Guanabara and Kooogan, Brazil, 1978.
15. Ell P.J., Langford, R.M., Pearce, P.C., Lui, D., Elliott A.T., Woolf N. and Williams E.S. Tc99m Imidodiphosphonate . A superior radiopharmaceutical for in vivo positive myo-cardial infarct imaging. I. Experimental Data. British Heart Journal, 40, 234-241, 1978.
16. Ell P.J. and Donaldson R.M. "Cardiovascular Nuclear Medicine and Intensive Care Medicine" Intensive Care Medicine, 4, 119-122, 1978.
17. Pereira-Prestes A.V., Donaldson R.M., Ell P.J., Brown, N.J.G., Jarritt, P.H, Al-Baghdadi T. and Elliott A.T. Mobile gamma cameras and 99mTc-labelled phosphates in acute myo-cardial infarction. Nuklearmedizin, 18, 73-78, 1979.
18. Joseph S.P., Pereira-Prestes A.V., Ell P.J., Donaldson R.M., Somerville W and Emanuel R.W. The value of positive myocardial infarction imaging in the coronary care unit. British Medical Journal, 1, 361-432, 1979.
19. Donaldson R.M., Jarritt, P.H, Liversedge S. and Ell P.J. Ventricular Pseudo-Aneurysm Demonstrated by Multiple Gated Cardiac Imaging. Nuklearmedizin, 18, 283-285, 1979.
20. Ell P.J. The role of 99mTechnetium labelled phosphate in the diagnosis of acute myo-cardial infarction. British Journal of Radiology, 53,178, 1980.
21. Donaldson R.M., Ell P.J. and Emanuel R.W. ECT Imaging in Acute Myocardial Infarction. British Heart Journal, 43,107, 1980.
22. Ell P.J. 201Thallium – clinical applications. Revista Latina de Cardiologia, 1, 123-126, 1980.
23. Ell P.J. and Khan O. The role of 99mTc-phosphates in the context of acute myocardial infarction. Progress in Radiopharmacology, Vol 2, 75-83. Ed. P.H. Cox, Elsevier, North Holland Biomedical Press.
24. Ell P.J. and Khan O. Emission Computerized Tomography, Clinical Application. Seminars in Nuclear Medicine, Vol II, 50-60, 1981.
25. Walton S., Jarritt, P.H, Brown, N.J.G., Ell P.J. and Swanton,R.H. Phase analysis of re-gional ventricular emptying in coronary artery disease. British Heart Journal, 45, 348-350, 1981.
26. Walton S., Brown, N.J.G., Ell P.J., Jarritt, P.H and Swanton. Phase analysis of the first pass radionuclide angiocardiogram. Nuclear Medicine Communications, 2, 93, 1981.

27. Walton S., Yiannikis S., Jarritt, P.H, Brown, N.J.G., Swanton, R.H., Ell P.J. Phasic abnormalities of left ventricular emptying in coronary artery disease. British Heart Journal, 96, 245-253, 1981.

28. Khan O., Ell P.J., Cullum I.D., Jarritt, P.H, Williams E.S.Clinical and pharmacological studies with 99mTc-plasmin. Progress in Radiopharmacology,Vol. 2, ed. Ed. P.H. Cox, Elsevier, North Holland Biomedical Press. 1981.

29. Walton S., Ell P.J., Jarritt, P.H, and Swanton, R.H. Phase analysis of the first pass radionuclide angiocardiogram. British Heart Journal, 48, 441-448, 1982.

30. Walton S., Brown, N.J.G., Jarritt, P.H, Ell P.J. and Emanuel R.W. Regional variation of left ventricular transit time in normal ventricles and those with abnormalities of contraction. British Heart Journal, 49, 388-392, 1983.

31. Underwood, S.R., Ell P.J., Jarritt, P.H., Emanuel R.W. and Swanton, R.H. ECG gated blood pool tomography in the determination of left ventricular volume, ejection fraction and wall motion. Nuclear Medicine Communications, 5, 258, 1984.

32. Underwood, S.R. and Ell P.J. La imagen de fase en la ventriculografia isotopica. Revista Latina de Cardiologia, 5, 139-146, 1984.

33. Underwood, S.R., Walton S., Laming, P.J., Ell P.J., Emanuel R.W, Swanton, R.H. Patterns of ventricular contraction in patients with conduction cbnormality studied by radionuclide angiocardiography. British Heart Journal, 51, 568-575, 1984.

34. Underwood, S.R., Walton S., Laming P.J., Jarritt, P.H, Ell P.J., Emanuel R.W, and Swanton, R.H. Three dimensional quantification of left ventricular wall motion by ECG gated blood pool emission tomography. British Heart Journal, 91, 1984.

35. Walton S., Underwood, S.R., Ell P.J., Swanton, R.H. and Emanuel R.W. Measurement of valvular regurgitation by first pass radionuclide angiocardiography. British Heart Journal, 91, 1984.

36. Walton S., Costa D.C., Ell P.J., Emanuel R.W. Myocardial Imaging with Iodine 123 Metaiodobenzylguanidine. British Heart Journal, 56, 617, 1985,

37. Underwood, S.R., Walton S., Laming, P.J., Jarritt, P.H, Ell P.J., Emanuel R.W., and Swanton, R.H. Left ventricular volume and ejection fraction determined by gated blood pool emission tomography. British Heart Journal, 53, 216-222, 1985.

38. Underwood, S.R., Walton S., and Ell P.J. Paradoxical phase changes induced by myocardial ischaemia. Nuclear Medicine Communications, 6, 225-228, 1985.

39. Underwood, S.R., Walton S., Ell P.J., Jarritt, P.H., Emanuel R.W and Swanton, R.H. Gated blood pool emission tomography: a new technique for the investigation of cardiac structure and function. European Journal of Nuclear Medicine, 10, 332-338, 1985.

40. Underwood, S.R., Campos-Costa D., Walton S., Laming, P.J., Ell P.J., Emanuel R.W., and Swanton, R.H. Stressed induced right ventricular dysfunction: an indication of reversible right ventricular ischaemia. British Heart Journal, 53, 685-686m 1985.

41. Mosley, J.G., Clark J.M.F, Ell P.J. and Marston A. Assessment of myocardial function before aortic surgery by radionuclide angiocardiography. British Journal of Surgery, 72, 886-887, 1985.

42. Smith, P.L.C., Joseph P.L.A., Newman, S.P., Ell P.J., Harrison, M.J.F. and Treasure T. Cerebral consequences of coronary artery surgery. British Heart Journal, 54, 639, 1985.

43. Smith, P.L.C., Newman, S.P., Ell P.J., Treasure T., Joseph S.P., Schneidan A., and Harrison M.J.G. Cerebral consequences of cardiopulmonary bypass. The Lancet, I, 823-825, 1986.

44. Ell P.J. and Underwood, S.R. Does it help to know the left ventricular ejection fraction. The Lancet I, 909, 1986.

Central Nervous System

45. Keeling D.H. Recent advances in brain scanning. Proc. Roy. Soc. Med. 64, 340, 1971.
46. Britton, K.E., Duplock G., and Vaughan-Hudson G. The prediction of strokes. European Surgical research 5, Suppl. 2., 3-4, 1973.
47. Vaughan-Hudson G. Carotid flow disorders in patients with cerebrovascular disease: Their atraumatic assessment by carotigraphy. British Journal of Surgery, 61, 873-877, 1974.
48. Ell P.J. and Meixner M. Non-invasive investigation of the brain. British Medical Journal, 40, 3, 1975.
49. Ell P.J., Lotritsch K.H., Hillbrand E., Meixner M., Barolin G. and Scholz H. Specific diagnosis of brain disease with double isotope brain scanning. Nuklearmedizin, XV, 1, 32-35, 1976.
50. Ell P.J., Lotritsch K.H. and Meixner M. Differential diagnosis of brain lesions with Tc-99m labelled pharmaceuticals. Nuclear Medicine, 17, 224, 976.
51. Meixner M. and Ell P.J. Brain Scanning: A step towards histological diagnosis with Tc-99m-labelled radiopharmaceuticals. European Journal of Nuclear Medicine, 1, 95, 1976.
52. Britton, K.E. and Williams E.S. E.M.I. and radioisotope brain imaging. The Lancet, I, 477-478, 1976.
53. Ell P.J. Isotope scans in chronic subdural haematoma. The Lancet, II, 592, 1979.
54. Harrison M.G.J. and Ell P.J. Ischaemic oedema in stroke. Stroke, 12, 888, 1981.
55. Ell P.J., Harrison M.G.J., Lui D. Cerebral blood flow with Iodine-123 labelled amines. The Lancet, I, 1348-1352, 1983.
56. Ell P.J., Williams E.S. and Deacon, M.J. Clinical efficacy study of ECAT and TCAT brain scans in 118 patients. Radioaktive Isotope in Klinik und Forschung, 1980, 14, 245-249.
57. Ell P.J., Deacon, M.J., Ducassou D. and Brendel A. Emission and transmission brain tomography. British Medical Journal, 3, 438-440, 1980.
58. Steiner, T.J., Ell P.J., Jewkes R and Clifford-Rose F. Cleon-710 cerebral blood flow tomography after acute cerebral infarction. Nuclear Medicine Communications, 5, 232m 1984.
59. Steiner, T.J., Jeweks R., Jones B., Ell P.J. and Clifford-Rose F. Cleon -710 cebreal blood flow (CBF) after acute cerebral blood flow (CBF) after Acute cerebral hemisphere infarction. Nuklearmedizin, 447-450, 1984.
60. Ell, P.J., Hocknell, J.M.L., Jarritt, P.H, Cullum I.D., Lui D., Campos-Costa D., Nowotnik, D.P., Pickett R.D., Canning L.R., and Neirinckx, R.D. A Tc-9m-labelled radiotracer for the investigation of cerebral vascular disease. Nuclear Medicine Communications 6, 437-441, 1985.
61. Ell P.J. Regional cerebral blood flow and Tc-99m. Editorial. Nuclear Medicine Communications 6, 435-436, 1985.
62. Ell P.J., Cullum I.D., Costa D.C. et al. Regional cerebral blood flow mapping with a new Tc-99m-labelled compound. The Lancet, II, 50-51, 1985.
63. Smith, P.L.C., Treasure T., Newman S.P., Joseph P.L.A., Ell P.J. and Harrison M.G.J. The cerebral consequence of coronary artery surgery. British Heart Journal, 54, 630, 1985.

64. Nowotnik, D.P., Canning L.R., Cumming S.A., Nechvatal G., Piper I.M., Pickett R.D., Neirinckx R.D., Ell P.J., Volkert W.A. and Holmes R.S. Tc-99m-HM-PAO: A new radio-pharmaceutical for imaging regional cerebral blood flow. J. Nucl.Med. All, Sco., 29, 3, 209, 1985.

65. Smith, P.L.C., Treasure T., Newman S.P., Joseph P.L.A., Ell P.J. and Harrison M.G.J. The cerebral consequence of coronary artery surgery. The Lancet, I, 823-825, 1986.

66. Ell P.J. and Costa D.C. Regional cerebral blood flow and Tc-99m: towards a routine SPET test, Diagnostic Imaging, 8, 112-117, 1986.

67. Hocknell, J.M.L., Cullum I.D., Smith, P.L.C., Costa D.C. and Ell P.J. Clinical studies using a new regional cerebral blood flow agent 99m-Tc-hexamethyl-propyleneamine oxime (HM-PAO). Nuclear Medicine Communications, 7, 295, 1986.

68. Costa D.C., Jones B.E., Steiner T.J., Aspey B.S., Ell P.J., Cullum I.D., Jeweks R.F. Experimental studies of Tc-99m HM-PAO with an rCBF model. Nuclear Medicine Communications, 7, 282, 1986.

Computer Applications

69. Ekins R.P. and Williams E.S. Computer assisted routine tracer tests. In Progress in Medical Computing. (Elliott Med. Aut) 1965.
70. Todd-Pokropek A.E. Methods of extracting digital data in radioisotope scanning. British Journal of Radiology, 40, 158, 1967.
71. Keeling D.H. and Todd-Pokropek A.E. Computer assisted parathyroid scanning, Proc. Symp. 'Medical Radioisotope scanning', IAEA, Vienna, 1, 765, 1969.
72. Todd-Pokropek A.E. Methods of developing a system of data analysis of the radioisotope. Proc. Symp. 'Radioactive isotopes in the localisation of tumours' (Heinmann, London), 50, 1969.
73. Todd-Pokropek A.E. and Newman G.B. The choice of a computer for on-line processing of radioisotope scans, British Journal of Radiology, 44, 76, 1971.
74. Todd-Pokropek A.E. Theoretical considerations when using various computer enhancing methods for the radioisotope scan, L'utilisation des ordinateurs en radiologie, (Karger, Basle), 291-296, 1971.
75. Berche C., Todd-Pokropek, A.E. and di Paola R. Preliminary results of the use of the Hadamard Transformation. Proc. 2nd Symp. Sharing of Computer Programs and Technology in Nuclear Medicine. USAEC CONF-720430, 429-437, 1972.
76. Todd-Pokropek A.E. Sharing of algorithms for scan processing in nuclear medicine. Proc. 2nd Symp. Sharing of Computer Programs and Technology in Nuclear Medicine. USAEC CONF-720430, 223-232, 1972.
77. Brown, N.J.G., Budd T., Britton, K.E. On the transmission of quantitative difference information via an interactive computer system to the clinical interpreter. Proc. IVth Int. Conf. on Information Processing in Scintigraphy. Ed. Raynaud E.C., Todd-Pokropek A.E. French Atomic Energy Commission, Orsay, Paris 1976.
78. Brown, N.J.G., Elliott A.T., Burns D., Ell P.J. Operating a Nuclear Medicine computer system with a remote mobile gamma camera. Physics in Medicine and Biology, 23, 981-985, 1978.
79. Ekins R.P., Malan P.G. Computerization in RIA and quality control. Proceedings of conference Computers in the Clinical Laboratory Dusseldorf, 19-20 November, 1979.
80. Edwards P.R. and Ekins R.P. Development of a microcomputer immunoassay RIA data processing programme for WHO laboratories. In Radioimmunoassay and Related Procedures in Medicine, 1982, IAEA, Vienna, 1982.

Endocrinology

81. Harvey R.F., Ekins R.P., Ellis S.M. and Williams E.S. Regulation of the serum free thyroxine fraction by thyroxine-binding globulin. Journal of Endocrinology, 43, ivoo-iviii, 1968.

82. Sonksen R.P., Ekins R.P., Stevens H.G., Williams E.S. and Nabarro J.D.N. Serum levels of protein bound iodine and thyroxine after a course of clioquinol. The Lancet, II, 425, 1968.

83. Williams E.S., Ekins R.P. and Ellis S.M. Thyroid stimulation test with serum thyroxine concentration as index to thyroid response, British Medical Journal, 4, 336-338, 1969.

84. Williams E.S., Ekins R.P., Ellis S.M. Thyroid suppression test with serum thyroxine concentration as index of suppression. British Medical Journal 4, 338-340, 1969.

85. Harvey R.F., Williams E.S., Ellis S.M. and Ekins R.P. Changes in thyroxine-binding globulin levels in thyrotoxicosis and in healthy subjects after triiodothyronine administration. Acta Endocrinologica, 63, 527-532, 1970.

86. Jacobs H.S. and Williams E.S. Effect of propranolol on serum thyroxine. The Lancet, II, 829, 1970.

87. Lawton N.F., Ekins R.P. and Nabarro J.D.N. Failure of pituitary response to thyrotrophin-releasing hormone in euthyroid Graves'disease. The Lancet, II, 14, 1971.

88. Williams E.S., Ekins R.P. and Ellis S.M. Thyroid hormone concentration in serum after thyroid stimulation. J. Endocrin. XI, 49, 1971.

89. Williams E.S. and Keeling D.H. Changes in the normal range of thyroidal radioiodine uptake. Journal of Clinical Pathology, 25, 863-866, 1972.

90. Chan V., Landon J., Besser G.M. and Ekins R.P. Urinary triiodothyronine excretion as index of thyroid function. The Lancet, II, 253, 1972.

91. Eastman C.J., Corcoran J.M., Jaquier A., Ekins R.P. and Williams E.S. Triiodothyronine concentration in cord and material sera at term. Clinical Science, 45, 251-255, 1973.

92. Pharoah P.O.D., Lawton N.F., Ellis S.M., Williams E.S. and Ekins R.P. The role of Triiodothyronine (T-3) in the maintenance of euthyroidism in endemic goitre. Clinical Endocrinology, 2, 1934, 1973.

93. Jacobs H.S., Eastman C.J., Ekins R.P., Mackie D.B., Ellis S.M. and McHardy-Young S. Total and free Triiodothyronine and thyroxine levels in thyroid storm and recurrent hyperthyroidism. The Lancet, II, 236-238, 1973.

94. Lawton N.F., Williams E.S., Pharoah P.O.D., Ekins R.P. and Ellis S.M. Serum Triiodothyronine concentrtion in subjects from an area of endemic goitre. Acta Endocrinologica, (Kbh), Suppl. 177, 214, 1973.

95. Britton, K.E. and Ell P.J. Thyroid scanning. British Medical Journal, 2, 728, 1973.

96. Jacobs H.S., Vanthuyne C. and Ekins R.P. Immunological cross-reactions of LH and HCG: Contributions of the subunits and of the conformation of the native hormone. In: Radioimmunoassay and Related Procedures in Medicine, Vol. 1, 237-243. IAEA, Vienna, 1974.

97. Ell P.J., Todd-Pokropek A. and Britton, K.E. Useful results from computer assisted parathyroid scanning. British Journal of Surgery, 62, 553, 1975.

98. Ell P.J. Terapeutica pelo 1-31. Revista Portuguesa de Clinica e Terapeutica, 5, 227-234, 1975.

99. Britton, K.E., Quinn V., Ellis S.M., Cayley A.C.D., Miralles J.M., Brown B.L., and Ekins R.P. Is T-4 toxicosis a normal biochemical finding in elderly women? The Lancet, I, 141, 1975.

100. Eastman C.J., Corcoran J.M., Ekins R.P., Williams E.S. and Nabarro J.D.N. The radioimmunoassay of Triiodothyronine and its clinical application. Journal of Clinical Pathology, 28, 225-230, 1975.

101. Ell P.J. and Lotritsch K.H. Importancia do Tc-99m em medicina. II. O Tc-99m-pertecnetato nas provas de funcao tiroideia. Medicina Universal, 18, 5-6, 1975.

102. Ell P.J., Todd-Pokropek, A.E. and Britton, K.E. Localization of parathyroid adenomas by computer assisted parathyroid scanning. British Journal of Surgery, 62, 553-555, 1975.

103. Britton, K.E., Quinn V., Brown, B.L. and Ekins R.P. A strategy for thyroid function tests. British Medical Journal, 3, 350, 1975.

104. Rocha A.F.G. and Ell P.J. Estudo da funcao tiroideia. Medicina Nuclear, Rocha, Guanabara-Koojan, 253-271, Brazil, 1976.

105. Pharoah P.O.D., Ellis S.M., Ekins R.P. and Williams E.S. Maternal thyroid function, iodine deficiency and fetal development. Clinical Endocrinology, 5, 159-166, 1976.

106 Marshall N.J., von Borcke S. and Ekins R.P. Independence of β-adrenergic and TSH receptors linked to adenylate cycles in the thyroid. Nature, 261, 603, 1976.

107. Schrey M.P., Brown B.L. and Ekins R.P. Relationship between calcium and cylic AMP during stimulated TSH and prolactin secretion. Acta Endocrinologia 85, (S212) 78, 1977.

108. Marshall N.J., von Borcke S., Christensen A. and Ekins R.P. Propranolol increases binding of thyroropin to thyroid membranes. Nature, 268, 58-60, 1977.

109. Gill D.L., Marshall N.J. and Ekins R.P. Binding of thyrotrophin to membranes from adipose tissue. Biochem. Soc. Trans., 569th Meeting, 1064, 1977.

110. Schrey M.P., Brown B.L. and Ekins R.P. Studies on the control and dynamics of thyrotrophin secretion from isolated adenohypophyseal cells. Molecular & Cellular Endocrinology, 8, 271-282, 1977.

111. Edwards P.R., Britton, K.E., Carson E.R., Ekins R.P. and Finkelstein L. A control system approach to thyroid health care in Medinfo 77. Proceedings of the 2nd World Conference on Medical Informatics, Toronto 1977. Amsterdam: North Holland Publishing Co. 507-511.

112. Britton, K.E. A control system approach to the management of thyroid disease. In: A link between science and the application of automatic control, ed. Niemi, A. Proc. 7th IFAC Congress, Helsinki 1978. Oxford: Pergamon pp. 541-548.

113. Edwards P.R., Malan G., Ekins R.P., Carson E.R., Britton, K.E. and Finkelstein L. Improved data handling for thyroid health care. British Journal of Radiology, 51, 640-643, 1978.

114. Ekins R.P. Euthyroid high total T4, normal T3 syndrome. The Lancet, I, 1191, 1979.

115. Kurtz A.B., Dwyer K. and Ekins R.P. Serum free thyroxin in pregnancy. British Medical Journal, 2, 550, 1979.

116. Kurtz A.B., Dwyer K., Capper S.J., von Borcke S. and Ekins R.P. Free thyroid hormone concentrations in serum from patients on thyroxine replacement therapy. Nuclear Medicine Communications, 1, 28, 1980.

General Topics

117. Williams E.S. The use of isotopes in medicine as an investigative technique. Proc. Roy. Soc. Med., 54, 791, 1961.
118. Ekins R.P. and Sgherzi A.M. Serum vitamin B-12 and chlorpromazine. The Lancet , I, 931-932, 1966.
119. Williams E.S. Desarrollo de las technicas del contaje in vivo con especial referencia a la labor desarrollada en el Insituto de Medicine Nuclear de la Escuela edical del Hospital Middlesex Londres. Anal. de Med. Barcelona, 52, 236, 1966.
120. Williams E.S. Radioactive isotopies. In Scientific Foundations of Surgery. (Heinemann) 1967.
121. Williams E.S. Diagnostic uses of radioisotopes: Body Composition. Hospital Medicine, 2, 81, 1967.
122. Keeling D.H. and Yacoub M.H. Chronic haemolysis following the insertion of ball valve prostheses. British Heart Journal, 30, 676, 1968.
123. Sonksen P.H., Ekins R.P., Stevens H.G., Williams E.S. and Nabarro J.D.N. Serum levels of protein-bound iodine and thyroxine after a course of clioquinol. The Lancet, II, 425-426, 1968.
124. Britton, K.E. and Brown, N.J.G. The use of the radioactive renogram in the reticuloses. British Journal of Radiology, 42, 34-43, 1968.
125. Williams E.S. Nuclear Medicine. Radiography, 57, 1968.
126. Williams E.S. Body composition studies. In Diagnostic uses of radioisotopes in medicine, Hospital Medical Publications Limited, 1969.
127. Keeling D.H., Yacoub M.H., Kothari M., Patterson M and Ross D.N. Red cell survival after homograft replacement of the aortic valve. Thorax, 24, 283, 1969.
128. Keeling D.H. and Crossland-Taylor P. Comparison of iron absorption from ferrous succinate and ferrous sulphate. Proceedings of the 'Symposium on Iron', Arosa, 1969.
129. Keeling D.H. Nuclear Medicine. In Diagnostic Methods. Ed. J.W. Mills, Butterworths, London, 1968.
130. Williams E.S. Scintillography. Trans. Med. Soc. Lond. 85, 166-172, 1969.
131. Keeling D.H. The use of 113mIn in Nuclear Medicine. In 'Isotope Information'; AB Atomenergi, Isotopservice, Studsvik, Sweden, 16, 1969.
132. Keeling D.H., Harvey R.F., Brown, N.J.G., Mackie D.B. and Davies T.G. Measurement of gastric emptying time with a gamma camera. The Lancet, 1, 16, 1970.
133. Keeling D.H., Newman G.B., Baker J.T. and Millett Y.L. Estimation of splenic volume "in vivo". British Journal of Radiology, 44, 403, 1971.
134. Brown B.L., Salway J.G., Albano J.D.M., Hullin R.P. and Ekins R.P. Urinary excretion of cyclic AMP and manic-depressive psychosis. British Journal of Psychology, 120, 405-408, 1972.
135. Williams E.S. Nuclear Medicine. Middlesex Hospital Journal, 72, 92-97, 1972.
136. Williams E.S. The future development of Nuclear Medicine. British Journal of Radiology, 46, 808-810, 1973.
137. Williams E.S. Adverse reactions to radiopharmaceuticals: a preliminary survey in the United Kingdom. British Journal of Radiology, 47, 54-59, 1974.
138. Williams E.S. Nuclear Medicine. In Scientific Foundations of Surgery, Heinemann, 1974.

139. Ell P.J. A cintigrafia em medicina. Alguns aspectos recentes. Revista de Terapeutica Medica, 6, 3-4, 1974.
140. Ell P.J. Importancia do Tc-99m em medicina. Medicina Universal, 17, 124-128, 1974.
141. Reuben A., Narasimha K., Myers M.J., Wood T.P. and Britton, K.E. An approach to the diagnosis of liver disorders using 123I-BSP. Gut, 15, 837, 1974.
142. Britton, K.E., Suwanik R., Tuntawiroon C. Premoydin M., Reuben A., Narasimha K., Myers M., Wood T.P. and Brown, N.J.G. Computer Assisted Blood Background Subtraction (CABBS) hepatography with 131I and 123I Bromosulphthalein. In Dynamic Studies with Radioisotopes in Clinical Medicine and Research, International Atomic Energy Agency (SM185) Vienna, 1974, 157-171.
143. Thompson N. and Ell P.J. Dermal and overgrafting in the treatment of venous stasis ulcers and as a substitute for skin flap repair in injuries of the extremities. A 10-year survey. Plastic and Reconstructive Surgery, 54, 290-299, 1974.
144. Hughes, S.P.F. and Ell P.J. An appraisal of bone scanning in clinical practice. Journal of the Irish College of Physicians and Surgeons, 4, 154-157, 1975.
145. Ell P.J. The clinical role of skeletal scanning. Annals of the Royal College of Surgeons of England, 57, 313-325, 1975.
146. Britton, K.E., Quinn V., Brown B.L. and Ekins R.P. A strategy for thyroid function tests. British Medical Journal, 3350-3352, 1975.
147. Williams E.S. Nuclear Medicine, University of London Bulletin, No. 23, 5-8, 1975.
148. Williams E.S. Organisation of the specialty of Nuclear Medicine. In Recent Advances in Clinical Nuclear Medicine, Churchill Livingstone, 1975.
149. Britton, K.E. The clinical value of the gamma camera. British Journal of Clinical Equipment, 1, 5, 1975.
150. Williams E.S. Postgraduate training in Nuclear Medicine in the United Kingdom. In Report of IAEA/WHO Seminar, 1975, ref: RAD 75.2. Annexe B4.
151. Williams E.S. Complications of isotope techniques. In Complications in Diagnostic Radiology, Blackwell, 1976.
152. Ell P.J. and Neto A.D. Medidas in vivo. Medicine Nuclear, Rocha, Guanabara-Koojan, 148-185, Brazil, 1976.
153. Ell P.J. Importancia do Tc-99m em medicina. III. O. Tc-99m no estudo do sistema nervoso central. Novos aspectos. Medicina Universal, 18, 13-16, 1976.
154. Ell P.J. Estudo das patologias osseas. Medicine Nuclear, Rocha, Guanabara-Koojan, 368-388, Brazil, 1976.
155. Ell P.J., DashJ. and Raymond J. Bone Scanning: A review on purpose and method. Skeletal Radiology, 1, 33-45, 1977.
156. Ell P.J., Beck E. and Meixner M. Liver and spleen scans as a useful diagnostic test in the management of liver trauma in young patients. Fortschritte auf dem Gebiet der Roentgenstrahlen und der Nuklearmedizin, 127, 123, 1977.
157. Stokes T., Ell P.J. and Deacon, M.J. Hypertrophic pulmonary osteoarthropathy. British Medical Journal, 2, 1151, 1977.
158. Williams E.S. Radioactive isotopes and their use as diagnostic agents. In Scientific Foundations of Obstetrics and Gynaecology, Heinemann, 1977.
159. Brown, N.J.G., Cruz F.B., Britton, K.E. Realising the quantitative potential of the radioisotope image. Medical Radioisotope Scintigraphy, International Atomic Energy Agency Vienna, 1977.

160. Williams E.S. Revisor of two sections and contributor of additional items to Butterworth's Medical Dictionary, 1978.
161. Cotton P.B., Britton, K.E., Hazra D.K., Stern R.B., Ponder B.A.J., Croft D.N. Is pancreatic isotope scanning worthwhile? British Medical Journal, 1, 282-283, 1978.
162. Ell P.J., Todd-Pokropek A.E. and Williams E.S. The clinical use of diagnostic imaging. British Journal of Hospital Medicine, 20, 119-127, 1978.
163. Ell P.J., Deacon J. and Al-Baghdadi T. Isotope scanning of bone. British Journal of Hospital Medicine 20, 140-154, 1978.
164. Ell P.J., Todd-Pokropek A.E. and Williams E.S. The future of Nuclear Medicine imaging. Fortschritte auf dem Gebriet der Rontgenstrahlen und der Nuklearmedizin, 128, 486-490, 1978.
165. Ell P.J., Jarritt, P.H., Langford, R.M. and Pearce, P.C. Is there a future for single photon emission tomography? Fortschritte auf dem Gebiet der Rontgenstrahlen und der Nuklearmedizin, 130, 499-507, 1979.
166. Ell P.J., Deacon J.M., Jarritt, P.H. and Williams E.S. Emission computerized tomography. Clinical Science, 56, 24, 1979.
167. Deckart H., Ell P.J., Pfitzmann A., Blottner A., Brunhober J.R., Janiszewski R. and Weiland,J. Experimentelle und Klinische Ergebnisse der Gallenwegsszintigraphie mit 99m-Tc-Diaethyl-IDA. Radiologie und Radiotherapie, 122-123, 1979.
168. Dunn E.C, Ebringer R.W. and Ell P.J. Scintigraphy in the early diagnosis of sacroilitis. British Journal of Radiology, 52, 249, 1979.
169. Dunn E.C, Ebringer R.W. and Ell P.J. Quantitative scintigraphy in the early diagnosis of sacroilitis. Rheumatology and Rehabilitation, 19, 69-75, 1980.
170. Lawaetz O., Ralphs D.N.L., Brown, N.J.G., Jarritt, P.H., Hobsley M. and Ell P.J. Does a pyloroplasty influence the gastric reservoir function? Nuklearmedizin, 19, 888-889, 1980.
171. Deacon J.M., Ell P.J., Anderson A. and Khan O. 99m-Tc-Plasmin: a new test for the detection of deep vein thrombosis. British Journal of Radiology, 53, 673-677, 1980.
172. Ell P.J. Clinical implications of emission computerized tomography. Emirates Medical Journal, 2, 177-180, 1980.
173. Ell P.J., Khan O., Jarritt, P.H. and Radia R.G. SPET II: The clinical role of single photon emission tomography. In Medical Radionuclide Imaging – Vol. 1 Proceedings of IAEA Symposium, September 1980 (pp. 255-261) ISBN 91-0-0/0081-3.
174. Ell P.J., Khan O. and Williams E.S. The management of disease and radionuclide section scanning. British Journal of Hospital Medicine, 225-231, 1980.
175. Khan O., Ell P.J. and Palmer J.G. Emission computerized tomography in the diagnosis of splenic trauma: a clinical report. Nuclear Medicine Communications, 1, 239-242, 1980.
176. Ell P.J. and Khan O. Radioisotope section scanning. Cancer Research, 40, 3059-3065, 1980.
177. Williams E.S. Medical training in Nuclear Medicine. Nuclear Medicine Communications, 1, 107-109, 1980.
178. Williams E.S. The place of Nuclear Medicine in a modern diagnostic service. Emirates Medical Journal, 1, 168-170, 1980.
179. Ekins R.P. The use of radioisotopes in clinical chemistry. J. Clin. Chem. Clin. Biochem, 19/8, 546, 1981.

180. Khan O., Cullum I.D., Jarritt, P.H. and Williams E.S. Clinical and pharmacological studies with 99m-Tc-Plasmin. Progress in Radiopharmacology, Vol. 2, 157-171, 1981.
181. Khan O. and Ell P.J. Radionuclide section scanning of the lungs in pulmonary embolism. British Journal of Radiology, 54, 586-591, 1981.
182. Hoflin F., Ell P.J., Rosler H. and Meier C. Acute muscular pain and positive bone scans. Nuclear Medicine Communications, 3, 30-34, 1982.
183. Ell P.J. Emissions tomographie. In Neue Aspekte Radiologicher Diagnostik und Therapie, 216-240. Ed. by Bessler W., Fuchs W.A., Locher J., Paunier J., Hans Huber, Bern, 1982 (pp 289).
184. Donaldson R.M., Khan O., Raphael J., Jarritt, P.H. and Ell P.J. Emission tomography in embolic lung disease: angiographic correlations. Clinical Radiology, 33, 389-393, 1982.
185. Ell P.J. Single photon emission tomography. Editorial, The Lancet, II, 138, 1982.
186. Ell P.J., Lui D., Cullum I.D. and Jarritt, P.H. Low dose I-123 HIPDM and I-123 IMP biodistribution study. British Journal of Radiology, 56, 506, 1983.
187. Rowles P.M. and Williams E.S. Abnormal red cell morphology in venous blood of men climbing at high altitude. British Medical Journal, 286, 1396, 1983.
188. Ell P.J. Editorial:Arquivos de Reumatologia, 5, 125-132, 1983.
189. Ell P.J. Liver Emission tomography with conventional radiopharmaceuticals. In:Diagnostic Methods in Hepatology, Ed. Lutz H. and Demling N.G.L.,MTP Press, 149-150, 1984.
190. Ell P.J. A review of the clinical value of single photon emission tomography. British Journal of Radiology, 57, 945, 1984.
191. George S.L., Flink K.C., Dawson P., Manhie A., Ell P.J. and Johnson N.Mc.I. Comparison of digital subtraction angiography and radionuclide ventilation-perfusion imaging in the diagnosis of pulmonary embolism.Nuclear Medicine Communications, 5, 246, 1984.
192. Ell P.J. Imaging with lipophy lic tracers: clinical implications. Physics in Medicine and Biology, 30, 605, 1985.
193. Ell P.J. Non-invasive assessment of oesophageal transit. Invited Editorial. Acta Medica Portuguesae, 6, 67-69, 1985.
194. Ell P.J. Comparison of intravenous digital subtraction angiography with radionuclide V/Q lung scanning in patients with suspected pulmonary embolism. Thorax, 40, 576-580, 1985.
195. Ell P.J. Task groups and the European Society of Nuclear Medicine, Editorial. Nuclear Medicine Communications, 7, 81-82, 1986.
196. Ell P.J. Nuclear Medicine Practice, cost benefit and risk – an introdution. "Report – CEIR Forum on the microdosimetry of radiopharmaceuticals". International Journal of Radiation Biology. In Press, 1986.
197. Williams E.S. Nuclear Medicine. In Training to be a Physician. Royal College of Physicians, 1986.
198. Watkin G.T. and Ell P.J. Radionuclide Venography – how accurate an examination? Nuclear Medicine Communications, 7, 322, 1986.
199. Jarritt, P.H., Pagtakhan E. and Ell P.J. A quantitative study of biliary dyskinesia using 99mTc-EHIDA. Nuclear Medicine Communications, 7, 280, 1986.
200. Williams E.S. The appropriate use of diagnostic services: (ix) Nuclear Medicine. Health Trends, 18, 4-6, 1986.

Nephrology

201. Ekins R.P., Nashat F.S, Portal R.W. and Sgherzi A.M. Determination of glomerular filtration rate. The Lancet, II, 109, 1966.
202. Ekins R.P., Nashat F.S and Portal R.W. The measurement of glomerular filtration rate by double isotope technique employing vitamin B-12. Journal of Physiology, 184, 26-28, 1966.
203. Ekins R.P., Nashat F.S and Portal R.W. Measuring glomerular filtration rate. The Lancet, I, 364, 1966.
204. Brewin E.G., Ekins R.P., Nashat F.S. and Portal R.W. Concealed glomerular filtration. Journal of Physiology,187, 603-614, 1966.
205. Ekins R.P., Nashat F.S., Portal R.W. and Sgherzi A.M. The measurement of glomerular filtration rate using radioactive and/or stable vitamin B-12. In: Radioaktive Isotope in Klinik und Forschung, VII,451-460, Urban und Schwarzenberg, Munich, 1967.
206. Britton, K.E. and Brown, N.J.G. Clinical use of Computer Assisted Blood Background Subtraction (CABBS) renography. British Journal of Radiology, 41, 570-579, 1968.
207. Brown, N.J.G. and Britton, K.E. The renogram and its quantitation. British Journal of Urology, 41, Supplement 15-25, 1969.
208. Keeling D.H. and Harvey R.F. Investigations of ureteric function by isotope renography. The Lancet, I, 847, 1969.
209. Britton, K.E. and Brown, N.J.G. The use of Hippuran renogram modified by Computer Assisted Blood Background Subtraction. Proceedings of 1st International Symposium on Radioisotopes in the Diagnosis of the Kidneys and Urinary Tract, Liege, 1967. Excerpta Med. Foundation, Amsterdam, 491-507, 1969.
210. Britton, K.E. and Brown, N.J.G. Computer Assisted Blood Background Subtraction (CABBS) Renography in Obstructive Nephropathy. Proc. Roy. Soc. Med. 63, 1246-7, 1970.
211. Britton, K.E. and Brown, N.J.G. Mobile CABBS renography. Computers in Radiology. S.A. Karger, Basel, 454-458, 1970.
212. Britton, K.E. The value of the Hippuran output curve in obstructive nephropathy in dynamic studies with radioisotopes in medicine. 263-275. International Atomic Energy Agency, SM 136/122, Vienna, 1971.
213. Brown, N.J.G. and Britton, K.E. The theory of renography and analysis of results. Radionuclides in Nephrology. Ed. Balufo M.D. and Funck-Bretano J.L. pp. 315-324. 1972. Grune and Stratton, New York.
214. Britton, K.E. and Brown, N.J.G. The current status of renography. La Ricerca II, 503-507, 1972.
215. Cage P.E., Britton, K.E. and Carson E.R. A 'Bootstrap' model of water conservation by Juxta Medullary Nephrons. Clinical Science, 46,29, 1974.
216. Britton, K.E. The measurement of renal blood flow in man. In Clinical Blood Flow Measurement, ed. Woodcock J. Sector Publishing Ltd., London, 1974, pp 77-84.
217. Britton, K.E., Corfield J.R. and Bluhum M.M. The measurement of individual renal function. In Radionuclides in Nephrology. Ed. Zum Winkel K., Blaufox M.D., Funck-Bretano J.L. George Thieme Verlag Stuttgart, 68-71, 1975.

218. Wilkinson S.P., Bernardo M., Britton, K.E., Brown, N.J.G., Pearce, P.C., Jenner R. and Williams E.S. Validation of transit renograpy as a method for determining the intrarenal distribution of blood flow. Clinical Science, 50, 13p 1976.

219. Britton, K.E., Cage P.E. and Carson E.R. A 'Bootstrap' model of the renal medulla. Postgraduate Medical Journal, 52, 279, 1976.

220. Britton, K.E. Renal radionuclide technique in their clinical context. Medical Radionuclide Imaging. II, pp 401-419. International Atomic Energy Agency, Vienna, 1977.

221. Britton, K.E., Khokar A.M., Brown, N.J.G., Davidson A. and Slater J.D.H. A non-invasive test for receptor binding applied to nephrogenic diabetes insipidus. Postgraduate Medical Journal, 53, 374-377, 1977.

222. Cage P.E., Carson E.R. and Britton, K.E. A model of the renal medulla. Computers in Biomedical Research, 10, 561-584, 1977.

223. Neyer U., Maehr G., Ell P.J., Meixner M and Bloor F. Die Knochenszintigraphie in der diagnostik der renalen osteopathie. Deutsche Medizinische Wochenschrift, 103, 451, 1978.

Oncology

224. Centi-Colella A., Reith W.S. and Williams E.S. The radioactive triolein test in malignant disease. British Journal of Cancer, 15, 848, 1961.
225. Keeling D.H., Jelliffe A.M., Millett Y.L., Marston J.A.P., Bennett M.H., Farrer-Brown G. and Kendall B. Laparotomy and splenectomy as routine investigations in the staging of Hodgkins Disease before treatment. Clinical Radiology, 21, 439, 1970.
226. Britton, K.E. and Brown, N.J.G. Advances in renography in relation to radiology and radiotherapy. Proc. Roy. Soc. Med., 64, 342-344, 1971.
227. Britton, K.E., Brown, N.J.G., Smith L.A., Glover G., Myers M.J., Goodwin T.J. and Bluhm M.M. Early adrenal tumour localisation. In Quality Factors in Nuclear Medicine, 1, p29. Ed. Munkner T. Fadl.s.Forlag, Copenhagen 1975.
228. Ell P.J., Britton, K.E., Farrer-Brown G., Keeling D.H., Jelliffe A.M. and Wood T.P. An assessment of he value of spleen scanning in the staging of Hodgkins disease. British Journal of Radiology, 48, 590-593, 1975.
229. Ell P.J. and Lotritsch K.H. O despiste precoce de metastase osseas e a cintigrafia do esqueleto pelos fosfatos marcados com on Tc-99m. Revista Portuguesa de Clinica e Terapeutica, 2, 83-90, 1976.
230. Ell P.J., Bretfellner A. and Meixner M. Tc-99m-EHDP concentration in calcified myoma. Journal of Nuclear Medicine, 17, 323-324, 1976.
231. Hughes S.P.F., Benson M.K.D., Ell P.J. and Britton, K.E. The use of Tc-99m-EHDP as a scanning agent in the detection of metastases from osteosarcoma. Font. Roent. und Nuclearm. 126, 551-555, 1977.
232. Ell P.J., Knittel B., Maehr G. and Meixner M. Whole body scans in patients with plasmacytoma. Typical pattern of hot spots in the rib cage. Nuklearmedizin, XV1, 195, 1977.
233. Ell P.J. Early diagnosis and space occupying disease; an ever increasing complex problem. Acta Medica Portuguesa, 1, 109-116, 1979.
234. Ell P.J., Dixon J.H., Sweetnam D.R. and Abdullah A.Z. Unusual spread of paraosteal osteosarcoma. Journal of Nuclear Medicine, 21, 190-191, 1980.
235. Stokes T., Belcher J.R., Ell P.J. and Williams E.S. Hypertrophic osteoarthropathy in lung cancer detected by skeletal imaging. Nuclear Medicine Communications, 1, 87-93, 1980.
236. Khan O., Ell P.J., MacLennann K.A., Kurtz A.B. and Williams E.S. Thyroid carcinoma in an autonomously hyperfunctioning thyroid nodule. Postgraduate Medical Journal, 57, 39-42, 1981.
237. Khan O. and Ell P.J. Emission and transmission tomography in the detection of space occupying disease of the liver. Journal of Nuclear Medicine, 22, 35, 1981.
238. Ell P.J. Clinical aspects of detection and imaging of brain tumours. In Nuclear Medicine in Clinical Oncology, Ed. E.C., Winkler, Springer-Verlag, 55-60, 1986.

Physiology

239. Ayres P.J, Hurter R.C., Williams E.S. and Rundo J. Aldosterone excretion and potassium retention in subjects living at high altitude. Nature, 191, 78-80, 1961.
240. Williams E.S. Salivary electrolyte composition at high altitude. Clinical Science, 21, 37-42, 1961.
241. Williams E.S. Electrolyte regulation during the adaptation of humans to life at high altitude. Proc. Roy. Soc. B., 165, 266-280, 1966.
242. Slater D.J.H., Williams E.S., Ekins R.P., Sonksen P.H., Beresford C.H. and Edwards R.H.T. Reduced aldosterone secretion during hypoxia and its relationship to potassium balance, cortisol secretion and plasma renin. Excerpta Medica, International Congress Series No. 157, 1968.
243. Britton, K.E. Renin and renal autoregulation. The Lancet, II, 329-333, 1968.
244. Slater D.J.H., Williams E.S., Edwards R.H.T., Ekins R.P., Sonksen P.H., Beresford C.H. and McLaughlin M. Potassium retention during the respiratory alkalosis of mild hypoxia in man: its relationship to aldosterone secretion and other metabolic changes. Clinical Science, 37, 311-326, 1969.
245. Slater D.J.H., Tuffley R.E., Williams E.S., Beresford C.H., Sonksen P.H., Edwards R.H.T., Ekins R.P., and McLaughlin M. Control of aldosterone secretion during acclimatization to hypoxia in man. Clinical Science, 37, 327-241, 1969.
246. Tuffley R.W., Rubenstein D., Slater D.J.H. and Williams E.S. Serum renin activity during exposure to hypoxia. Journal of Endocrinology, 49, 497-510, 1970.
247. Brown B.L., Ekins R.P., Price I., Tait S.A.S., Tait J.F. The effect of increased K+ concentration and serotonin on cyclic AMP and corticosterone output by dispersed adrenal zona glomerulosa cells. Journal of Endocrinology, 58, xi, 1973.
248. Eastman C.J., Corocoran JM., Jequier A., Ekins R.P. and Williams E.S. Triiodothyronine concentration in cord and maternal sera at term. Clin.Sci. and Mol. Med., 45, 251-255, 1973.
249. Albano J.D.M., Brown B.L., Ekins R.P., Mee M., Tait S.A.S. and Tait J.F. Effect of angiotensin II on cyclic AMP and corticosterone output by purified zona glomerulosa and zona fasciculate cells of the rat adrenal cortex. Journal of Endocrinology, 61, 1xxiii, 1974.
250. Eastman C.J., Ekins R.P., Leith I.M. and Williams E.S. Thyroid hormone response to prolonged cold exposure in man. Journal of Physiology, 241, 175-181, 1974.
251. Albano J.D.M., Brown B.L.,Ekins R.P., Tait S.A.S. and Tait J.F. The effects of potassium, 5-hydroxytryptamine adrenocorticotrophin and angiotensin II on the concentration of adenosine 3':5'-cyclic monophosphate in suspension of dispersed rat adrenal zona glomerulosa and zona fasciculate cells. Biochemical Journal, 142, 391-400, 1974.
252. Williams E.S. Mountaineering and the endocrine system. In Mountain Medicine and Physiology, Alpine Club, 1975.
253. Chapman R.S., Malan P.G. and Ekins R.P. Influence of dietary iodine on thyroid hormone levels secreted from mouse thyroid lobes in vitro. Journal of Endocrinology, 60, 6-7P, 1976.
254. Chapman R.S., Malan P.G. and Ekins R.P. The effects of microunit doses of thyrotrophin on iodothyronine release from mouse thyroid lobes in vitro. In: Thyroid Re-

search, 217-220. Jacob Robbins and Lewis E. Braverman, eds. Excerpta Medica, Amsterdam, 1976.

255. Schrey M.P., Brown B.L. and Ekins R.P. Thyrotrophin secretion from superfused fat anterior pituitary cells. In: Thyroid Research, 617-620 Jacob Robbins and Lewis E. Braverman, eds. Excerpta Medica, Amsterdam, 1976.

256. Milledge J.S., Halliday D., Pope C., Ward P., Ward M.P. and Williams E.S. The effect of hypoxia on muscle glycogen resynthesis in man. Quarterly Journal of Experimental Physiology, 62, 237-245, 1977.

257. Gard T.G., Brown B.L., Atkinson D. and Ekins R.P. Effects of thyrotrophin releasing hormone on cyclic AMP concentrations in preparations of enriched mamotrophs and thyrotrophs from rat pituitary gland. Journal of Endocrinology, 72, 67P-68P, 1977.

258. Gard T.G., Brown B.L., Atkinson D. and Ekins R.P. Studies on the role of calcium and cyclic nucleotides in the control of TSH secretion. Molecular and Cellular Endocrinology, 11, 249-264, 1978.

259. Barnes G.D., Brown B.L., Gard T.G., Atkinson D. and Ekins R.P. Effects of TRH and dopamines on cyclic AMP levels in enriched mammotroph and thyrotroph cells. Molecular and Cellular Endocrinology, 12, 273-284, 1978.

260. Gill D.L., Marshall N.J. and Ekins R.P. Binding of thyrotrophin to receptors in fat tissue. Molecular and Cellular Endocrinology, 10, 89-102, 1978.

261. Gill D.L., Marshall N.J. and Ekins R.P. Thyrotrophin receptors in the human adipose tissue. Journal of Endocrinology, 79, 57-58, 1978.

262. Gill D.L., Marshall N.J. and Ekins R.P. Characterization of thyrotrophin binding to specific receptors in human fat tissue. Molecular and Cellular Endocrinology, 12, 41-51, 1978.

263. Williams E.S., Taggart P. and Carruthers M. Rock Climbing: Observations on heart rate and plasma catecholamine concentrations and the influence of Propranolol. British Journal of Sports Medicine, 12, 125-128, 1978.

264. Dickson J.G., Malan P.G. and Ekins R.P. The association of actin with a thyroid lysosomal fraction. European Journal of Biochemistry, 97, 471-479, 1979.

265. Williams E.S., Ward M.P., Milledge J.S., WitheyW.R., Older M.W.J. and Forsling, M.L. Effects of the exercise of seven consecutive days hill-walking on fluid homeostasis. Clinical scoence, 56, 305-316, 1979.

266. Williams E.S. Exercise and Altitude. Postgraduate Medical Journal, 55, 492-495, 1979.

267. Bidey S.P., Marshall N.J. and Ekins R.P. Characterizationof thyrotrophin stimulation of the accumulation of cyclic AMP in himan thyroid slices and its modification by immunoglobulins derviced from normal serum. Journal of Endocrinology, 83, 53, 1979.

268. Gill D.L., Bidey S.P., Marshall N.J. and Ekins R.P. The effects of calcium and local anaesthetics on thyrotrophin binding to membrane associated receptors. Proc. XIth Int. Congress of Biochemistry, Toronto, 1979.

269. Bidey S.P., Marshall N.J. and Ekins R.P. Release of cyclic AMP from normal human thyroid slices in response to thyrotrophin and thyroid-stimulating antibodies. Journal of Endocrinology, 85, 26-27P, 1980.

270. Bidey S.P., Marshall N.J. and Ekins R.P. Cyclic AMP accumulation in monolayer cultures of normal human thyroid cells: comparative responses to thyrotrophin and thyroid-stimulating antibodies. Proceedings Society for Edocrinology, 49, 25, 1980.

271. Ealey P.A., Marshall N.J., Bidey S.P., Botazzo G.F., Dandona P. and Ekins R.P. Changes in thyroid stimulating antibody levels with plasmapharesis as detected by the cyto-chemical section bioassay. Proceedings Society for Endocrinology, 52, 26, 1980.

272. Bidey S.P., Marshall N.J. and Ekins R.P. Inhibition by normal immunoglobulins of thy-rotrophin-stimulated production of cyclic AMP in slices of normal human thyroid.

273. Bidey S.P., Marshall N.J. and Ekins R.P. Cyclic AMP release from normal human thyroid slices in response to thyrotrophin. Acta Endocrinologica, 95, 335, 1980.

274. Bidey S.P., Marshall N.J. and Ekins R.P. Thyrotrophin-stimulated release of cyclic AMP from normal human thyroid slices. Journal of Endocrinology, 85, 26, 1980.

275. Gill D.L., Marshall N.J. and Ekins R.P. Effects of immunoglobulins upon the interaction of thyrotrophin with receptors in human fat tissue. Endocrinology, 107, 1813-1818, 1980.

276. Pharoah P.O.D. Connolly K., Hetzel B., and Ekins R.P. Maternal thyroid function and motor competence in the child. Develop. Med. Child Neurol. 23, 76-82, 1981.

277. Ekins R.P. The biological significance and measurement of "free" hormones in blood. In: Recent Advances in Endocrinology and Metabolism, 2. ed. J.H.L. O'Riordan, Churchill Livingstone, Edinburgh, 287, 1981.

278. Ealey P.A., Marshall N.J. and Ekins R.P. Time related thyroid stimulation by TSH and thyroid stimulating antibodies as measured by the cytochemical section bioassay. Journal of Clinical Endocrinology and Metabology, 52, 483-487, 1981.

279. Bidey S.P., Marshall N.J. and Ekins R.P. Characterisation of the cyclic AMP response to thyrotrophin in monolayer cultures of normal human thyroid cells. Acta Endo-crinologica, 98, 370-376, 1981.

280. Bidey S.P., Marshall N.J. and Ekins R.P. Adenylate cyclase activity and the accumula-tion and release of adenosine d'5'-monophosphate in normal human thyroid tissue slice preparations: responses to thyrotrophin and thyroid stimulating antibodies. Journal of Clinical Endocrinology & Metabology, 53, 264-253, 1981.

281. Pennisi F., Becker C., Caarayon P., Chopra I.J., Ekins R.P., Ermans A., Faglia G., Kohler H., Larsen R., Lewis M., Mornex R., Pinchera A., Ross H.A., Weeke J. and Salvaore G. International collaborative study on the assessment of normal values for free thyroid hormones. In: A. Albertini and R.P. Ekins (Eds) Free Hormones in Blood. Elsevier Bio-medical Press (1982).

282. Bidey S.P., Marshall N.J. and Ekins R.P. A characterisation of AMP release from monolayer cultures of normal human thyroid cells. Acta Endocrinologica, 101, 359, 1982.

283. Ekins R.P., Edwards P.R., and Newman B. The role of binding proteins in hormone delivery. In: A. Albertini and R.P. Ekins (Eds) Free Hormones in Blood. Elsevier Bio-medical Press, Amsterdam, 1982.

284. Ekins R.P. The physiological significance and measurement of free hormones in blood. In: Radioimmunoassay and Related Procedures in Medicine, 1982, IAEA, Vienna, 1982.

285. Withey W.R., Milledge J.S., Williams E.S., Minty B.D., Bryson E.I., Luff N.P., Older M.W.J. and Beeley J.M. Fluid and electrolyte homeostasis during prolonged exercise at altitude. Journal of Applied Physiology, 55, 409-412, 1983.

286. Milledge J.S., Catley D.M., Williams E.S., Withy W.R. and Minty B.W. Effects of pro-longed exercise at altitude on the renin-aldosterone system. Journal of Applied Phys-iology, 55, 413-418, 1983.

287. Milledge J.S., Catley D.M., Ward M.P., Williams E.S. and Clarke C.R.A. Renin-aldosterone and angiotensin-converting enzyme during prolonged altitude exposure. Journal of Applied Physiology, 55, 699-702, 1983.
288. Milledge J.S., Catley D.M., Williams E.S., Ward M.P., Clarke C.R.A., West J.B., and Blume F.D. The effect of chronic hypoxia on the renin-aldosterone system in man. In: Hypoxia, Exercise and Altitude, 456-466, New York, Alan R. Liss, 1983.

Radiation Protection

289. Williams E.S. Radiation hazards and isotope tests. Middx. Hosp. J. 65, 15, 1965.
290. Williams E.S. The safe use of radioactive materials. Pharmaceutical Bulletin, 16, 26 and 44, 1967.
291. Elliott A., Britton, K.E. and Constable A.R. Dosimetry of current radiopharmaceuticals used in renal investigations. Proc. Conf. Oak Ridge. 1977. Q.J. Exp. Physiol. 62, 237-245, 1977.
292. Williams E.S. Protection problems in the use of radioactive materials in medical diagnosis. Rad. Protect. Bull.No. 20, 5-9, 1977.
293. Elliott A.T. and Britton, K.E. A review of the physiological parameters in the dosimetry of 123I and 131I-labelled hippuran. Int. J. Appl. Rad. Isotopes, 29, 571-5723, 1978.
294. Williams E.S. Radiation dosimetry in the routine medical investigation of patients using radiopharmaceuticals. Rad. Protect. Bull. No. 22, 12-15, 1978.
295. Williams E.S. and Halnan K.E. Risks from radioiodine treatment of thyrotoxicosis. Brit. Med. J. 287, 1882, 1983.

Radioimmunoassay and Related Topics

296. Barakat R.M. and Ekins R.P. The assay of vitamin B-12 in blood: a simple method. The Lancet, 2, 25-26, 1961.
297. Ekins R.P. Saturation analysis: a microanalytical technique for assaying some compounds of biological importance. In. Radioaktive Isotope in Klinik und Forschung, V, 211-220, Urban und Schwarzenberg, 1963.
298. Ekins R.P. and Samols E. Immunoassay of insulin with insulin antibody precipitate. The Lancet 2, 202, 1963.
299. Barakat R.M. and Ekins R.P. An isotope method for the determination of vitamin B-12 levels in blood. Blood, 21, 7-79, 1963.
300. Ekins R.P. and Sgherzi A.M. The microassay of vitamin B-12 in human plasma by the saturation assay technique. In: Radioaktive Isotope in Klinik und Forschung, VI, 446-473, Urban und Schwarzenberg, 1965.
301. Ekins R.P. and Sgherzi A.M. The microassay of vitamin B-12 in human plasma by the saturation assay technique. Proc. Int. Symp. on Radiochemical methods of analysis, Vol. II, IAEA, Salzburg, 1964, Vienna 1965.
302. Ekins R.P. Microanalysis of some vitamins and hormones in blood. Brit. J. Radiol. 37, 723, 1964.
303. Ekins R.P. and Sgherzi A.M. Intrinsic factor assay. The Lancet 2, 1242-1243, 1964.
304. Ekins R.P., Newman G.B. and O'Riordan J.L.H. Theoretical aspects of 'Saturation' and radioimmunoassay. In Radioisotopes in Medicine: In Vitro Studies, R.L. Hayes, F.A. Goswitz, B.E.P. Murphy, eds, U.S.A.E.C., Oak Ridge, Tenn, 59-100, 1968.
305. Ekins R.P., Newman G.B. and O'Riordan J.L.H. Saturation Assays. Statistics in Endocrinology, 345-378, 1968.
306. Ekins R.P. and Newman G.B. The optimisation of precision and sensitivity in the radioimmunoassay method. In: Protein and polypeptide hormones, 2, M. Margoulies, Ed., Exceprta Medica Foundation, Amsterdam, 329, 1968.
307. Ekins R.P. Specificity of radioimmunoassay: hormonal non-specificity. In: Protein and polypeptide hormones, 3, M. Margoulies, Ed., Excerpta Medica Foundation, Amsterdam, 575, 1968.
308. Ekins R.P. Problems of sensitivity with special reference to optimal conditions. In: Protein and polypeptide hormones, 3, M. Margoulies, Ed., Excerpta Medica Foundation, Amsterdam, 672, 1968.
309. Albano J.D.M. and Ekins R.P. The fundamental principles governing the attainment of high sensitivity and precision in radioimmunoassay techniques and their exemplification in a method for the assay of serum insulin. Acta Endocrinologia Supply 138, 61, 2, 1969.
310. Santos M., Poshyachinda V., Brown B.L., Sgherzi A.M., and Ekins R.P. A simple and sensitive assay of plasma testosterone by saturation (displacement) analysis. Acta Endocrinologica Supply, 138, 61, 16, 1969.
311. Ekins R.P. Theoretical aspects of saturation analysis. Proc. Int. Symp. on In vitro procedures with radioisotopes in Medicine, IAEA, Vienna, 1969, Printed in Vienna, 1970.
312. Albano J., and Ekins R.P. Attainment of high sensitivity and precision in radioimmunoassay techniques in a simple assay of serum insulin. Proc. Int. Symp. on In vitro

procedures with radioisotopes in Medicine, IAEA, Vienna, 1969, Printed in Vienna, 1970.

313. Brown B.L., Ekins R.P., Ellis S.M. and Reith W.S. A specific saturation assay technique for serum Triiodothyronine. Proc. Int. Symp. on In vitro procedures with radioisotopes in Medicine, IAEA, Vienna, 1969, Printed in Vienna, 1970.

314. Vyzantiades A., Ekins R.P. and Slater D.J.H. The characterisation and localisation of high-energy-binding sites in mammalian and amphibian kidney and amphibian bladder; preliminary studies for the assay of aldosterone by saturation analysis. Proc. Int. Symp. on In vitro procedures with radioisotopes in Medicine, IAEA, Vienna, 1969, Printed in Vienna, 1970.

315. Ekins R.P. Immunoassay. British Journal of Hospital Medicine, 930, 1969.

316. Ekins R.P., Williams E.S. and Ellis S.M. The sensitive and precise measurement of serum thyroxine by saturation analysis (competitive protein binding assay). Clin. Biochem., 2, 253-288, 1969.

317. Cotes, P.M., Mussett M.V., Berryman I., Ekins R.P., Glover S., Hales N., Hunter W.M., Lowy C.N.R.W.J., Samols E. and Woodward P.M. Collaborative study of estimates by radioimmunoassay of insulin concentrations in plasma samples examined in groups of 5 or 6 laboratories. Journal of Endocrinology, 45, 557-569, 1969.

318. Ekins R.P. Saturation analysis. Clinical Science, 570, 1969.

319. Brown B.L., Ekins R.P., Ellis S.M. and Reith W.S. Specific antibodies to Triiodothyronine hormone. Nature, 226, 359, 1970.

320. Ekins R.P. and Newman G.B. Theoretical aspects of saturation analysis. Acta Endocrinologica, 64, Suppl. 147, 11-30, 1970.

321. Ekins R.P. Radioimmunoassay of thyroid and steroid hormones. British Journal of Radiology, 43, 828, 1970.

322. Brown B.L., Ekins R.P. and Tampion W. The assay of adenosine3'5'-cyclic monophosphate by saturation analysis. Biochemical Journal, 120, 8,1970.

323. Brown B.L., Albano J.D.M., Ekins R.P. and Sgherzi A.M. A simple and sensitive saturation assay method for the measurement of adenosine 3'5'-cyclic monophosphate. Biochemical Journal, 121, 561, 1971.

324. Ekins R.P. Radioimmunoassay protein-binding assay and other saturation assay techniques. The Prationer, 207, 312-321, 1971.

325. Piyasena R.D.M., Ekins R.P. and Slater D.J.H. The determination of corticosterone levels in human plasma by saturation analysis.

326. Brown B.L., Ekins R.P., Sgherzi A.M. and Tampion W. Saturation analysis of cyclic AMP. Journal of Endocrinology, 49, xvii, 1971.

327. Banks P., Ekins R.P. and Slater D.J.H. Development of a rapid, sensitive and specific method for the measurement of aldosterone by radioimmunoassay. Acta Endocrinologica, (Kbh) Suppl. 155, 94, 1971.

328. Ekins R.P. and Brown B.L. Cyclic nucleotides and thyroid hormones: radioimmunoassay or protein-binding assay? Biochemical Journal, 126, No. 3, 1, 1971.

329. Brown B.L.,Ekins R.P., Ellis S.M. and Williams E.S. The radioimmunoassay of Triiodothyronine. In: Further advance in thyroid research, 1107-1120, 1971. K. Fellinger and R. Hofer, eds.

330. Albano J.D.M., Ekins R.P., Martiz G. and Turner R.C. A sensitive precise radioimmunoassay of serum insulin relying on charcoal separation of bound and free hormone moieties. Acta Endocrinologica, 70, 487-509, 1972.

331. Ekins R.P., Newman G.B., Piyasena R., Banks P. and Slater D.J.H. The radioimmuno-assay of aldosterone in serum and urine: theoretical and practical aspects. Journal of Steroid Biochemistry, 3, 289-304, 1972.

332. SufiS.B., Toccafondi R.S., Malan P.G. and Ekins R.P. Binding of thyroid hormones to a soluble fraction from porcine anterior pituitary. Journal of Endocrinology, 58, 41-52, 1973.

333. Ekins R.P. and Newman G.P. Optimisation of radioimmunoassay, proteinbinding and other saturation assay techniques. Journal of Endocrinology, 58, xxi, 1973.

334. Corcoran J.M., Eastman C.J., Ekins R.P. and Paul W. The production of antisera for the radioimmunoassay of thyroxine. Journal of Endocrinology, 58, xxii, 1973.

335. Eastman C.J., Corcoran J.M., Millar J.G.B., Weschler N., Lawton N.F., Ekins R.P. and Nabarro J.D.N. Radioimmunoassay of serum triiodothyronine in patients with thyroid disease. Journal of Endocrinology, 58, xxii, 1973.

336. Malan P.G., Newman G.B. and Ekins R.P. Non-linear curve fitting to radioimmunoassay standard curves. Acta Endocrinologica, (Kbh), Suppl. 177, 99, 1973.

337. Ellis S.M. and Ekins R.P. The direct measurement by radioimmunoassay of the free thyroid hormone concentrations in serum. Acta Endocrinologica (Kbh), Suppl. 177, 106, 1973.

338. Ekins R.P. Automation in radioimmunoassay. Acta Endocrinologica, (Kbh), Suppl. 177, 383, 1973.

339. Jowett T.P., Slater D.J.H., Piyasena R.P. and Ekins R.P. Radioimmunoassay of aldoster-one in plasma and urine: validation of a novel separation techniqe and a rapid urine assay. Clin. Sci. and Mol. Med., 45, 607, 1973.

340. Ellis S.M. and Ekins R.P. The radioimmunoassay of free (diffusible) T3 and T4 concen-trations in serum. Journal of Endocrinology, 59, xiii, 1973.

341. Ekins R.P. Saturation analysis of vitamin B12 and data processing associated with this and similar assays. British Journal of Haematology, 25, 541, 1973.

342. Brown B.L., Albano J.D.M., Barnes G.D. and Ekins R.P. The saturation assay of adeno-sine 3':5'-cyclic monophosphate in tissues and body fluids. Biochemical Society Transaction, 338, 1974.

343. Ekins R.P. Automation of radioimmunoassay and other saturation assay procedures. In: radioimmunoassay and related procedures in medicine. Vol. 1, 91-109, IAEA, Vienna.

344. Albano J.D.M., Barnes G.D, Maudsley D.V., Brown B.L. and Ekins R.P. Factors affecting the saturation assay of cyclic AMP in biological systems. Analytical Biochemistry, 60, 130-141, 1974.

345. Ekins R.P. Basic principle and theory. British Medical Bulletin (Radioimmunoassay and Saturation Analysis), 30, 3, 1974.

346. Eastman C.J., Corcoran J.M., Ekins R.P., Williams E.S. and Nabarro J.D.N. The radio-immunoassay of triiodothyronine and its clinical radioimmunoassay sample counting employing a microprocessor application. Journal of Clinical Pathology, 28, 225, 1975.

347. Ekins R.P. Automation and standardisation of radioimmunoassay. In: Proceedings of the 12th International Society of Nuclear Medicine, 636, Munich, 1974, F.K. Schattauer Verlag, Stuttgart, New York, 1975.

348. Ekins R.P. Radioimmunoassay Design. In: Radioimmunoassay in Clinical Biochemistry, 3-13, C.A. Pasternak, ed. 1975.

349. Ellis S.M. and Ekins R.P. The radioimmunoassay of serum free Triiodothyronine and thyroxine. In: Radioimmunoassay in Clinical Biochemistry 187-194, C.A. Pasternak, ed. 1975.

350. Sufi S.B., Malan P.G. and Ekins R.P. Interactions of thyroxine with a pituitary cytosol fraction. In: Thyroid Hormone Metabolism, 105-123. W.A. Harland and J.S. Orr, Eds. Academic Press, 1975.

351. Ekins R.P. and Ellis S.M. The radioimmunoassay of free thyroid hormones in serum. In: Thyroid Research, 597-600. Jacob Robbins and Lewis E. Braverman, eds, Excerpta Medica, Amsterdam, 1976.

352. Ekins R.P. ELISA: A replacement for radioimmunoassay? The Lancet, II, 569, 1976.

353. Brown B.L., Albano J.D.M., Barnes G.D., Maudsley D.V. and Ekins R.P. The assay of cyclic AMP in biological material. In Eukaryotic cell function and growth: Regulation by intracellular cyclic nucleotides, 285-25. Eds. Jacques E. Domont, Barry L. Brown and Nicholas J. Marshall. Plenum Press, New York and London 1976.

354. Milutinovic P., von Borcke S., Chapman R.S., Marshall N.J., Malan P.G. and Ekins R.P. Comparison of two methods for free thyroxine determination: equilibrium dialysis and immobilised antibody phase assays. Radiol. Jugosl. 12, 429-433, 1978.

355. Ekins R.P. and Marshall N.J. Radioassays – Developments and Trends. Proceedings of the 15th Annual Meeting of Society of Nuclear Medicine, Groningen, The Netherlands. 1977.

356. Ekins R.P. The future development of immunoassay. In: Radioimmunoassay and related procedures in medicine 1977.Procedings of a Symposium in Berlin, 1977, IAEA, Vienna. 1, 241-275, 1978.

357. Hazra D.K., Ekins R.P., Edwards P.R. and Williams E.S. Labelled antibody techniques in glycoprotein estimation. In: Radioimmunoassay and related procedures in medicine 1977. IAEA, Vienna, 1, 329-346.

358. Malan P.G., Cox M.G., Long E. and Ekins R.P. A multi-binding site model-based curve-fitting program for the combination of RIA data. In: radioimmunoassay and related procedures in medicine. IAEA, Vienna, 1, 425-436, 1977.

359. Ekins R.P., Sufi S. and Malan P.G. An 'intelligent' approach to controlled sample counter. In: Radioimmunoassay and related procedures in medicine 1977. IAEA, Vienna, 1, 437-455, 1978.

360. Ekins R.P. Basic concepts in quality control. In: Radioimmunoassay and related procedures in medicine 1977. IAEA, Vienna Vol II, 6-20, 1978.

361. Ekins R.P. Quality control and assay design. In: Radioimmunoassay and related procedures in medicine 1977. IAEA, Vienna Vol II, 39-56, 1978.

362. Bidey S., Gill D., Ackroyd B., Malan P., Marshall N.J. and Ekins R.P. Optimisation of TSH radioligand receptor assays. Annales d'endocrinologie: 9th Annual Meeting of the European Thyroid Association, Berlin p. 4A, 1978.

363. Hazra D.K., Jain R.K., Bharti A., Ekins R.P. and Williams E.S. Labelled antibody techniques in communicable diseases. Proceedings of II International Congress of the World Federation of Nuclear Medicine and Biology, Washington, U.S.A., 17-21 September, 1978.

364. Ekins R.P., Malan P.G. Identification of outliners. Annals of Clin. Biochem. 15, 125-126, 1978.

365. Malan P.G., Cox M.G., Long E.M.R. and Ekins R.P. Curve-fitting to radioimmunoassay standard curves: spline and multiple binding – site models. Annals of Clin. Biochem. 15, 132-135, 1978.

366. Ekins R.P. Methods for the measurement of free thyroid hormones. In: Free Thyroid Hormones. Ed. R. Ekins, G. Faglia, F. Penisi and A. Pinchera. Excerpta Medica Amsterdam, 72-92, 1979.

367. Milutinovic P., von Borcke S., Chapman R.S., Marshall N.J., Malan P.G. and Ekins R.P. Comparison of equilibrium dialysis and immobilized antibody phase assays for free thyroxine determination. In: Free Thyroid Hormones. Ed. R. Ekins, G. Faglia, F. Penisi and A. Pinchera. Excerpta Medica Amsterdam, 253, 1979.

368. Malan P.G. , Chapman R.S., Redford C.R. and Ekins R.P. Results from the UK National Quality Control Schemes for T3 and T4. Annales d'Endocrinologie, 9A, 1979.

369. Mathur H., Ekins R.P., Brown B.L., Malan P.G. and Kurtz A.B. Correction for the presence of cross-reactants in saturation assays: application to thyroxine cross-reactivity in 3,3;,5'-(reverse)- Triiodothyronine radioimmunoassay. Clinica Chimica Acta, 19, 317-327, 1979.

370. Ekins R.P. Commercial radioimmunoassay for free thyroxine. The Lancet, I, 1190, 1979.

371. Ekins R.P. The Corning Immophase Free T4 Kit.Ligand review, 1, 7-9, 1979.

372. Ekins R.P. Radioassay methods. In: Radiopharmaceuticals II: Proceedings 2nd International Symposium on Radiopharmaceuticals, March 19-22, 1979, Seattle, Washington, 219-240, 1979.

373. Ekins R.P. Assay design and quality control. In: Radioimmunology 1979: Proceedings of the IVth International Sympoisum on Radioimmunology, Lyon, France, April 1979. Ed. Ch. A. Bizollon, 239-255, 1979.

374. Ekins R.P. and Kurtz A.B. Measurement of free ligands. UK Patent Application 7906526, 1979.

375. Ekins R.P., Filetti S., Kurtz A.B. and Dwyer K. A simple general method for the assay of free hormones (and drugs): its application to the measurement of serum free thyroxine levels and the bearing of assay resultson the "free thyroxine" concept. Journal of Endocrinology, 85, 29-30, 1980.

376. Ekins R.P. More sensitive immunoassays. Nature, 284, 14, 1980.

377. Ekins R.P. Merits and disadvantages of different labels and methods of immunoassay. In: Immunoassays for the 90s. Ed. A. Voller A. Bartlett and D. Bidwell. 5-16, 1980. MTP Press.

378. Bidey S.P., Marshall N.J. and Ekins R.P. The stimulation of cAMP accumulation in human thyroid slices: a study of its use as an assay for thyroid stimulating antibodies. Journal of Endocrinology, 87, 36, 1980.

379. Ealey P.A., Bidey S.P., Marshall N.J. and Ekins R.P. Use of the section cytochemical bioassay for the measurement of thyroid stimulators. Journal of Endocrinology, 87, 35, 1980.

380. Ekins R.P. Measurement of free ligands. USA.European Patent Applications, 123, 328/80300514.9, 1980.

381. Ealey P.A., Marshall N.J. and Ekins R.P. Comparison of the responses to the thyrotrophin and thyroid stimulating antibodies in the section cytochemical bioassay. Proceedings 163rd Meeting Society for Endocrinology, p.15, 1981.

382. Bidey S.P., Marshall N.J. and Ekins R.P. A bioassay for thyroid stimulating immunoglobulins based on the cyclic AMP response of cultured human thyrocytes. Proceedings 163rd Meeting Society for Endocrinology, p.15, 1981.

383. Ekins R.P. Free hormones and drugs: Their physiological significance and direct measurement by radioimmunoassay. In: Radioimmunology 1981, Lyon, France, 9-11 April,

1981. Ed. Ch.A. Bizollon. Elsevier/North Holland Biomedical Press. Amsterdam, p. 191-214, 1981.

384. Ekins R.P. The "Precision Profile": Its use in RIA assessment and design. Ligand Quarterly, 4, 33-44, 1981.

385. Ekins R.P. Towards immunoassays of greater sensitivity, specificity and speed: An overview. In: Monoclonal antibodies and developments in immunoassay. Ed. A. Albertini and R. Ekins. Elsevier/North Holland, Amsterdam, 3-23, 1981.

386. Ealey, P.A., Marshall N.J., Ekins R.P., Lightman S., Lawton N.F. and Fells P. Application of an ultrasensitive cytochemical bioassay to detect thyroid stimulating immunoglobulins (TSI) in dysthyroid eye disease. Society for Endocrinology 164th Meeting, 26-27, November 1981.

387. Bidey S.P., Marshall N.J. and Ekins R.P. Cyclic AMP release from human thyroid cells in culture: implications for the bioassay of the thyroid stijulators. Society for Endocrinology 164th Meeting, 26-27, November, 1981.

388. Ekins R.P. Misunderstanding about assay sensitivity and precision. Ligand Quarterly, 4, 60-65, 1981.

389. Marshall N.J., Dakubu S., Jackson T. and Ekins R.P. Pulse-light, time-resolved fluoroimmunoassay. In: Monoclonal antibodies and developments in immunoassay. Ed. A. Albertini and R.P. Ekins. Elsevier/North Holland, Amsterdam, 101-108, 1981.

390. Ekins R.P. The radioimmunoassay of free hormones in blood. In: A. Albertini and R.P. Ekins (Eds). Free Hormones in Blood. Elsevier Biomedical Press, Amsterdam, 1982.

391. Ekins R.P. RIA: Past, present and future: A personal view. World Federation of Nuclear Medicine and Biology, Third World Congress, Paris 29 August – 2 September, 1982.

392. Ekins R.P. Radioimmunoassay is not dead – yet. Robert S. First Inc. Intern. Conf. Tarrytown, New York, 10-11 May, 1982.

393. Ealey P.A., Marshall N.J., Valente W., and Ekins R.P. Characterisation of monoclonal antibodies raised against solubilised TSH receptors, in a cytochemical bioassay for thyroid stimulators. Annales d'Endocrinologie, 43, Abs, 100, 1982.

394. Ekins R.P. Measurement of analyte concentration. UK Patent Application 8224600, 1982.

395. Ekins R.P. Method and composition for free ligand assays. UK Patent Application 8208043, 1982.

Technical Applications

396. Reith W.S., Thomas N.J. and Williams E.S. The 131I-Triolein fat absorption test. The Lancet, II, 1229, 1961.
397. Bannerjee R.N. and Ekins R.P. A simple microdiffusion technique for the radioiodination of proteins. Nature, 192, 746-747, 1961.
398. Bannerjee R.N., Ekins R.P., Ellis J., Lowry C. and O'Riordan J.L.H. Iodination of proteins to high specific activity. Proc. Euratom Conf. on 'Methods of preparing and storing marked moleculars', Brussels, 1093.
399. Ekins R.P. Simultaneous sodium and potassium space measurements and computer analysis of data. British Journal of Radiology, 38, 558, 1965.
400. Todd-Pokropek A.E. and Williams E.S. A simple approach to the visualisation of radio-isotopes in vivo. British Journal of Radiology, 35, 756-957, 1966.
401. Ekins R.P., Nashat F.S., Portal R.W. and Sgherzi A.M. The use of labelled vitamin B-12 in the measurement of glomerular filtration rate. Journal of Physiology, 186, 347-362, 1966.
402. Ekins R.P. Sample measurement techniques. British Journal of Radiology, 30, 712, 1966.
403. Brown, N.J.G. and Williams E.S. Use of a tape recorder in the interpretation of the radioisotope renogram. Abstract: Physics in Medicine and Biology, 11, 338, 1966.
404. Edwards R.H.T., Fluck D.C., Burgess P.A. and Williams E.S. Permanently attached electrodes for high altitude electrocardiograms. Biomedical Engineering, 2, 544, 1967.
405. Keeling D.H. and Williams E.S. Problems in the visualization of the pancreas. British Journal of Radiology, 40, 798, 1967.
406. Keeling D.H. and Bryant T.H.E. The preparation of technetium-99m for clinical use. Radioaktive Isotope in Klinik und Forschung, VII, Urban and Schwarzenberg, 1967.
407. Todd-Pokropek A.E. Adaptive techniques for classification in image recognition. Physics in Medicine and Biology, 13, 128, 1968.
408. Ekins R.P. Labelling and separation: limitations of specific activity. In: Protein and polypeptide hormones, 3, M. Margoulies, Ed. Excerpta Medical Foundation, Amsterdam, 612, 1968.
409. Ekins R.P. Labelling and separation: separation methods (charcoal). In: Protein and polypeptide hormones, 3, M. Margoulies, Ed. Excerpta Medical Foundation, Amsterdam, 633, 1968.
410. Brown, N.J.G. and Britton, K.E. A new method of separation of renal and non-renal components of the hippuran renogram. In: Proc. 1st Int. Symp. on Radioisotopes in the Diagnosis of Diseases of the Kidney and Urinary Tract, Liege 1967. Excerpta Med. Foundation, Amsterdam, 491-498, 1969.
411. Brown, N.J.G. and Britton, K.E. The renogram collimator maze. Design of counting systems for dynamic studies and uptake measurement. (Ed. Trtt N.G., Williams H.S. and Brown, N.J.G. British Journal of Radiology, Series III, British Institute of Radiology, London, 1969.
412. Brown, N.J.G. and Britton, K.E. A new system of renography. Biomedical Engineering, 4, 268-275, 1969.

413. Britton, K.E. A feasibility study of a screening test for abnormalities of carotid blood flow using technetium 99m. J. Neurol. Neurosurg. Psych., 33, 379-382, 1969.

414. Keeling D.H. Some experience with indium generators and compounds. British Journal of Radiology, 42, 236, 1969.

415. Todd-Pokropek A.E. An intercomparison of several display methods. Proc. Symp. 2nd Eur. Congress of Radiology. (Excerpta Medica, Amsterdam, 1971).

416. Todd-Pokropek A.E. Tomographic reconstruction, Proc. Symp. 2md Eur. Congress of Radiology (Excerpta Medica, Amsterdam), 572, 1971.

417. Cradduck, T.D., MacIntyre W.J. and Todd-Pokropek A.E. Contrast efficiency and FWHM. Journal of Nuclear Medicine, 12, 322, 1971.

418. Todd-Pokropek A.E. Display systems in clinical practice. In: Quantitative organ visualization. Eds. Kenny P.J. and Smith E.M. (U. of Miami Press, Miami), 717-730, 1971.

419. Todd-Pokropek A.E. Problems of band pass filtering. In: Quantitative organ visualization. Eds. Kenny P.J. and Smith E.M. (U. of Miami Press, Miami), 619-650, 1971.

420. Ekins R.P. Methods of data acquisiton and analysis. Journal of Endocrinology, 54, x-xi, 1972.

421. Todd-Pokropek A.E. Formation and display of section scans. In: Radioaktive Isotope in Klinik und Forschung, 10, (Urban and Schwarzenberg, Munchen), 396-401, 1973.

422. Ell P.J. As provas de fixacao da tiroideia. Novo metodo para a captacao de Tc-99m pertecnetato. Journal da Sociedade das Ciencias Medicas de Lisboa, CXXXVIII, 191-285, 1974.

423. Ell P.J. and Keeling D.H. A new pertechnetate thyroid uptake technique. Clinical Radiology, 25, 217-220, 1974.

424. Britton, K.E., Hall F.M., Webb P., Cox N.J., Goodwin T.J. and Bluhm M.M. The measurement of individual renal function: A comparison of a gamma camera-computer-light-pen system with background subtraction renography. Radioaktive Isotope in Klinik und Forschung, 11, 186-195, 1974.

425. Malan P.G., Jayaram L., Marshall N.J. and Ekins R.P. An electrolytic procedure for iodination of glycoprotein and protein hormones. Journal of Endocrinology, 61, xiiii, 1974.

426. Ell P.J. A cintigrafia em medicina. Detector movel (cintigrafo) vesrsus detector fixo (gamma camera). Revista Portuguesa de Terapeutica Medica, 6, 120-126, 1975.

427. Ell P.J. and Myers M.J. Intercomparison of recent instrumentation used in Nuclear Medicine imaging based on a new realistic phantom. Proceedings of the Congress Tertius Societatis Radiologicae Europae, Edinburgh, 1975.

428. Brown, N.J.G., Budd T., and Britton, K.E. Quantitation of difference using an interactive display system with reference to brain scanning. In: Quality factors in Nuclear Medicine. Vol. 2, 107.1. Ed. Munkner T. Fadls, Forlag, Copenhagen, 1975.

429. Ell P.J. and Myers M.J. A new whole body scanner. A comparison with a large crystal scanning camera in organ and whole body mode. European Journal of Nuclear Medicine, 1, 75, 1976.

430. Britton, K.E., Brown, N.J.G., Cruz F.B., Chang H.C., Reuben A. and Ralphs D. Deconvolution analysis of dynamic studies. Proc. IVth Int. Conf. on Information Processing in Scintigraphy. Ed. Raynard C. and Todd-Pokropek A.E. p. 244. French Atomic Energy Commission, Orsay, Paris, 1976.

431. Ell P.J. and Myers M.J. A comparison of a new whole body scanner with a large crystal scanning camera in whole body imaging. European Journal of Nuclear Medicine, 2, 281-284, 1977.

432. Constable A.R., Rothwell D.L., Ell P.J. and Elliott A.T. Radionuclide cystography. British Journal of Radiology, 50, 606, 1977.

433. Ell P.J., Al-Eid M., Lui D., Pearce, P.C., Elliott A.T. and Brown, N.J.G. High quality, high throughput, early whole body scanning. Nuklearmedizin, xvi, 238-240, 1977.

434. Wilkinson S.P., Vernardi M., Pearce, P.C., Britton, K.E., Brown, N.J.G., Poston L., Clarke M., Jenner R. and Williams R. Validation of transit renography for the determination of the intrarenal distribution of plasma flow: comparison with the microsphere method in the anaesthetized rabbit and pig. Clinical Science, 55, 277-283, 1978.

435. Ell P.J., Elliott A.T., Sanyal B., McSweeney F. and Lovell J. An improved whole body bone scanning technique. Skeletal Radiology, 3, 24-29, 1978.

436. Ell P.J., Jarritt, P.H., Deacon J., Brown, N.J.G. and Williams E.S. Emission computerized tomography. A new diagnostic imaging technique. The Lancet, II, 608-610, 1978.

437. Jarritt, P.H., Ell P.J., Myers M., Brown, N.J.G. and Deacon J.M. A new transverse section brain imager for single-gamma emitters. Journal of Nuclear Medicine, 20, 319-327, 1979.

438. Jarritt, P.H. and Ell P.J. Quantitation of 99m-Tc-phosphate uptake by emission tomography. British Journal of Radiology, 52, 252, 1979.

439. Ell P.J., Deacon J.M., Jarritt, P.H., Pearce, P.C. and Allan A. A comparison between 99m-Tc-Plasmin and 125I-Fibrinogen in the detection of deep vein thrombosis. Journal of Nuclear Medicine, 20, 633, 1979.

440. Jarritt, P.H., Ell P.J., Myers M.J. and Brown, N.J.G. Spezifikationen des Cleon-710 emissions tomographen. Nuc. Compact. 10, 202-206, 1979.

441. Jarritt, P.H. and Ell P.J. A new emission tomographic body scanner. Nuclear Medicine Communications, 1, 94-101, 1980.

442. Jarritt, P.H., Cullum I.D. and Ell P.J. SPET I: figures of merit for two multiple detector (single slice) and one area detector (multiple slice) single photon emission tomographic instruments. In: Medical Radionuclide Imaging – Vol. I. Proceedings of IAEA Symposium, September 1980 (pp. 243-253).

443. Khan O., Ell P.J., Jarritt, P.H., Cullum I.D. and Williams E.S. A comparison between emission and transmission computed tomography of the liver. British Medical Journal, 283, 1212-1219, 1981.

444. Ell P.J. Present trends of single photon radionuclide tomography. Fortschritte auf dem Gebiet der Rontgenstrahlen und der Nuklearmedizin, 130, 499-507, 1982.

445. Ell P.J., Cullum I.D., Jarritt, P.H and Lui D. The skull uptake test. A new investigative and perhaps diagnostic tool. Nuclear Medicine Communications, 5, 215-216, 1984.

446. Nowotnik D.P., Canning L.R., Cumming S.A., Nechvatal G., Piper I.M., Pickett R.D., Neirinckx R.D., Ell P.J., Volkert W.A. and Holmes R.S. 99mTc-HM-PAO: A new radiopharmaceutical for imaging regional cerebral blood flow. J. Nucl.Med. All. Sci. 20, 3, 209, 1985.

Part II: Growth and Progress
1986–2011

Bone Densitometry and Osteoporosis

For many years measurements of bone density were considered important in the assessment and hopefully management of patients presenting with osteoporosis.

Osteoporosis has major health implications – fractures caused by reduced bone density represent a major economic burden. It has been described as the most common of all diseases, one in three post menopausal women are at risk of osteoporosis, a risk which increases with the greater longevity of the untreated population, and there is a 20 fold increase in expected mortality for untreated women over the age of 40 years, sustaining a fracture of the neck of femur. Then as today, prevention and early recognition of this condition are major strategic options to be pursued and developed. Early on it had been stated that in order to recognise hypertension one would need to measure blood pressure – what was preventing us to apply the same consideration to the measurement of bone density for the definition of osteoporosis?

Osteoporosis can affect the entire skeleton, but it may also affect it at different sites and rates of intensity. First instruments were used to measure specific sites only, often the forearm, but soon a need emerged to investigate the entire axial skeleton. Bone density at the forearm is not predictive of bone density in the spine, site of frequent fractures and associated morbidity. Approximately 50% of all fractures caused by osteoporosis are to be found in the spine, 15% in the forearm, 20% at the hip, the remaining fraction at other sites.

Initially the instruments available were mostly based on the use of low photon flux radionuclides, such as I-125 and Am-241 for single photon absorptiometry measurements. These were mostly applied to the measurement of the forearm. The technique of dual photon absorptiometry was developed, making use of the different energies and spectrum emitted by Gd-153 and thus the first whole body scanners emerged.

Despite the progress achieved over the years, the measurement precision of these devices was poor, rarely better than 2 to 3%, in fact insufficient to allow these data to be used in the context of the longitudinal follow up of patients, and especially, the assessment of patient and disease response post therapy. In addition, the radiation burden was somewhat higher than one would like to see in an instrument which would have been used in the same patient, over several years.

It is in the context of using radionuclides for these measurements, that it came to being that worldwide most of these techniques and instruments were housed in nuclear medicine departments. And so it also was at the Institute of Nuclear Medicine. A clinical Bone Density service emerged at the Institute, based on dual photon absorptiometry devices.

A clear step change in performance was needed. There were no solutions in sight, involving radionuclide approaches. There was a limit of the strength of the source which could be used, a limit of the radiation exposure of patients, many of which, could be of child bearing age.

The answer was to be given by a small (at the time) USA company, called Hologic. Shrewd physicists determined that a stable X-Ray source might offer the required photon flux for such studies. Rumours told the tale of X ray sources being used in airports to scan baggage and cargo – why could these not be modified for a whole body 2D imaging device ? So it came to pass that Hologic in 1988 introduced this first X ray based dual photon absorptiometry device at the major meeting of the Radiological Society of North America (RSNA). With good due diligence, staff at the Institute attended the meeting, and the first such instrument to arrive in the UK, came to us later in the year. It must be said that this technology was a disruptive event in this field. It offered fast scanning, low radiation dose and precision at or below the 1% - precisely the figure needed for patient follow-up.

We received this instrument in late 1988, and in a short period of time, a seminal and first UK study on this topic was published in the British Journal of Radiology: X ray dual photon absorptiometry: a new method for the measurement of bone density (Cullum, Ell and Ryder, 62, 587-592, 1989).

Scanning time of 4 lumbar vertebrae was reduced to 10 minutes from previous 30 minute studies, allied with a reduced radiation exposure. Modern equivalent systems now in use at the Institute offer scanning times of the lumbar spine in 5 to 30 seconds.

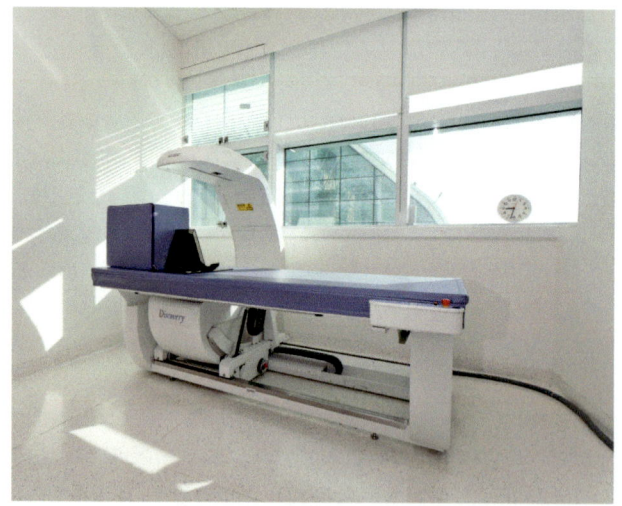

A number of publications were to follow, amongst others, investigating the range of bone density in norma british women (1990), the variation between femurs as measured by dual energy X-ray absorptiometry (DEXA) (1990), the effect of disease activity on bone density on rheumatoid arthritis (1990), investigating the 3rd and 4th generation of bone densitometry and the impact of fan beam technology (1995 and 1996).

A clinical routine service now investigates approximately 3500 patients each year. Typical follow up entails a review every two years.

Brain Blood Flow
and Neuroreceptor Imaging

In 1985, scientists working at Amersham, UK, developed a first agent (hexamethylpropylenamine oxime – HMPAO - Ceretec) capable of traversing the intact blood brain barrier, with cerebral distribution according to blood flow (CBF).

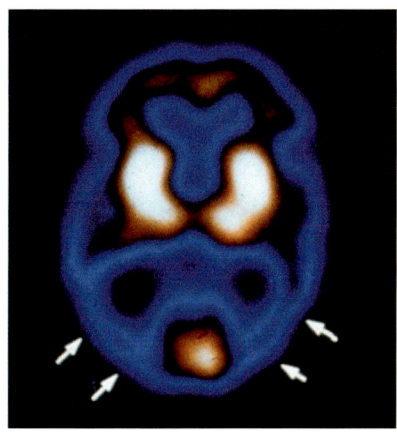

Capable of being labelled with Tc-99m, this discovery represented a major step in the development of imaging agents for single photon emission tomography. A first in man study was performed at the Institute of Nuclear Medicine and reported at a meeting of the British Institute of Radiology in February 1985. We show typical patterns of impaired blood flow in a patient with dementia of the Alzheimer type (see white arrows pointing to bilateral parietal impaired flow).

This development, for which Amersham twice received H. M. Queen Industry Awards, led to a significant clinical program at the Institute. First patterns of regional cerebral blood flow were published (Lancet 1985), cerebral damage in HIV infection was studied (Lancet 1987), the patterns of CBF in dementia investigated (J Cerebral Blood Flow and Metabolism 1988 and J. of Neurology, Neurosurgery and Psychiatry, 1989). Patients with focal epilepsy were investigated (Lancet 1989 and Neurology 1992), stroke (Lancet 1989), follow up studies in dementia published (Journal of Nuclear Medicine 1989, J. Neurology, Neurosurgery and Psychiatry 1991 and BMJ 1992),in traumatic intracerebral haematoma (J. of Neurology, Neurosurgery and Psychiatry 1991). A start in neuroactivation imaging was made (European J Nuclear Medicine 1991 and J. of Neural Transmission 1992), and the effect of depression on CBF investigated (J. of Affective disorders 1993). We show an image of simple motor activation with a finger opposition task, the activated image is subtracted from the resting study, revealing the expected activated area with increased flow.

This development led to one of the most productive research periods of the Institute, with a long list of peer reviewed publications. A clinical service

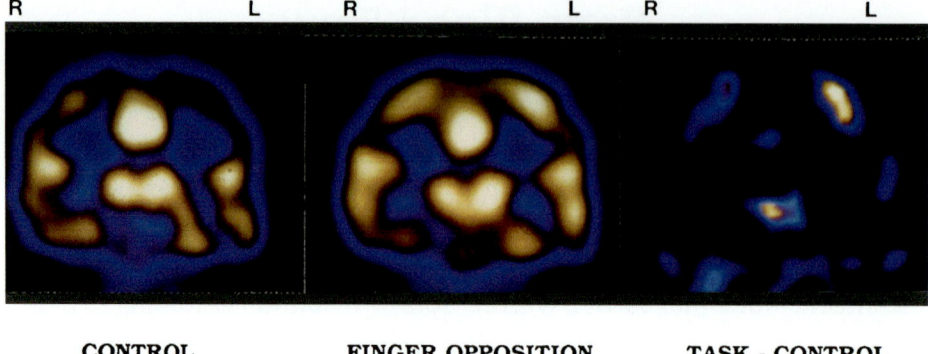

R   L   R   L   R   L

CONTROL   FINGER OPPOSITION   TASK - CONTROL
TASK

was initiated, world wide HMPAO SPET is still the most common nuclear medicine imaging procedure for CBF studies, and renewed the interest of the community to brain imaging procedures. Soon labelled probes would be introduced to image a number of neuroreceptors of the human brain.

The advent of PET would of course play a big role, even with the simple use of labelled glucose, a metabolic marker acting as a surrogate marker for brain blood flow, in most circumstances where the brain blood barrier is not impaired (such as epilepsy, the dementias, for example). This has now led to a routine clinical activity in the investigation of non lesional patients with focal epilepsy (namely patients with normal or equivocal MR studies), where with FDG PETCT we can in one third of all referrals (in this difficult population) offer clinical information with management utility.

Evolution of Brain Imaging with Nuclear Medicine Probes

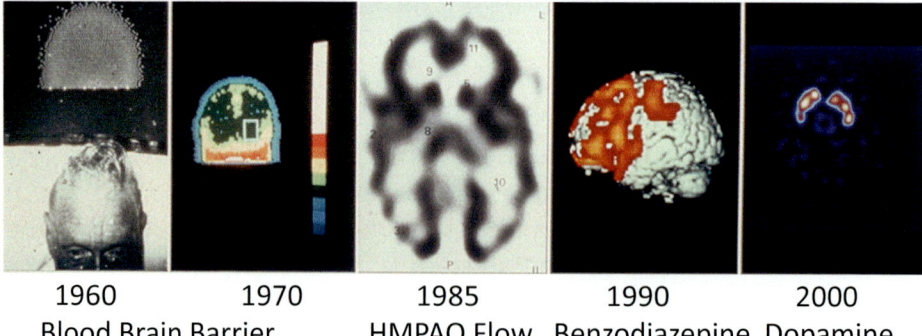

1960	1970	1985	1990	2000
Blood Brain Barrier		HMPAO Flow	Benzodiazepine	Dopamine

Neuroreceptor Studies

With single photon emission tomography being at the time the only practical tomographic imaging technology for radiolabeled probes, Costa and staff at the Institute published very early on an important study, characterizing in vivo an I-123 labelled neuroreceptor for the D2/D3 dopaminergic system – 3-iodo-6-methoxybenzamide – IBZM (European J Nuclear Medicine 1990). We show an IBZM study in a normal and a medicated patient, over a period of time, and the different degrees of receptor blockade in the striatum.

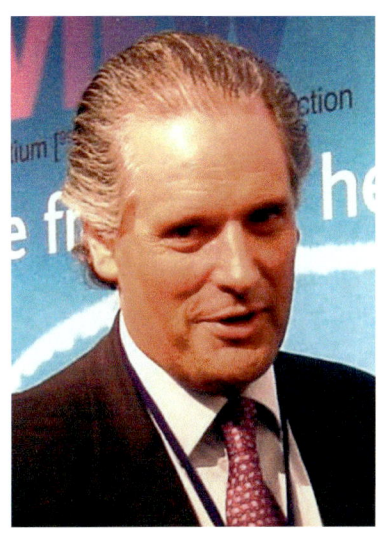

D.C. Costa

This was important work, and attracted to the Institute a young psychiatrist, from the Institute of Psychiatry at Denmark Hill (the late Lyn Pilowsky). Lyn was an enthusiastic researcher and soon obtained a Fellowship from the Medical Research Council (MRC).

Lyn was especially interested in managing patients with schizophrenia. There was indisputable pharmacological evidence for dopaminergic dysfunction in schizophrenia. Dopamine receptor blockade was shown to be an invariate requirement for the activity of antipsychotic drugs. The administration of clinical doses of antipsychotic medication resulted in a substantial degree of striatal D2 dopamine receptor occupancy in humans.

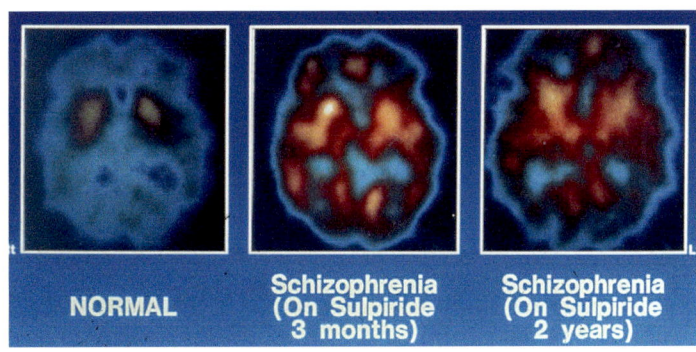

NORMAL

Schizophrenia (On Sulpiride 3 months)

Schizophrenia (On Sulpiride 2 years)

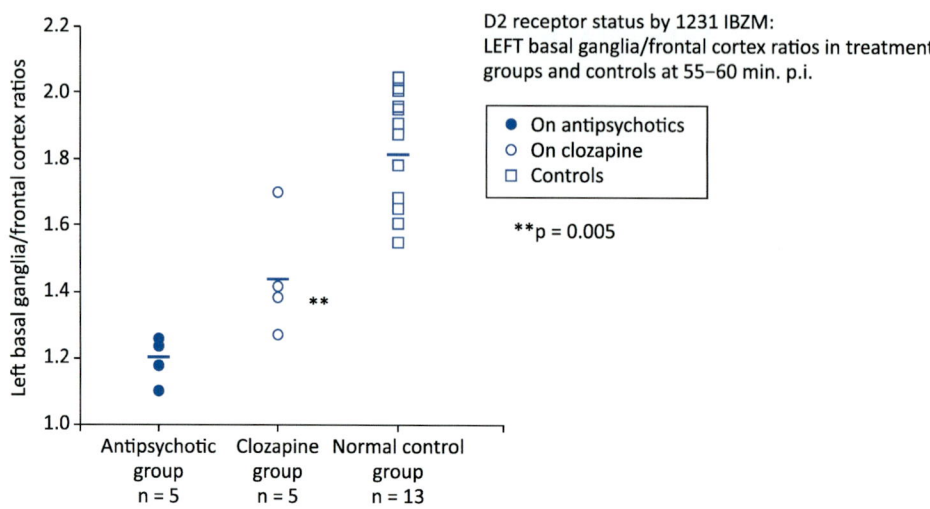

D2 receptor status by 1231 IBZM:
LEFT basal ganglia/frontal cortex ratios in treatment groups and controls at 55–60 min. p.i.

- ● On antipsychotics
- ○ On clozapine
- □ Controls

**p = 0.005

Antipsychotic group n = 5   Clozapine group n = 5   Normal control group n = 13

Lyn wished to test the hypothesis that the D2 imaging ligand IBZM would be able to identify differences in D2 receptor activity in a population of schizophrenic patients (untreated drug naïve patients compared to controls, antipsychotic treated responders compared with non responders, and treated schizophrenic patients with tardive dyskinesia, compared with those without.

A seminal publication in The Lancet presented her findings: clozapine, single photon emission tomography, and the D2 dopamine blockade hypothesis of schizophrenia (Lancet 340, 199-202, 1992). The study showed beyond doubt that patients on typical antipsychotics showed poor response, despite D2 receptor blockade. Significant clinical improvement occurred in all patients on clozapine, but at a lower level of D2 blockade by the drug. These findings suggested a more complex relation (rather than the hitherto suspected linear relation) between D2 blockade and clinical efficacy! In an important review in The Lancet, reviewing the 10 most important publications of that decade in psychiatry, Lyn's contribution was clearly acknowledged (Flaum and Andreasen, 1997)

Between 1985 and 1990, some 40+ peer reviewed publications emanated from the Institute in respect to brain imaging. Whilst HMPAO became the most widely imaging probe used for

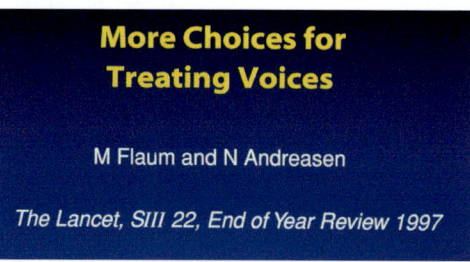

More Choices for Treating Voices

M Flaum and N Andreasen

The Lancet, SIII 22, End of Year Review 1997

blood flow SPET studies of the brain, other probes and approaches were investigated.

A further area of interest developed, with major input from the cardiac surgeons and psychologists. It was known for some time, that patients undergoing coronary bypass surgery, often presented with a degree of cognitive impairment. If you were an excellent chess player pre-operatively, you may not be performing as well in the post operative period. To investigate organ function prior interventions, had met with recent success. One of our studies showed the clinical relevance of assessment cardiac ejection fraction prior aortic surgery. It was clearly possible to stratify patients into different risk categories (Mosley et al Brit J Surgery 1985, Ell The Lancet 1986)

And so it was decided to investigate brain blood flow, during and after 8 days and 8 weeks post coronary bypass surgery. Labelled xenon-133 was used for this purpose. A series of publications assessed the effect of surgery on this patients, the time required for their recovery and the modifications needed during surgery to minimise this risk (Smith et al, the Lancet 1986, Venn et al The Brit Heart J 1987 and 1988, Treasure et al, Europ J Cardio Thoracic Surgery 1989).

Early studies with labelled HMPAO in patients with refractory and focal epilepsy showed the potential of interictal and ictal imaging. Again a number of publications emerged and a limited clinical service developed. In recent times a service has developed based on FDG PETCT and the investigation of MR non lesional patients with refractory and focal epilepsy. We show below a typical example where FDGPET aids in the localization of the epileptic focus.

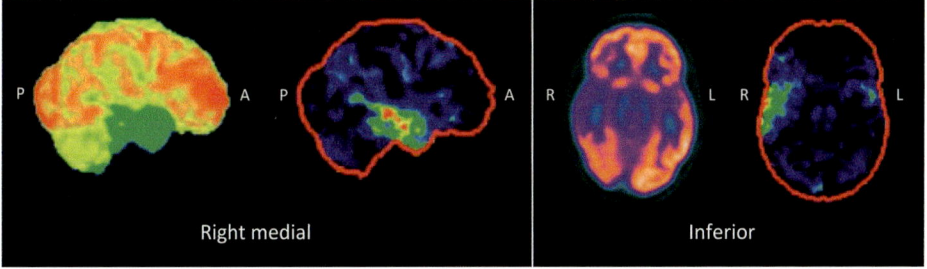

Refractory epilepsy. Scalp video EEG telemetry suggests this comes from right frontal or temporal lobes. MRI is unremarkable. For intracranial EEG planning. There is focal right temporal lobe hypometabolism. Localization to right temporal lobe

The Sentinel Node

In 1998 a young surgeon joined the Institute of Nuclear Medicine, for a 3 year program leading to a PhD. It became the most successful collaboration between Nuclear Medicine and Surgical Oncology, in a field which barely a few months later, had been baptised by a most eminent Dutch surgeon, S. Meijers as "the most significant advance in surgical oncology – 1st International SLN Congress-Amsterdam 1999". The young surgeon was Mohammad Keshtgar, now an eminent breast specialist, his profile recently reviewed in Lancet Oncology July 2011.

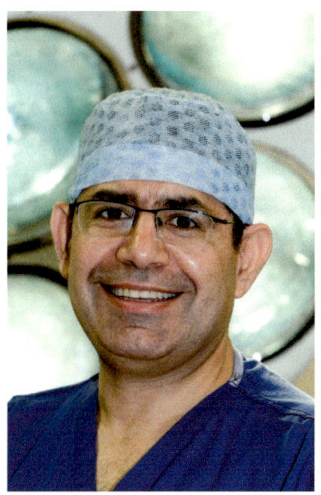

M. Keshtgar BSc, MBBS,
FRCSI, FRCS (Gen), PhD
Reader and Consultant
Surgical Oncologist
Department of Surgery
Royal Free Hospital

The routine management of patients presenting with carcinoma of the breast invariably required the excision of the tumour and a more or less complete excision of the axillary lymph nodes. Interestingly, whilst the removal of the primary breast cancer was the least difficult intervention, it was the dissection and removal of the axillary lymph nodes (ALND) which took time, skill and caused the greatest patient morbidity. It was nevertheless thought that this operation was essential: it would clarify whether regional lymph nodes were either free or invaded by tumour (considered a most important prognostic factor) and (to some extend),allowed for the reduction of tumour burden to the patient. Apart from the significant morbidity which many patients endured, it became apparent over the years, that in some 65% of patients presenting with early primary breast disease, the local lymph nodes were not involved – they were free from disease!

Breast cancer spreads via two main routes: distant spread can occur with metastasis travelling via the circulation, or, most often, breast metastasis travel to regional lymph nodes, such as those present in the axilla and the internal mammary lymph node chain. Whilst blood borne metastasis behave in an entirely unpredicted manner, opinion was split as to whether lymph born metastasis from breast carcinoma could have a predictable pattern of distribution. Such patterns had been observed in other cancers, such as penile cancers, where this was first observed by a Paraguayan surgeon (Ramon Cabanas) working in the USA (1976). Could a predictable pattern of lymphatic spread in breast cancer be detectable by imaging, and could Nuclear Medicine provide the solution? This was the subject of the PhD project of Keshtgar with support of the staff at the Institute.

The term Sentinel Node, from the roman soldier posted to the watch, was defined as any lymph node directly receiving draining lymph from the primary tumour. And so it was postulated that if the Sentinel Node was seen to be free of tumour, the more distant draining lymph nodes would also be free from metastasis. This hypothesis was extensively tested at the Institute and proven to be correct.

A simple technique was developed to administer Tc-99m labelled colloid particles to the site of the breast tumour, image the site of injection and the progressive spread of the particles to the neighbouring nodes, identifying the sentinel nodes/s (often if not always, less than 2), detecting the sentinel node with an appropriate radiation probe during surgery, removing the sentinel node, and rapidly obtaining histological proof of the status of the node in terms of presence or absence of metastasis. And indeed it turned out that if the Sentinel Node was free of disease, the regional axillary nodes were also proven to be free of disease.

This simple technique proved to be extraordinarily effective, sparing invasive axillary surgery in 2 out of 3 patients presenting with early breast cancer. Many refinements of the technique ensued, but the overall message was clear: Nuclear Medicine and expert surgeons delivered major improvements in the management of patients with breast cancer.

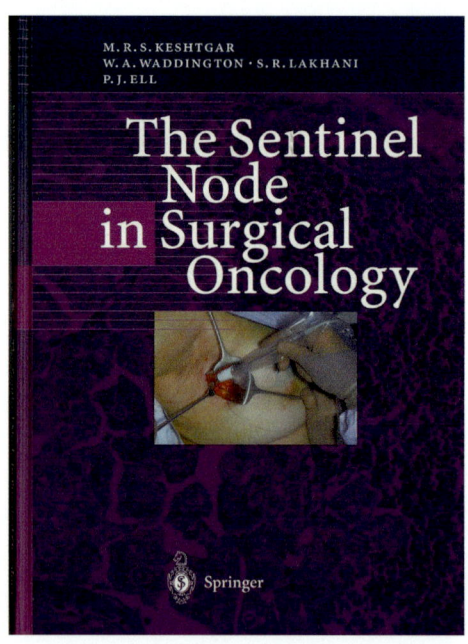

A series of publications underlined the progress achieved, the first Text book and CD on the subject published, and a training program initiated, teaching in the clinical skills lab, this new technique to many teams from the UK. Keshtgar and Ell became involved in joint discussions with the Royal College of Surgeons concerning the training of surgical and nuclear medicine teams interested in adopting this new technique, a new phantom was developed to aid in this training, educational lectures delivered nationally and overseas, the International Atomic Energy Agency in Vienna became interested in extending this training program. Training workshops in developing countries some of them sponsored by IAEA (India, Pakistan, Egypt, Saudi Arabia, Iran) were held. The Annual British Surgery year Book quotes: "Educational materials and theory day structure was adapted from those developed by M Keshtgar".

Some of the peer reviewed data appeared in The Lancet, 352, 1471-1472, 1998, in European J Nuclear Medicine 26, 57-68, 1999, The Lancet 355, 1410-1411, 1999, The Lancet 354, 773, 199, the European J Nuclear Medicine 27, 377-391, 2000, the European Journal of Surgical Oncology 27, 113-122, 2001, Lancet Oncology 3, 105-110, 2002, the European J of Surgical Oncology 30, 480-483, 2004 and several others of note. A major impact had been made.

A randomized multicenter trial of sentinel lymph node in breast cancer confirmed all the initial hopes and was published in the Journal of the National Cancer Institute, 98, 599-609, 2006.

THE UCL TRAINING SIMULATOR FOR SENTINEL NODE BIOPSY

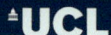

WA Waddington, MRS Keshtgar, DW Chicken, PJ Ell.
Collaboration with the Academic Department of Surgery, UCL

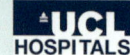

Introduction – the Sentinel Lymph Node Concept

Breast cancer is the most common malignancy affecting women in the Western World, and its incidence is rising. Surgery entails both therapeutic tumour resection and axillary staging, traditionally by axillary lymph node dissection (ALND). This carries a morbidity often exceeding that of the primary tumour surgery, and whilst staging information allows patients at risk of distant metastases to be selected for systemic therapy, there is no benefit for patients without axillary disease. Heightened public awareness and effective screening programmes now result in earlier diagnosis and the majority of patients presenting with node negative disease.

The Sentinel Lymph Node (SLN) concept states that the pattern of lymphatic drainage from an intradermal injection of a suitable radioactive colloid administered appropriately local to the tumour site will reflect that of the lymph-borne spread of metastatic cells from a tumour, and that it will thereby permit identification of those 'sentinel' lymph nodes receiving drainage directly from the tumour. The concept has been validated, its techniques optimised and the first randomised comparison of SLN biopsy versus ALND in early breast cancer has confirmed that SLN biopsy is an accurate staging investigation with significantly less morbidity. The recent UK ALMANAC trial was called to an early close due to the overwhelming quality of life benefit conferred by SLN biopsy. The technique is therefore being adopted both within the US and Europe as the standard of care, and patients are increasingly demanding this accurate and minimally invasive procedure.

Optimal SLN Biopsy Technique

Intra-operative identification requires a gamma probe to localise the sentinel node, a skill that is unfamiliar to many surgeons. It has been shown that the procedure is associated with a significant learning curve, and so appropriate training is essential to ensure that a consistently high identification rate and a low false negative rate is reached as soon as possible. Additionally, surgeons need to be equipped with the appropriate new practical skills required to handle radioactive materials in the operating theatre. Recognising the need for a realistic model for training purposes, we have designed and built a model that can be used for training surgeons in all aspects of the technique.

Simulator Concept and Design

The simulator consists of an anatomically accurate torso lying with its arm extended in the operating position. The breast and axilla are constructed from a hotmelt thermoplastic elastomer which closely matches the physical properties and radiation attenuation characteristics of human tissue. Hollow, injection moulded PVC beads filled with a ^{99m}Tc solution and sealed are then inserted into the breast and axilla to simulate the injection site and one or more radioactive sentinel nodes. ^{99m}Tc is used for the sentinel node biopsy procedure, and so by using this the clinical situation is accurately simulated. ^{99m}Tc is readily available in any nuclear medicine department, and by manipulating the concentration of solution used to fill the beads the activity within both the "injection site" and the "node" can be varied. The short half-life of ^{99m}Tc (6 hrs) also greatly simplifies the regulatory requirements for its use.

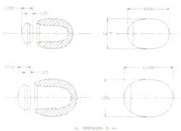
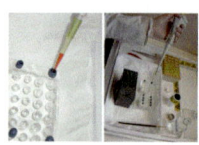

Moulds for two PVC beads have been produced (35ul and 70ul internal capacity). The beads are filled using a pipette, sealed with a separate cap and glued using a PVC solvent such as cyclohexanone. By varying the ^{99m}Tc solution concentration the radioactivity of the injection site or sentinel node bead(s) can be varied individually to realistically simulate injection protocols and the range of lymph node uptakes clinically encountered. These are further modified to mimic the radioactive decay due to the interval period between ^{99m}Tc colloid administration and the SLN biopsy procedure.

Bead "nodes" can be placed almost anywhere within the breast or axilla, simulating both usual locations and the more unusually encountered intramammary or internal mammary nodes. In particular, configurations known to lead to difficult detection using a gamma probe, such as that when two nodes are in close proximity, or when a node lies close to the injection site, may be expressly created by using this simulator, and the trainee instructed in the correct techniques and strategies for overcoming these difficulties.

Teaching Exercises Utilizing the Model

Several practical aspects of sentinel node biopsy can be effectively demonstrated and practiced using the model.

Probe-guided sentinel node mapping

By setting up the model phantom in various configurations, trainees may gain practice at probing strategies and sentinel node mapping, and deciding on the most appropriate site to place a surgical incision. The model presents an excellent opportunity for trainees to become familiar with the performance and operating characteristics of gamma probes, and principles such as scanning techniques, the effects of angulation of the probe, and line of sight dissection can be demonstrated and practiced (below).

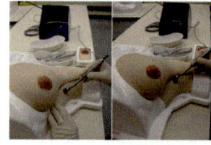
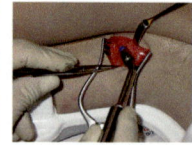

Probe-guided removal of nodes

The model accurately simulates the physical characteristics of the axilla. After making an appropriate incision, trainees can dissect down to the radioactive node, using the gamma probe for guidance (above). As more than one radioactive node can be placed within the model, after removal of the first radioactive node, the presence of residual radioactivity within the axilla enables trainees to continue dissecting until additional radioactive nodes are identified and removed. Any combination of blue stained and non stained nodes, as well as radioactive ("hot") and non-radioactive ("cold") nodes may be placed within the axilla, as appropriate for the simulation.

Injection techniques

As the elastomer is oil-based, water-based dyes may be injected intradermally, peri-areolarly or peritumourally, without causing staining. All aspects of the handling of radioactive injectate, and related radiation protection issues are taught (below).

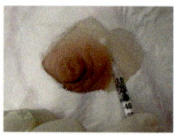
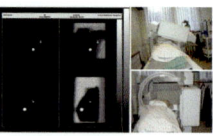

Imaging techniques

As the attenuation characteristics of the model are very similar to that of the human body, the model may be imaged with a gamma camera, producing standard two view static images. These images may be provided to trainees to later assist in node localization (above).

Conclusion

We strongly believe that training for sentinel node biopsy should begin in the skills laboratory setting. The model we have developed provides an accurate simulation of the many new practical skills required, and is thus an important aid to training in the procedure for ca. breast. We have now used the model on the many UCL 'New Start' sentinel node biopsy training courses run to date. Candidates are given an opportunity to practice all the technical aspects of the procedure, and to record their findings. Their response has been overwhelmingly favourable.

Acknowledgment

We wish to acknowledge the assistance and technical expertise of Anthony Rollason and Matt Pilston of Pharmabotic medical model makers in the production of the trainer.

INSTITUTE OF NUCLEAR MEDICINE

UCL 'NEW START' SENTINEL LYMPH NODE TRAINING COURSE

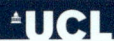

MRS Keshtgar, DW Chicken, WA Waddington, PJ Ell
Collaboration with the Academic Department of Surgery, UCL

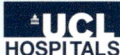

The Sentinel Lymph Node (SLN) Technique

Breast cancer is the most common female cancer in the western world, with increasing incidence. Traditional management is by tumour resection and staging through axillary dissection. This permits histological analysis of axillary lymph nodes but morbidity is often significant, and whilst patients at risk can receive systemic therapy most patients are now node negative due to earlier detection through greater awareness and screening.

The SLN technique was developed to reduce this morbidity. The physiological concept of the 'orderly flow' of lymphatic drainage from a tumour is used to identify these drainage paths to 'sentinel' lymph nodes so that the presence of metastatic cells within these nodes can be used to determine axillary status – if the SLN is negative then the whole axilla will be. The SLN is thus defined as 'any node which receives lymphatic drainage directly from the primary tumour'.

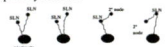

In practice SLNs are identified using a radiolabelled tracer injected along the drainage path immediately distal to the tumour. On migrating to the SLN most tracer particles are trapped by phagocytosis, with any travelling further trapped by secondary nodes. The radioactive SLNs can thus be imaged, excised using an intra-operative gamma-detecting probe and subject to sophisticated, more sensitive histological analysis.

The first study to randomise SLN biopsy vs ALND in early ca. breast confirmed it as an accurate staging investigation with significantly less morbidity, and the recent UK ALMANAC trial closed early due to the overwhelming quality of life benefit conferred. The technique has been adopted rapidly in the US and Europe as the standard of care, with patients increasingly demanding this accurate and minimally invasive procedure.

UCL Sentinel Lymph Node Training Course

The Institute of Nuclear Medicine and Department of Surgery began a joint UCL SLN programme in 1997; one of the first in Europe.

Recognising that success depends upon good communication across the entire team with each procedure performed optimally, we organised the UK's first SLN Training Course at UCL in 2004.

This 2-day course uniquely allowed registrants to watch a SLN biopsy via live link to the Operating Theatre and to use the newly developed Trainer (see separate poster and below).

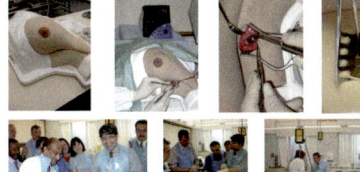

'New Start' Sentinel Lymph Node Training Programme

This DH aided programme organised by the Royal College of Surgeons was mandated in 2005 for all units in England and Wales introducing the technique. Drawing on UCL's experience and representing a new model for proctored surgical training, it incorporates:

One day theory course for the whole team. Run at 5 centres including UCL. Lectures and supporting material provide the knowledge base and introduce techniques and equipment required for the practical training.

Two day practical training involving a experienced SLN surgeon trainer visiting the trainees' own unit and directly supervising 5-6 cases in their hospital.

Validation phase comprising 25 further cases. A 95% identification rate is required with <5% false negative rate and at least 10 node positive cases. Audited centrally by RCS.

UCL New Start Course Content and Structure

Introduction of NEW START SLN Training Programme
Overview of current evidence for the SLN Technique

Patients Journey:
  Radiolabelled Colloidal Tracers
  Injection Methodology
  Sentinel Node Imaging
  Histopathological analysis of the SLN & Intra-Operative Analysis

Video presentation of Injection & Imaging
Intra-operative Radiation Detection
Video and discussion of Surgical Technique
Practical Radiation Protection Issues
Discussion

Practical Session At the UCL Clinical Skills Laboratory :
Demonstration of Injection and Surgical Techniques to All Participants
Break-out Sessions :
  Surgeons & Theatre Staff – Laboratory and Practical Exercises on SLN Trainer
  Radiologists & Nuclear Medicine – Laboratory and Demonstration of Technique
  Breast Care Nurses – Counselling Issues
  Pathologists – Practical Session : Interpretation of Histopathology & Cytology

Case Discussions & Current Controversies
Clinical Governance Issues : The Department of Health view
Local Service Issues & Formulation of Action Plan
Discussion and Feedback

UCL Course Statistics to Date (Mar 2004 – Nov 2006)

Total Participants	254
2 day courses held	6
1 day courses held	4

Attendees' Specialities

Surgeons	124	Teams	19
Radiologists	37	Individuals	113
Breast Care Nurses	34		
Nuclear Medicine	19		
Pathologists	14		
Theatre Nurses	20		
Other	6		

Centres Completed New Start Audit Phase (Proctoring and Validation)

UHW, Cardiff	Hull
Royal Marsden	Russells Hall Hospital
St James	Altnagelvin
King Edward II	Kings Lynn
Leeds General Infirmary	Royal Berkshire
Warwick	

Centres Proctored by UCL undergoing Validation

Altnagelvin Hospital	Northampton
Whittington	Pilgrim
Kettering	Darrent Valley
Barnet & Chase Farm	

Centres Waiting to be Proctored by UCL

Ashford & St Peters	St Margarets
Homerton	

Five UCL New Start SLN courses are planned for 2007
For further information please contact :

Mr Mohammed RS Keshtgar   m.keshtgar@ucl.ac.uk
Senior Lecturer in Surgery / Consultant Surgical Oncologist

PA and Course Organiser   julie.power@uclh.org   tel 020 7679 6491

INSTITUTE OF NUCLEAR MEDICINE

Nuclear Cardiology

By 1986, almost 25% of all diagnostic procedures carried out at the Institute of Nuclear Medicine, involved the investigation of cardiac function, such as the study of wall motion and ventricular ejection, and, importantly, of myocardial perfusion. Coronary artery disease remains a major pathology and intervention was in full swing, surgery involving the coronary arteries became the most frequent surgical procedure performed in the developed world. Dedicated imaging instrumentation had matured to meet our demand: dedicated cameras appeared to provide mobility (to the coronary and intensive care units) and tomographic Anger cameras were optimised to image the heart in 3D.

Programs developed to measure cardiac pump performance (inter alia left ventricular ejection fraction) and to assess the movement synchronicity of the 4 cardiac chambers. An early publication "quantitative phase analysis in the assessment of coronary artery disease" was published (British Heart Journal, 61, 14-22, 1989) Several methodologies were developed to investigate myocardial blood flow during pharmacologically induced stress, this intervention being more reproducible and applicable to a wider variety of patients. Pharmacological stress testing with adenosine and dobutamine was investigated, comparing the recent technology of magnetic resonance imaging (MRI) with nuclear cardiology (British Heart Journal 64, 362-369, 1990). Dobutamine stress testing was used with the original SPET tracer for myocardial perfusion, Tl201, and published in JACC 18, 1471-1479, 1991 and a contribution made to The Lancet 338, 1405-1406, 1991. A different form of stress testing using atrial pacing was investigated, and published in the American Heart Journal 122, 1559-1609, 1991. It was important to be able to study in a reproducible manner the coronary tree at rest and during maximal stress, only then could one hope to detect early disease. Many more publications arose from this technologies, a special mention is made here in respect of a comparison of two nuclear medicine probes with MRI in the investigation of hibernating myocardium, published in Circulation 98(18),1869-1874, 1998.

A landmark study was the first formal investigation of the cost and benefit of a nuclear medicine diagnostic procedure, and probably, one of the very few cost benefits studies published in the whole field of diagnostics in nuclear medicine. Led by Richard Underwood, collaborating with Arthur D Little, the European Nuclear Medicine Industry (represented by

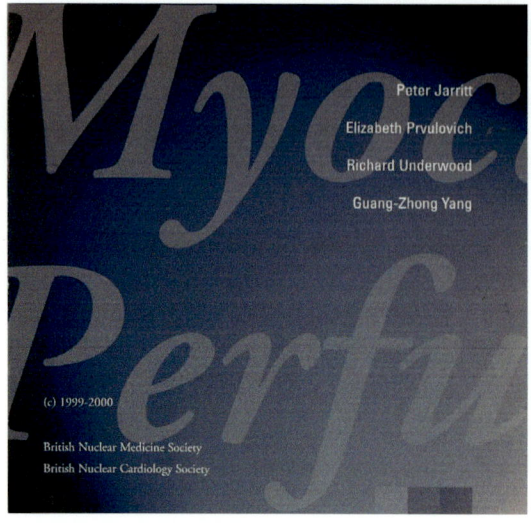

John Ogle from Amersham) and the European Association of Nuclear Medicine (Ell), the economics of myocardial perfusion in Europe was published as the Empire study (European Heart Journal 20(2), 157-166, 1999).

This proved to be an important publication. It formed the basis for European wide negotiations with Purchasers, and in the UK, formed the basis for final approval of NICE for myocardial perfusion studies in a wide range of clinical indications. Further evidence data was also published in the European J of Nuclear Medicine 31, 261-291, 2004.

Peter Jarritt (formerly at the Institute) and Consultant Physician Elizabeth Prvulovich, in conjunction with Richard Underwood (also formerly at the Institute) and Guang-Zhong Yang, produced in 1999-2000, and on behalf of the British Nuclear Medicine Society, a 5 CD ROM teaching aid, as a valuable tool for physicians, cardiologists and radiologists, providing experience and guidance on the reporting of myocardial perfusion studies. Each CD ROM

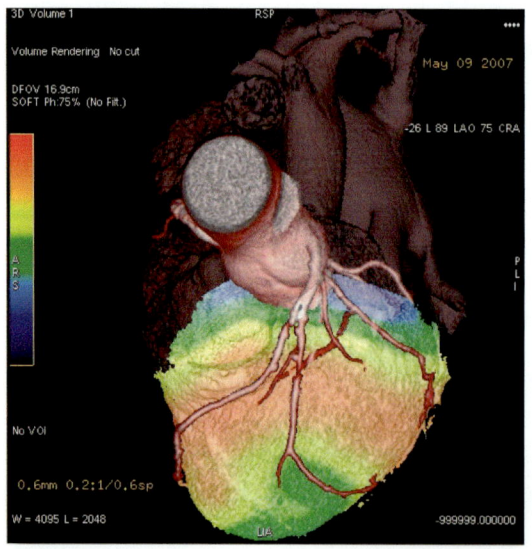

would contain 20 clinical cases, for self assessment and comparison with the formal approved clinical report. It was recognised for 20 credit hours for CME.

With the arrival of the 64 slice PETCT, again a first, the Institute was first in Europe to use Rubidium-82 and PETCT for myocardial perfusion studies. This novel approach had a huge impact on the patient journey, comfort of the procedure, at a much less reduced radiation

146

exposure. The initial European Experience was published by Ashley et al in the European Journal of Nuclear Medicine, 34, 1965-1972, 2007. Combining Rb-82 myocardial perfusion with adenosine stress testing and using the novel 64 slice CT component of the PETCT scanner to outline, non invasively, the coronary artery tree, provided for the fastest and most comprehensive documentation of cardiac function in man. Remarkable progress in CT scanning technology and the almost ideal properties of generator delivered Rubidium 82, allowed for a comprehensive Rb-82 perfusion and CTA study be offered to patients with minimal radiation risk.

Imaging technology is in constant evolution. How did this affect gamma camera technology, first conceived and brought to medicine in the early 60's?

A significant advance occurred with the move from sodium iodide scintillation detectors to solid state technology. A new chapter has opened in cardiac imaging – with a significant donation from industry (Spectrum Dynamics) the Institute has been at the forefront in the evaluation and optimisation of this novel approach. The following posters describe some of the recent advances achieved.

CARDIAC 82 RUBIDIUM PET/CT AND CT CORONARY ANGIOGRAPHY : First European Experience

A Groves, M Shastry, R Endozo, I Kayani, J Dickson, S Habobib, S Ben-Haim, E Prvulovich, S Hain, J Bomanji, W Waddington, C Townsend, P Blanchard, B Hutton, P Ell

INTRODUCTION:

There are only limited studies of combined positron perfusion CT angiography in the literature. We describe initial European experience of integrated Cardiac 82Rb-PET/CT angiography. We retrospectively analysed our first 4 patients that had undergone combined cardiac 82Rb-PET/CTA for clinical indications. Acquisitions were made on a GE-DST-16-detector PET/CT machine. Patients underwent PET imaging during adenosine infusion and at rest. Images were acquired over 5-minutes following 2200MBq of 82Rb. CT attenuation-correction scans were performed. CT images with a test bolus of contrast medium were then performed before a CT angiographic (140kV 150mAs 16x 0,625mm detectors, pitch 0.2-0.3) acquisition was made using 100ml of IV contrast medium in suspended respiration timed using the test-bolus data. PET images were reported by 6 consultants and CT images were reported by 3 consultants in consensus.

82Rb protocol

CT scout and CTAC (rest)

'Rest injection' 2200MBq 82Rb.

'Rest scan', 90-120 seconds after 82Rb inflows. Image acquisition for 5 mins

No delay

Adenosine Stress IV Adenosine @ 140 mcg/kg/min for 6 mins

'Stress injection' 2200 MBq 82Rb (infused 2 mins into Adenosine infusion).

'Stress scan', 90-120 seconds post 82Rb inflows completed. Image acquisition for 5 mins

CTAC (stress)

End of test. Total Time = 30 minutes

One patient had a normal angiogram and normal PET study. One patient had calcification in the left descending artery (LAD) making it difficult to assess significant stenosis, but the PET data was normal. One patient had mild apical ischaemia and a mildly stenosed LAD stent .

Some of the images are presented here.

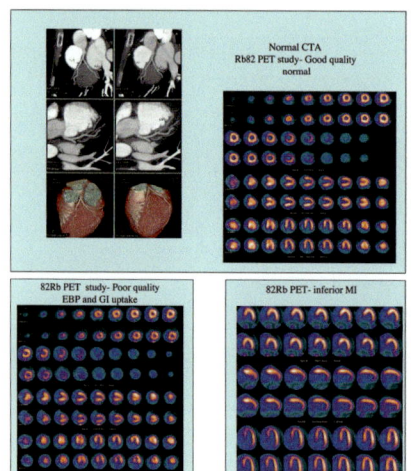

Normal CTA
Rb82 PET study- Good quality normal

82Rb PET study- Poor quality EBP and GI uptake

82Rb PET- inferior MI

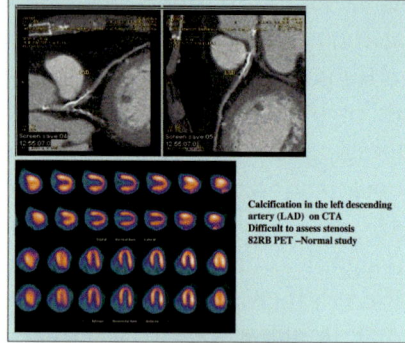

Calcification in the left descending artery (LAD) on CTA
Difficult to assess stenosis
82RB PET –Normal study

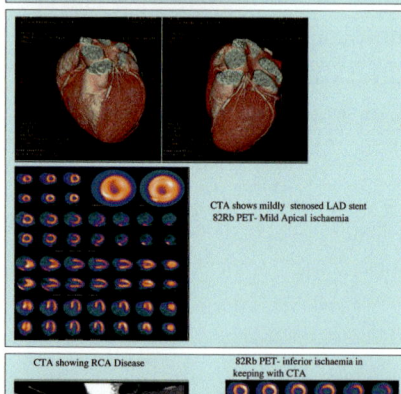

CTA shows mildly stenosed LAD stent
82Rb PET- Mild Apical ischaemia

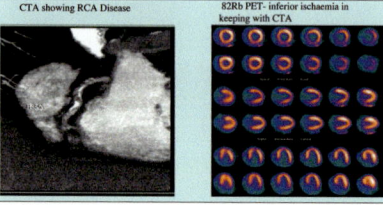

CTA showing RCA Disease

82Rb PET- inferior ischaemia in keeping with CTA

CONCLUSION:

Our initial experience confirms that combining cardiac 82Rb-PET/CT with 16-detector CT angiography is feasible and appears helpful for image interpretation.

INSTITUTE OF NUCLEAR MEDICINE

CLINICAL EVALUATION OF ULTRA RAPID SPECT FOR MYOCARDIAL PERFUSION IMAGING

S Ben-Haim, B Hutton, D Dickman, J Bomanji, E Prvulovich,
S Hain, A Groves, PJ Ell
Collaboration with Spectrum Dynamics, Tirat Hacarmel, Israel.

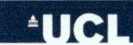

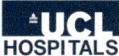

D-SPECT Cardiac Scanner System Configuration

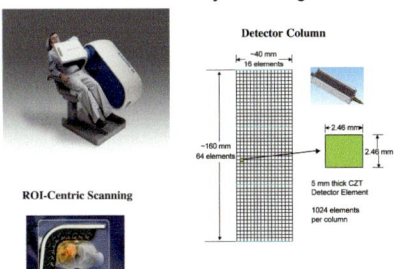

ROI-Centric Scanning

Detector Column

~40 mm
16 elements

2.46 mm

2.46 mm

~160 mm
64 elements

5 mm thick CZT
Detector Element

1024 elements
per column

Spatial Resolution NEMA NU1 2001

D-SPECT   A-SPECT

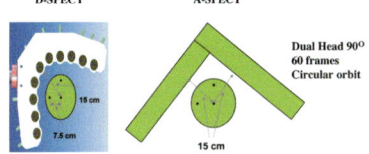

Dual Head 90°
60 frames
Circular orbit

15 cm

7.5 cm

15 cm

	Spatial Resolution (mm)			Spatial Resolution (mm)			Ratio A-SPECT/ D-SPECT	
Point #	X	Y	Point #	X	Y	Point #	X	Y
1-outer	4.7	5.2	1-outer	14.8	12.4	1-outer	3.1	2.4
2-outer	5.5	4.7	2-outer	12.8	12.4	2-outer	2.3	2.6
3-central	7.0	6.5	3-central	12.6	13.6	3-central	1.8	2.1
Average	5.7	5.5	Average	13.4	12.8	Average	2.3	2.3

Sensitivity

Co-57 line source 2.5 million counts measured at 100 mm

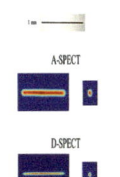

A-SPECT

D-SPECT

System	Spatial Resolution (mm)	Time (sec)
A-SPECT	10.4	600
D-SPECT	5.5	49
Ratio	1.9	12.3

Normal myocardial perfusion. Excellent quality of both sets of images.

AXIS, Philips Medical Systems   D-SPECT, Spectrum Dynamics

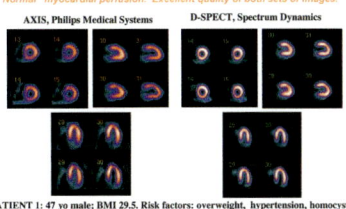

PATIENT 1: 47 yo male; BMI 29.5. Risk factors: overweight, hypertension, homocysteinemia. Atypical chest pain. One-day stress (treadmill)/ rest, Tc99m MIBI 400 Mbq (stress)+1000 MBq (rest). Exercise: 12min, MPHR 91%. Clinical and ECG response : non ischemic.
A-SPECT acquisition: Stress 30 sec/projection; total 15 min. Rest 25 sec/projection total 12.5 min
D-SPECT acquisition: Stress 2 sec/position; total 4 min. Rest 1 sec/position; total 2 min

Antero-apical MI. No inducible ischaemia. Excellent quality of both sets of images.

AXIS, Philips Medical Systems   D-SPECT, Spectrum Dynamics

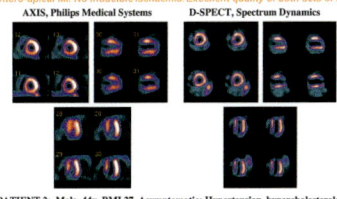

PATIENT 2: Male, 44y, BMI 27. Asymptomatic; Hypertension, hypercholesterolemia, past smoker, Ant. MI, PCI to LAD (7/2005). Treadmill exercise stopped (fatigue). One-day stress (Dipyridamole with low level treadmill)/ rest, Tc99m MIBI 400 Mbq (stress)+1000 MBq (rest). Clinical and ECG response: non-ischemic.
A-SPECT acquisition: Stress 30 sec/projection; total 15 min. Rest 25 sec/projection total 12.5 min
D-SPECT acquisition: Stress 2 sec/position; total 4 min. Rest 1 sec/position; total 2 min

Clinical Feasibility Study – high speed and high quality 2-minute gated SPECT acquisition

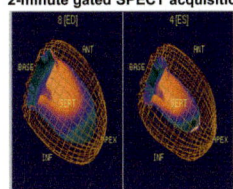

Spectrum Dynamics' Innovation: Molecular Imaging Platform

Improved sensitivity X10   Improved image quality
Improved energy resolution X2   Fast scanning
Reduced radiation dose   Improved patient comfort
Personalized diagnostic imaging   Novel imaging protocols
Novel radiopharmaceuticals

INSTITUTE OF NUCLEAR MEDICINE

The Institute and its European Impact

A DIFFICULT BUT EXCITING DELIVERY (06.09.1985)

The document shown in this rather brief account, represents the outcome of many hours and days burning the midnight oil, to call to senses those who were initially unable or unwilling to see the future vision for a unified European nuclear medicine organisation. Announced on September 6th, 1985, it made public the foundation of the European Association of Nuclear Medicine (EANM). As a precaution, this document contained a get out clause, over a period of two years, but it was never enacted upon.

In the early 80's, the atmosphere was not too different from the present squabble we have witnessed and is ongoing between the republicans and the democrats across the pond to achieve consensus for the common good. Now, we have well passed those tumultuous days and discussions, the EANM is an established reality, whose mission is well enshrined in its constitution and bye-laws.

Prior to the formation of the EANM, two aspiring European Societies, very different in their make up, maintained regular annual congresses and competed for industry funds and membership participation. The older and more established, was the result of a very strong, efficient and developed national society, the German Society of Nuclear Medicine (DGN). With a pre-dominant national membership base, it had conducted annual meetings over many years, in fact since 1963, and was rightly proud of its achievements and success. It had however real difficulty in claiming its "European character", since a membership based committee structure guaranteed a focussed national element in governance. Aiming at captivating a wider audience, it began inviting expert speakers from several nations, and at a late stage, as a consequence of what was happening to Europe as a whole, it changed its named in 1981 to the Society of Nuclear Medicine Europe (SNME).

A younger society, established a principled governance structure, based on national representation in the form of delegates from many European national societies – founded on June 8th, 1974 in Clermont-Ferrand, as the European Nuclear Medicine Society (ENMS), it had its first annual congress in 1974 in Lausanne under the chair of B. Delaloye. With a European credential, it had nevertheless a much smaller membership base, reflecting the language barriers which (even today) prevent the wider participation at European meetings of significant sections of the nuclear medicine workforce.

For many of us, then younger in years, it was difficult to understand the need for two, competing, European societies. Some thought that sponsors, such as Industry, would be able to guide or take a lead in such endeavours –funding issues were ever present-but clearly this was not the case, the lead would have to come from committed clinicians, with a fresh outlook. The reader can see that the seeds of conflict had been sown. Something had to be done for the future success of our field.

The Austrian spa resort of Bad Gastein, hosted every two years, under the chair of R Hoefer, a meeting where early advances in the field were discussed by experts around the world. The Bad Gastein Symposium started as early as in 1954, and became an international significant landmark for discussions relevant to the development of radioactive tracers in medicine. The most prominent scientists and clinicians in the field would have attended this meeting, at one time or another, which combined exciting science with the beauty of the Austrian mountains. Where best could the leaders of these two societies come together and meet in a perfect atmosphere for preliminary discussions?

And so it was that in January 1982, leaders from both Societies agreed to appoint a Linking Committee, to start a process of engagement and discussions, initially focussing on the need to join forces and to avoid two annual meetings with European ambitions (linkage meant something, and was aimed at). The annual meetings of the national societies were to remain sacrosanct (useful to recall that the Council of Europe (The Europe of the 2nd Vienna Congress in October 1993) described Europe as having 32 member states and 8 special guests parliaments...) – 40 national nuclear medicine annual meetings in Europe?

A further meeting in Paris took place on the 30th of August 1982, a third meeting in Ulm, on September 14th, 1983. The next meeting of the Linking Committee took place in Helsinki in 1984, where the SNME and ENMS would have their first joint annual congress chaired by Vauramo. The final composition of the Linking Committee was agreed: Donato (Italy), Rihiimaki (Finland) and Ell (UK) on be-

EUROPEAN NUCLEAR MEDICINE CONGRESS
LONDON, ENGLAND. SEPTEMBER 3-6, 1985

PARTICIPATING ORGANISATIONS
The Society of Nuclear Medicine-Europe: 23rd Meeting
The European Nuclear Medicine Society: 8th Meeting
The British Nuclear Medicine Society: 13th Meeting

half off the ENMS) and Hundeshagen (Germany), Riccabona (Austria) and Schmidt (Germany) on behalf of the SNME. A fifth encounter ensued in London in 1985, where the 2nd joint Congress was chaired by Britton, then at St. Bartholomew's.

Between 1982 and 1988, dozens of encounters, not all pleasant, took place, between different groups of engaged individuals, proffering different views and concepts as to what a single European Association should look like. There were significant issues to be debated, but also minor distractions which, consuming time, needed to be eliminated... Some quibbled about the word "association" versus "society", but most of the expressed differences related to the significant asymmetry which pertained to the larger national societies. Some of these placed great emphasis in membership participation, others underlined the need for scientific output, and education, but greatest worries were expressed about the mechanism of representation and election of officers. Concerns were also expressed about the appropriate representation of the non central European nations. Nevertheless, a general consensus began to emerge that something indeed had to be done.

In a fit of enthusiasm and urgency, Ell wrote in a weekend the outline of a constitution for the EANM. This was shown at an informal meeting between Ell as Secretary of the ESNM, Noesslin as President of the ESNM and Britton, instrumental as now President of the SNME. With skill and enthusiasm, Britton redrafted and clarified the original version, which met with approval of the Presidents of both societies. The rest is possibly known history. The staff of the Institute of Nuclear Medicine with Britton as President, Ell As Secretary and Jarritt as IT Co-ordinator and Administrator, organised this major London Congress, which, in today's prices, brought to the Exchequer, well over 2 M Sterling.

A contract was agreed upon (see Table I), presented to both Societies and at the joint meeting and members assembly of the joint Congress, submitted to vote. Rudolf Hoefer gave a skilled, balanced and reasoned plea to the membership, that time had come to take the plunge. The foundation of the EANM was approved (1985) and the Linking Committee disbanded in 1987.

Then first 3 Presidents of the EANM were G Riccabona (Austria) from 1988 to 1990, S. Askienazy (France) from 1991 to 1993 and P. Ell (UK) from 1994-1996. Now in 2012, the EANM is celebrating its Silver Jubilee. With over 3000 members, 35 national societies represented, a major scientific publication (EJNMMI) and regular annual congresses, it has gained an established reputation as the single European forum for Nuclear Medicine.

Relevant Dates:

1982: Start of 15 Meetings of the Linking Committee

06.09.1985: Foundation of the European Association of Nuclear Medicine (EANM)

1985: European

1984-1987: Joint European (SNME+ENMS) Congresses

1988: First EANM Annual Congress

30.10.1989: EC Directive recognizes Nuclear Medicine as Independent Medical Speciality

01.01.1990: European Journal of Nuclear Medicine (EJNM) starts a long road to become a major publication in the field edited by Peter Ell

EJNMMI Editor-in-Chief 1988-2003

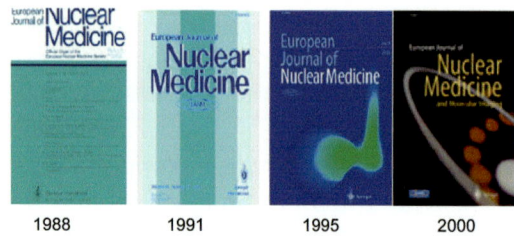

| 1988 | 1991 | 1995 | 2000 |

European Journal of Nuclear Medicine and Molecular Imaging

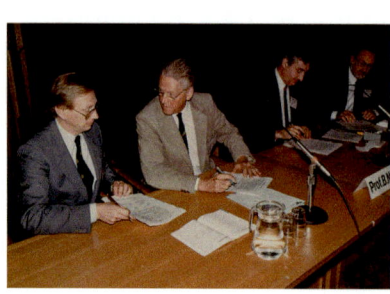 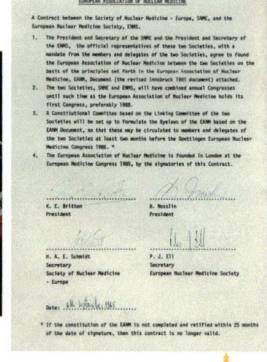

Signing the foundation document of the EANM

Recommended Reading:

The History of Nuclear Medicine in Europe. M. Feld and M. De Roo. Edited by H. Schicha, K. Bergdolt and P.J. Ell, Schattauer Verlag, 2003

The Institute and the Lancet

In the UK, Nuclear Medicine has long lingered as a Cinderella medical speciality. Here is not the place too discuss the origins and the effects of this development, these are manifold and significant. They contrast with the more rapid development of Nuclear Medicine in Europe (see Table) But the reader can find similar areas of contrast in other fields of medicine – whilst the UK is justly proud for its Nobel laureates G Hounsfield and P Mansfield for their invention of the X-RAY CT scanner and the MRI instrument respectively, for decades the UK has fallen behind in terms of the application of imaging technologies for the benefit of patients. Nothing new here. So what could be done?

2009/10 Data for PET Studies

	10^6 Population	Nr of Scanners	FDG Totals	FDG/10^3	Nr of Com. Sites	Trends
USA	308	2000	2,500,000	8.1		
Europe	239	800?	550,000	2.3		3% Growth by 2014
UK	65	59		0.9	8	
France	60	85		2.0	20	
Spain	44	54		1.4	12	
Italy	60	200		3.2	12	
Belgium	10	20		3.5	3	
Germany	82	158		1.4	?	

It was clear to us that the benefits of Nuclear Medicine were by en large, poorly understood. The specialist society (as often happens with these) would convene regular meetings, but these failed to attract enough senior clinicians to engage and be involved with the developments of the field. In view of this, staff at the Institute requested an audience with the Editor of the Lancet. There was a most favourable response, the problem we described was clearly appreciated. After some discussion, The Lancet graciously agreed to publish 6 articles, in subsequent weekly issues of the Journal, covering the main aspects of our clinical practice. The only require-

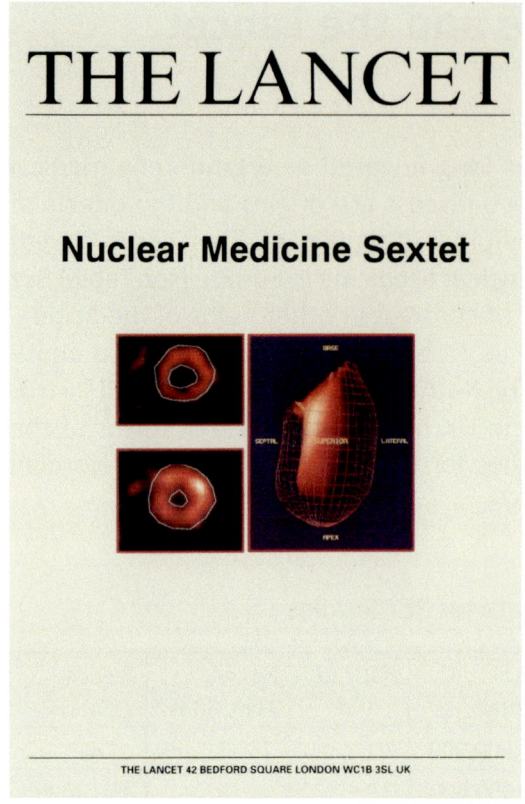

THE LANCET

Nuclear Medicine Sextet

THE LANCET 42 BEDFORD SQUARE LONDON WC1B 3SL UK

ment was that, whilst editing, we were requested to spread the author's net, so that only one of the 6 articles would be contributed by us. So the Nuclear Medicine Sextet was born.

A unique educational tool was developed to spread the message to a very wide audience. Whilst the European societies embraced this project with enthusiasm, and distributed this sextet widely, we were most disappointed with the lack of interest of our own British Nuclear Medicine Society. It was felt that our national Society should take an active role in distributing this Sextet widely throughout the UK but there was no interest! How odd — and what missed opportunity to disseminate this series so that in the UK, the benefits and clinical value of the practice of Nuclear Medicine could be fully appreciated.

Contents

Bright future for nuclear medicine

See page 661

It was my good fortune to meet one of the founders of nuclear medicine, the late Glenn Seaborg, at the annual meeting of the Society of Nuclear Medicine in June, 1996. He was keen as ever to discuss the future of nuclear medicine and was particularly interested in contacting the Commission on Nomenclature of Inorganic Chemistry, and not without reason. Glenn Seaborg was involved in the discovery of iron-59, iodine-131, cobalt-60, and technetium-99m. Element 106 is now named Seaborgium. In 1951, he, with Edwin McMillan, was awarded the Nobel Prize in chemistry. Several eminent scientists who applied the radioactive-tracer principle have also been Nobel laureates: Becquerel and the Curies (Physics, 1903); von Hevesy (Chemistry, 1943, for the first radiotracer study in animals); and Yalow (Medicine, 1977) for her work with Berson on the radioimmunoassay.

Development in nuclear medicine has always been along two lines—clinical service, for diagnosis and therapy, and basic research, aimed at unravelling disease mechanisms, pathways of drug interaction, and early assessment of individual organ function. The large variation in practice worldwide reflects this duality and, naturally, the funding of the specialty. In the bigger medical institutions, large teams branch out into the different areas of application and research. In smaller centres, a simple but effective clinical service emerges. There is a world of difference between the complexity of a bone scan and tomographic maps of receptors, and between treatment of thyroid diseases with radioiodine and specific treatment of a lymphoma with a labelled, monoclonal antibody. The availability of nuclear medicine is hence non-uniform; some European countries do more than 50 000 procedures per million population whereas the frequency in others is about 10 000 per million.

The attraction of nuclear medicine is strong. The detection of biological signals at the picomolar level, associated with specificity of the ligand in question, explains the interest and the potential. The methods are uniquely suited to tissue characterisation, to early assessment of the extent and severity of disease, and finally to treatment of disease with specific ligands. And yet over-regulation is posing possibly the biggest threat to its expansion. The estimation of risks involved is not proportional to the vast body of legislature that begins to impact on progress. The cost of registration of new radiopharmaceuticals is clearly deterring industry and sponsors alike. A tracer delivered once or twice to an individual in quantities of less than a milligram (often in the nano or picomolar range) will require, for registration purposes, the imprimatur of a body of legislation basically designed to monitor the side-effects of drugs, given commonly daily in doses of hundreds of milligrams.

The series of six articles on nuclear medicine that *The Lancet* begins today describe the wide clinical applications, potential, and future developments. Nuclear medicine has offered new insights in the understanding of the dementias, the spread of cancer, and the early detection of coronary-artery disease. Not all potential applications could be covered in this series. There is, however, ample food for thought.

Peter J Ell

Institute of Nuclear Medicine, University College London Medical School, Mortimer Street, London W1N 8AA, UK

157

PET/CT
Positron Emission Tomography

UCLH NHS Trust and INM-UCL
June 1999 – February 2006

Positron Emission Tomography - PET

Minimally Invasive Imaging

Linkage to Clinical, Molecular and Biology Medicine

Exquisite Anatomical Detail via Image Fusion with PETCT

Molecular PET Mapping

Cellular Proliferation
Apoptosis
Hypoxia
Angiogenesis
Metabolism
Alzheimer Plaque Localization
Atheroma Plaque Imaging
Neuroreceptor Imaging
Oncoreceptor Imaging
Infection/Inflammation

First UK 16 Slice PETCT

Discovery LS with RT table top

With the assistance of a generous grant from the Trustees for the University College London Hospitals Charity, a clinical and research programme was initiated at the Institute of Nuclear Medicine (INM) with respect to positron emission tomography (PET). A full ring top of the range PET scanner was commissioned in June 1999, this being the most modern scanner in the UK. The new facilities were inaugurated in September 1999. By mid 2000, a first formal peer reviewed publication had been accepted for publication in the British Journal of Surgery. With the delivery of F-18 labelled fluorodeoxyglucose (FDG), a clinical programme was commenced. Oncology was to be the focus of this programme. Initially, patients were scanned on a 3 day per week basis, but the service was soon expanded to 4 and then 5 days per week. By August 2000, 400 patients had been investigated, and by February 2001 the figure had reached 650. Complimentary letters from patients began to arrive, and in 2001 Lancet Oncology published an article from the INM. With a further grant from the Trustees, the PET scanner was upgraded to the first PET/CT scanner in the UK. The first UK patient to benefit from this new development was investigated on the 17th of January 2002! PET/CT led to a dramatic increase in the acceptance and utility of the PET clinical programme – in the 3 months of September, October and November 2002, 402 patients were investigated with this unique technology. A formal presentation was made to the North London Cancer Network.

PET technology has been described as the most advanced and accurate imaging methodology presently available. It is now felt that in oncology PET is the most accurate staging and re-staging method for 75% of all cancers. Over years, several Health Technology Assessment (HTA) reports have expanded the "approved" indications for PET in the assessment of patients with cancer.

PET/CT, on the other hand, is unique in that it combines metabolic and anatomical cross-sectional mapping into a single investigation. Image fusion is routinely and accurately obtained, patient throughput is enhanced by at least 30%, costs per case are contained if not reduced and a major impact on radiotherapy planning is expected in the near future.

The power of PET also resides in the ability to develop metabolic tracers that will map specific biological signals. A brief overview of F-18 labelled ligands is given in Table I . At the INM, exciting work is underway in developing F-18 labelled thymidine, a ligand which we have shown is able to image cellular proliferation (Fig. 1) and now most recently we are introducing new applications with ligands able to specifically image neuroendocrine tumours.

A number of clinical cases illustrate the current utility of PET and PET/CT as currently performed at the INM (Figs. 2-9).

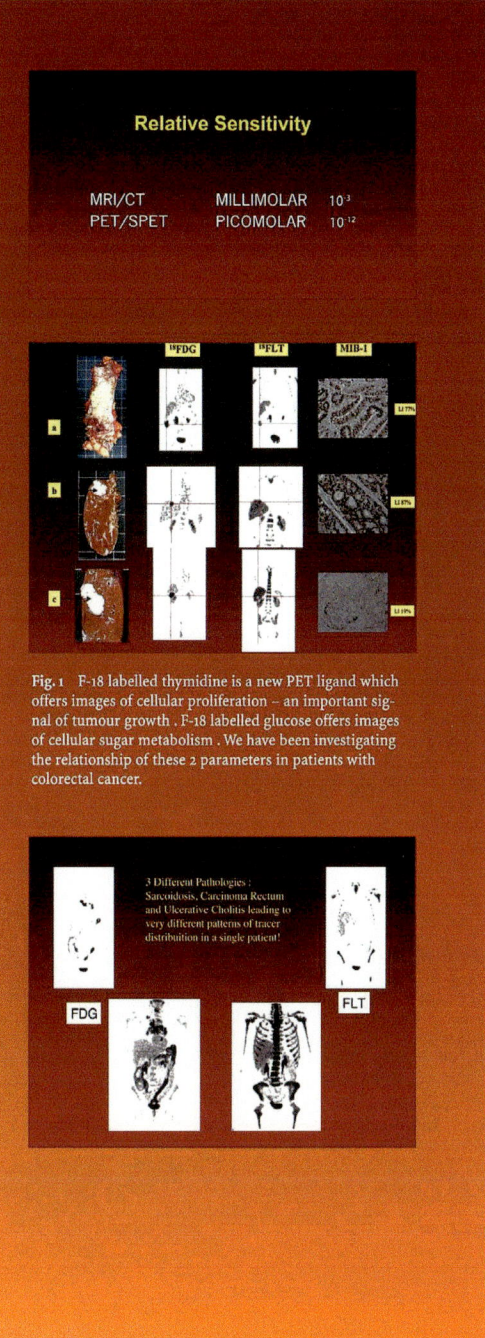

Fig. 1 F-18 labelled thymidine is a new PET ligand which offers images of cellular proliferation – an important signal of tumour growth . F-18 labelled glucose offers images of cellular sugar metabolism . We have been investigating the relationship of these 2 parameters in patients with colorectal cancer.

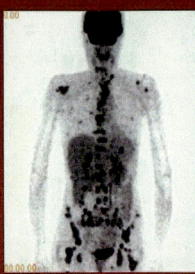 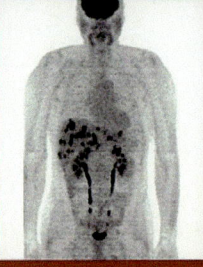 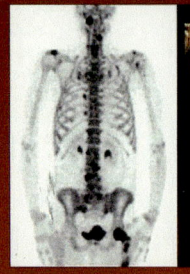 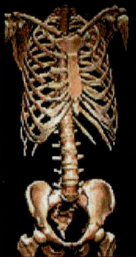

Fig. 2 Patients with advanced glucose avid metastasis not demonstrated on conventional CT or MR!

Fig. 3 F-18 labelled fluoride offers superior images of skeletal metabolism – the PET bone scan. Patient with multiple skeletal deposits.

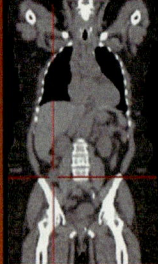 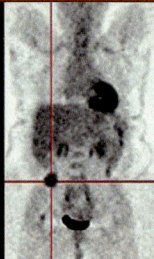 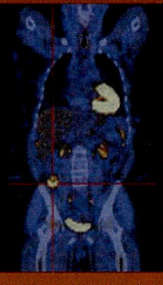 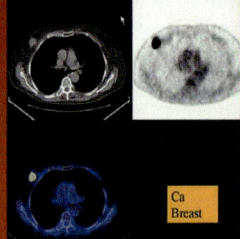

Fig. 4 75 year old female previous right hemicolectomy and chemotherapy. A PET/CT study shows increased sugar metabolism in a clearly localised recurrence in the right iliac fossa.

Fig. 5 Primary breast tumours can be intensely glucose avid, as in this patient shown by PET/CT. The transaxial section clearly depicts the tumour. In general, tumour response to chemotherapy as seen by PET serial studies correlates well with outcome.

PET/CT : a new imaging tool
Enhances Patient Acceptance
Enhances Referrer's Acceptance
Enhances PET Only
Enhances CT Only
Improves PET Throughput
Will Impact on IMRT
May replace CT Simulator
Very fast throughput in the future

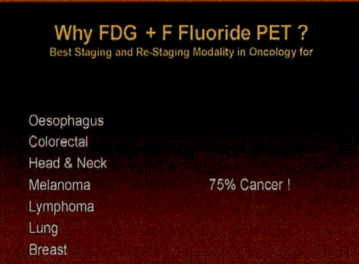

Why FDG + F Fluoride PET ?
Best Staging and Re-Staging Modality in Oncology for

Oesophagus
Colorectal
Head & Neck
Melanoma   75% Cancer !
Lymphoma
Lung
Breast

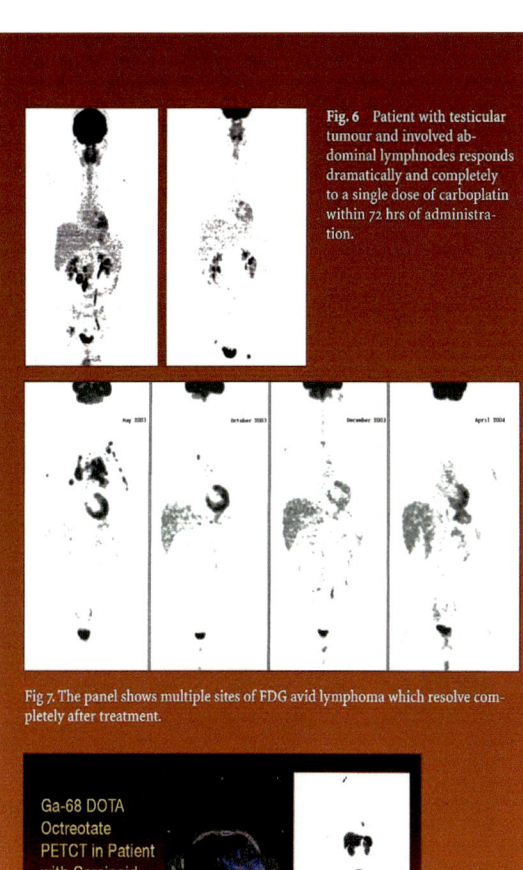

Fig. 6 Patient with testicular tumour and involved abdominal lymphnodes responds dramatically and completely to a single dose of carboplatin within 72 hrs of administration.

Fig 7. The panel shows multiple sites of FDG avid lymphoma which resolve completely after treatment.

Ga-68 DOTA Octreotate PETCT in Patient with Carcinoid

Note very different information and tracer distribution between these 2 studies

FDG PETCT in same patient

Typical FDG Pattern in Patient with Arturitis

The PET programme has made a significant impact on the day-to-day management of patients at UCLH NHS Trust. A peer-reviewed, prospective and published clinical audit demonstrated that PET investigations altered the staging of 39% of all patients referred to the INM. In 25% of patients, disease was upstaged and in a further 14%, disease was downstaged. The issued PET clinical report was deemed by the referrers to be helpful in more than 75% of cases. As a result, a change in management occurred in a third of patients and a change of treatment in 10%.

Routine referrals now include patients with head and neck, lung, skin, oesophageal, colorectal and gynaecological cancer, as well as patients with lymphoma and paraneoplastic syndromes. PET studies are now routinely discussed at UCLH Trust at multidisciplinary and clinical meetings, and are no longer perceived as "research only" investigations.

The ligands listed under Biological PET Mapping can all be labelled with F-18, which has become the ubiquitous tracer for PET investigations. These and others still under development can, when studied with PET, deliver with unique sensitivity and specificity new information on cellular metabolism – they are ushering in what has been described as the birth of molecular imaging. One exciting area will be the investigation of the response of cancer to treatment. As an example, Fig. 6 shows two FDG PET studies performed 48 hours apart in a patient with a testicular cancer, treated by a single dose of carboplatin. Significant disease present in the abdominal lymph nodes showed a complete response to the treatment within this short period of time. Definition of the metabolic profile of tumours over time and in response to novel therapeutic agents will be immensely aided by PET technologies. Another example is given in Fig 7. We are now investigating the role of PETCT in the evaluation of response to T-cell infusion treatment in follicular lymphoma. Most encouraging data will shortly appear in the literature, showing that PETCT is useful in determining when and if at all treatment is to be commenced.

An exciting period lies ahead. During 2006 and the following years we see PETCT gaining major relevance in the cardiovascular field. This will now become the fastest growing area for PETCT. The INM, again assisted by generous support from the Trust and its Trustees has been able to create the necessary infrastructure for this development. We have commenced work with the first 16 slice PETCT scanner in the UK and a first patient was investigated on the 6th of January 2006.

The future is bright!

February 2006
Professor Peter Josef Ell FMedSci Dr HC AΩA,
Clinical Director Nuclear Medicine
UCLH NHS Foundation Trust Hospitals

161

POSTGRADUATE SUCCESSES

MD Thesis
T Arulampalam: 2002
D Francis: 2003
A. Engledow : In progress 2006

MS Thesis
N Hyde: 2003
F Pakzad: Submission 2006

ACADEMIC OUTPUT
1999 – 2006 : PET and PETCT
PROGRAMME

Published Original Papers

1. Multiresolution analysis of emission tomography images in the wavelet domain. Turkheimer F, Brett M, Visvikis D and Cunningham V. *Journal of Cerebral Blood Flow and Metabolism*. 1999: 19, 1189-1208.

2. Modelling dynamic PET-SPET studies in the wavelet domain. Turkheimer F, Banati R, Visvikis D, Aston J, Gunn RN and Cunningham V. *Journal of Cerebral Blood Flow and Metabolism*. 2000: 20, 879-893.

3. The impact of FDG-PET on the management algorithm for recurrent colorectal cancer. Arulampalam THA, Costa DC, Visvikis D, Boulos P, Taylor I and Ell PJ. *European Journal of Nuclear Medicine*. 2001: 28(12), 1758-1765.

4. Influence of OSEM and segmented attenuation correction in the calculation of standardised uptake values for 18FDG-PET. Visvikis D, Cheze-Le Rest, C, Costa DC, Bomanji JB, Gacinovic S and Ell PJ. *European Journal of Nuclear Medicine*. 2001: 28, 1326-1335.

5. Functional imaging of malignant paragagliomas and carcinoid tumours. Cheze-Le Rest, C, Bomanji JB, Costa DC, Visvikis DC and Ell PJ. *European Journal of Nuclear Medicine*. 2001: 28, 475-479.

6. Positron emission tomography in colorectal cancer. Arulampalam THA, Costa DC, Loizidou M, Visvikis D, Ell PJ and Taylor I. *British Journal of Surgery*. 2001: 88, 176-189.

7. FDG PET in clinical oncology: The referrer's perspective. Gopalan D, Griffiths D, Townsend CE, Prvulovich EM, Bomanji JB, Costa DC and Ell PJ. *Nuclear Medicine Communications*. 2002: 23, 1041-1046.

8. Glucose utilisation and cell proliferation in colorectal cancer. Visvikis D, Francis DL, Costa DC, Mulligan RS, Townsend CE, Arulampalam THA, Islam MS, Taylor I and Ell PJ. *European Journal of Nuclear Medicine and Molecular Imaging*. 2002: 29(2), 280.

9. CT based attenuation correction in the calculation of semi-quantitative indices of 18FDG uptake in PET. Visvikis D, Costa DC, Croasdale I, Lonn AHR, Bomanji JB, Gacinovic S and Ell PJ. *European Journal of Nuclear Medicine and Molecular Imaging*. 2003: 30(3), 344-353.

10. Positron emission and computed x-ray tomography: a coming together. Costa DC, Visvikis D, Croasdale I, Pigden I, Townsend CE, Bomanji JB, Prvulovich EM, Lonn A and Ell PJ. *Nuclear Medicine Communications*. 2003: 24(4), 351-358.

11. A new approach to pre-treatment assessment of the No neck in oral squamous cell carcinoma: the role of sentinel node biopsy and positron emission tomography. Hyde NC, Prvulovich EM, Newman L, Waddington WA, Visvikis D and Ell PJ. *Oral Oncology*. 2003: 39, 350-360.

12. In vivo imaging of cellular proliferation in colorectal cancer using Positron Emission Tomography. Francis DL, Freeman A, Visvikis D, Costa DC, Luthra SK, Novelli M, Taylor I and Ell PJ. *GUT*, 52, 1602-1606, 2003

13. Does 18FDG-PET/CT as compared to dedicated CT alter management of pancreatobiliary tumours? Pakzad F, Syed R, Nagabushan N, Shankar A, Taylor I, and Ell PJ. *Journal of Nuclear Medicine*. 45, 87, 2004

14. A comparison of FDG PET/CT and MRI versus histology for staging of primary head and neck cancers and detection of recurrent disease. Hughes SJ, Prvulovich EM, Witherow H, Kalavrezos N and Ell PJ. *Journal of Nuclear Medicine*. 45, 80, 2004.

15. Impact of 18F-FDG PET/CT in the management of pancreatobiliary tumours. Syed R, Pakzad F, Nagabhushan N, Groves A, Copland C, Taylor I, Ell PJ and Bomanji JB. *Journal of Nuclear Medicine*. 45, 344, 2004.

16. FDG-PET for the pre-operative staging of colorectal liver metastases. Arulampalam THA, Francis DL, Visvikis D, Taylor I and Ell PJ. *European Journal of Surgical Oncology*. 30, 286-291, 2004.

17. Assessment of recurrent colorectal cancer following 5-fluorouracil chemotherapy using both 18FDG and 18FLT PET. Francis DL, Visvikis D, Costa DC, Croasdale I, Arulampalam TH, Luthra SK, Taylor I, and Ell PJ. *European Journal of Nuclear Medicine and Molecular Imaging*. 31, 928, 2004.

18. The role of PET imaging in lymphoma. Burton C. Ell PJ and Linch D. *British Journal of Haematology*. 126, 772-784, 2004.

19. How often do patients undergo repeat PET or PET/CT examinations? Experience from a UK Institution. Groves AM, Cullum ID, Syed R, Nagabhushan N, Kayani I, Pakzad F and Ell PJ. *Nuclear Medicine Communications*. 26, 2, 137-139, 2005.

20. Imaging bronchial carcinoma in situ: possible roles for combined positron emission tomography – PET/CT. Kayan I, Groves AM, Ell PJ, George PJ and Bomanji J. *Lancet Oncology*. 6(3), 190, 2005.

21. Oral contrast medicine in PET/CT: should you or shouldn't you? Groves AM, Kayani I, Dickson JC, Townsend C, Croasdale I, Syed R, Nagabhushan N, Hain S and Ell PJ. *European Journal of Nuclear Medicine and Molecular Imaging*. 32, 1160-1166, 2005.

22. Clinical evaluation of 2D versus 3D whole body PET image quality using a dedicated BGO PET scanner. Visvikis D, Griffiths D, Costa DC, Bomanji J and Ell PJ. *European Journal of Nuclear Medicine and Molecular Imaging*. 32, 1050-1056, 2005.

23. Impact of combined 18F-FDG PET/CT in head and neck tumours. Syed R, Bomanji JB, Nagabhushan N, Hughes S, Kayani I, Groves AM, Gacinovic S, Hydes N, Visvikis D, Copland C and Ell PJ. *British Journal of Cancer.* 92(6), 1046-50, 2005.

24. 18F-FDG PET scanning and lymphoma. Bomanji JB and Ell PJ. British *Journal of Cancer Management.* 2, 8-11, 2005.

25. Use of 18F-FDG positron emission tomography following allogeneic transplantation to guide adoptive immunotherapy with donor lymphocyte infusions. Hart DP, Avivi I, Thomson KJ, Peggs KS, Morris EC, Goldstone AH, Linch DC, Ell PJ, Bomanji JB and McKinnon S. *British Journal of Haematology.* 128(6), 824-829, 2005.

26. Anti-CD20 monoclonal antibody (rituximab) as an adjunct in the treatment of giant cell arteritis. Bhatia A, Ell PJ and Edwards JC. *Ann Rheum Dis.* 64(7), 1099-100, 2005.

27. Molecular imaging in animal models of disease – every detail counts. Pakzad F, Ell PJ and Carrio I. *European Journal of Nuclear Medicine and Molecular Imaging.* 32, 899-960, 2005.

28. The contributions of PET/CT to improved patient management. Ell PJ. *British Journal of Radiology.* 79, 32-36, 2006.

Invited Lectures

1. PET for the few or for the many. Ell PJ. *World Congress of High Technology Medicine.* Berlin 2000.

2. PET/CT and SPET/CT: A meeting of minds or a fortunate coincidence. Ell PJ. *International Cancer Imaging Society.* London 2001.

3. The role of PET in oncology. Principles and impact. Ell PJ. *International Cancer Imaging Society.* London 2001.

4. PET in colorectal cancer. Francis DL. *North Middlesex Hospital Oncology Forum.* March 2002.

5. Use of PET in colorectal cancer. Francis DL. *Trent Regional Joint Oncology / Palliative Medicine Study Day.* April 2002.

6. Imaging cellular proliferation in colorectal cancer. Francis DL. *UK PET group meeting.* April 2002.

7. The further evaluation of PET scanning in colorectal cancer. Francis DL. *The General Surgical Forum (Middlesex Hospital) Masterclass.* July 2002.

8. The role of PET scanning in upper gastrointestinal cancer. Francis DL. *Association of Upper Gastrointestinal Surgeons of Great Britain & Ireland.* September 2002.

9. PET in clinical oncology. Ell PJ. *42nd Meeting, Japanese Society of Nuclear Medicine.* Kobe 2002.

10. PET in oncology. Ell PJ. *Turkish Society of Nuclear Medicine, Kusadasi.* Turkey 2002.

11. F-18 FDG PET. A clinical tool. Ell PJ. *Belgium Society of Nuclear Medicine.* Brussels 2002.

12. Gamma camera PET. Is it worthwhile. Ell PJ. *Royal College of Radiologists.* London 2003.

13. PET. Ell PJ. *PETCT – a new technology Advanced Medicine Conference. Royal College of Physicians.* February 2003

14. Where are we with PET/CT? Ell PJ. *International Cancer Imaging Society.* London, October 2003.

15. PET/CT: Present and Future, Merits and Constraints. Ell PJ. *FORUM 2003.* Barcelona, October 2003.

16. Overview of PET in Oncology. Ell PJ. *Scottish Radiological Society,* Glasgow, November 2003.

17. PET in Surgical Oncology. Ell PJ. *European Society of Surgical Oncology.* Budapest, March 2004.

18. PET/CT in Abdominal Tumours. Ell PJ. *European Congress of Radiology.* Vienna, March 2004.

19. PET/CT in Oncology. Ell PJ. *The 8th Annual International Cancer Symposium on PET/CT in Oncology.* Taiwan, October 2004.

20. PET/CT in Clinical Oncology. Ell PJ. *Royal College of Radiologist.* London. January 2005.

21. Imaging: Blind Without a Target. Ell PJ. *Honoris Causa Lecture. University of Barcelona.* April 2005.

22. The contribution of PET/CT to improved patient management. Ell PJ. *BIR President's Conference.* London, May 2005.

23. Activation of thymidine salvage pathway measured with FLT PET, as a potential indicator of response to 5FU in colorectal cancer. Pakzad F, Loizidou M, Ell PJ and Taylor I. *American Society of Clinical Oncology.* Florida, May 2005.

Published Book Chapters

1. PET in the measurement of cerebral cancer. Francis DL, Costa DC and Ell PJ. In: *Clinical Molecular Imaging. PET, PET/CT and SPET/CT.* Ed. Von Schulthess GK. Lippincott Williams and Wilkins, Philadelphia 2003.

2. Atlas of PET/CT in Oncology. Francis DL, Costa DC and Ell PJ. In: *Nuclear Medicine in Clinical Diagnosis and Treatment.* Ed. Ell and Gambhir, Churchill Livingstone. 3rd Ed, 503-538, 2004.

3. PET and PETCT of the oesophagus, stomach and large intestine. Francis,DL,Arumpalam,THA,Costa, DC and Ell,PJ. In: *Clinical Molecular and Anatomic Imaging.* Ed. G von Schulthess, Lippincott Williams & Wilkins, 318-333,2003

Published Abstracts

Over 40

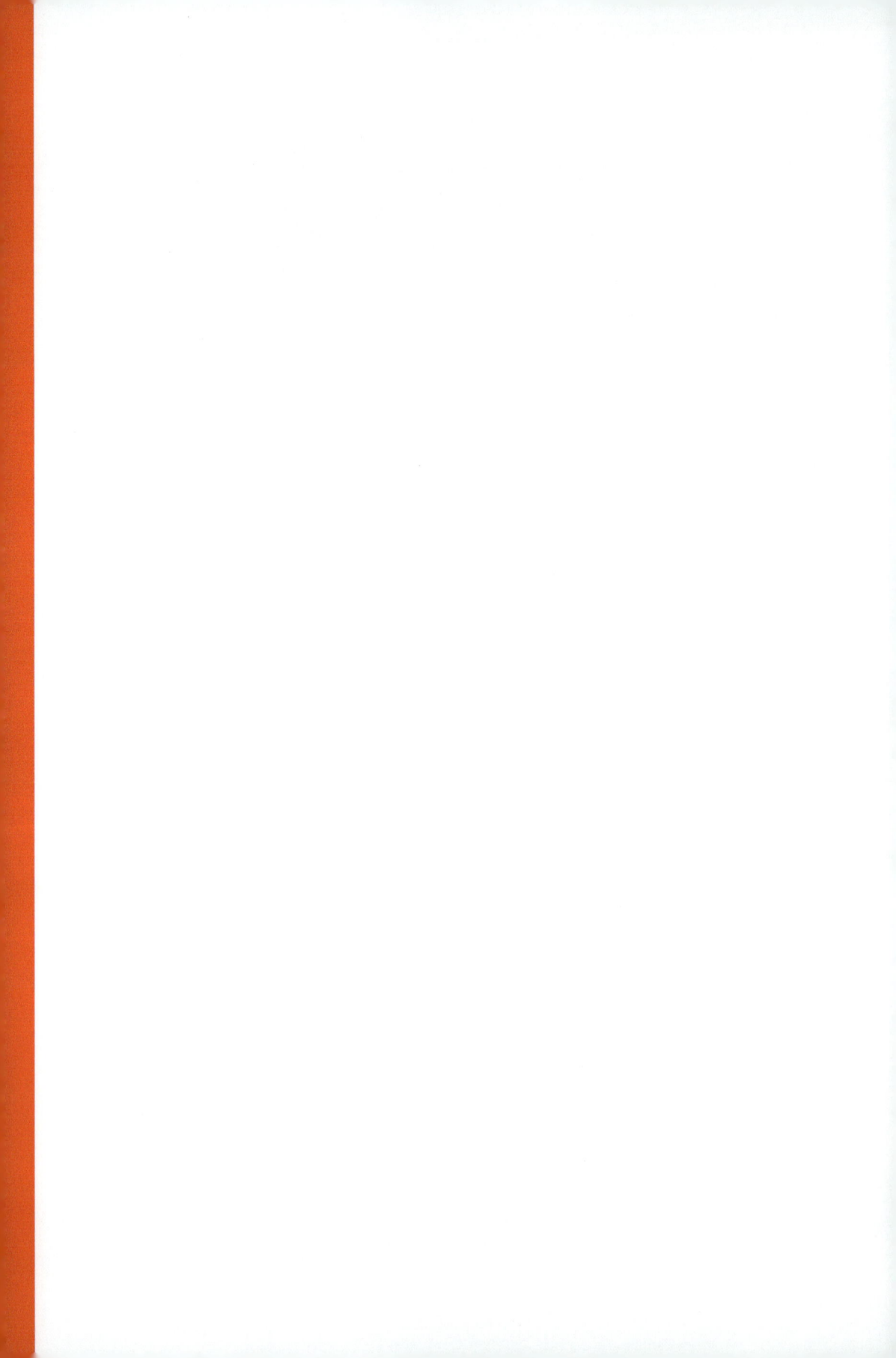

The new UCLH Hospital and the Institute of Nuclear Medicine

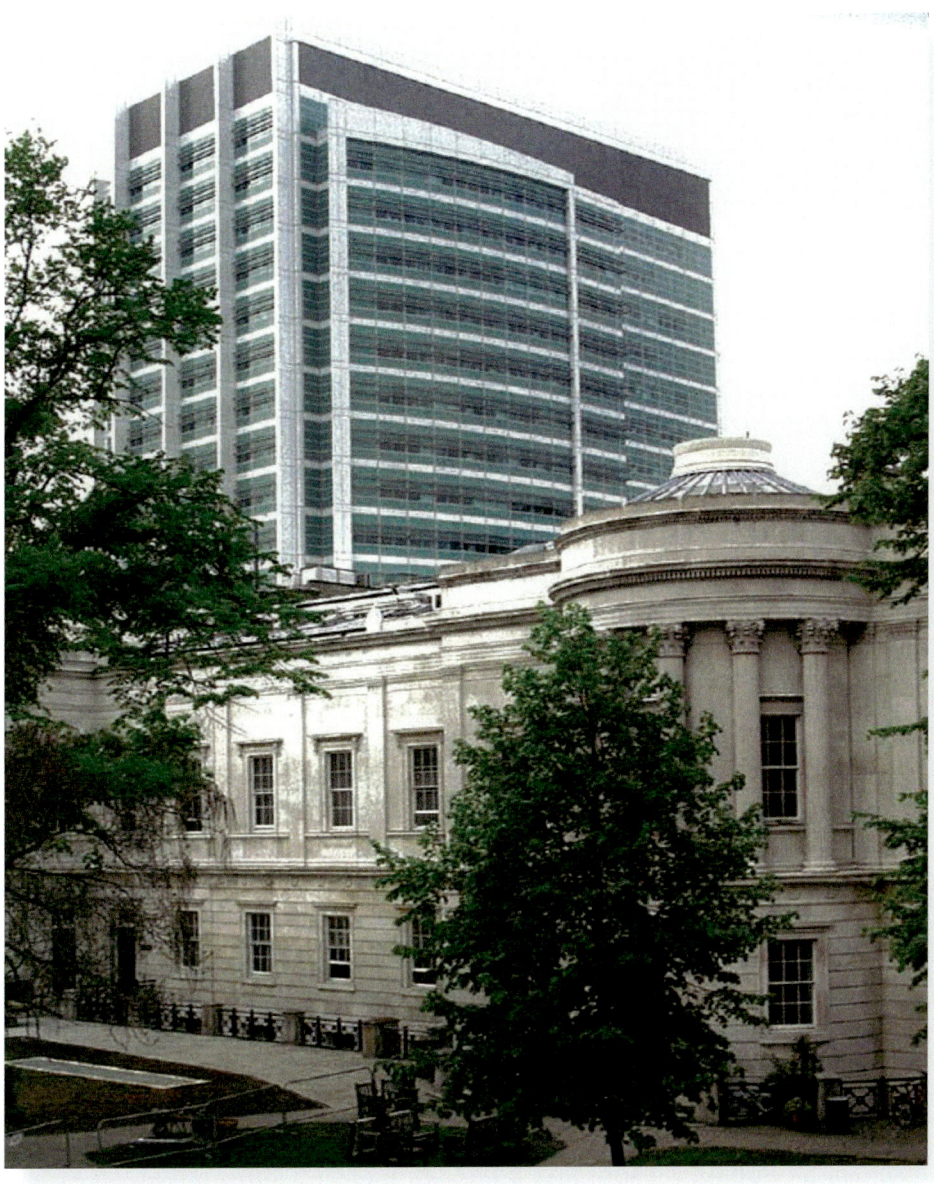

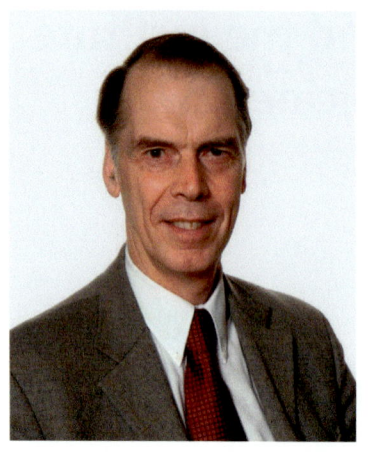

P.H. Jarritt

Since its Foundation, the Institute of Nuclear Medicine, as an academic unit, was housed in what was then Middlesex Hospital Medical School space. It had moved twice already, within the old envelope, a significant enlargement was planned by Ell and Jarritt (now Clinical Director of Medical Physics and Clinical Engineering Cambridge at University Hospitals NHS Foundation Trust). One of the most significant organisational developments was the early introduction of e-mail and the use of the internet and in particular the patient information system in 1987, which integrated the reception, radiopharmacy and reporting functions, and allowed a rapid expansion of the throughput of the Institute to exploit the new technology. This stood the test of time for over 15years.

The Institute's new premises opened on the 5th of February 1993. The great and the good attended, the then President of the Royal College of Physicians, the late Professor L A Turnberg presided. Guests included the then Provost of UCL Sir Derek Roberts, Sir Roben Ibbs as Chairman of UCL Council, Professor J R Pattinson as Dean of the Medical School, Professor Dame June Lloyd, Scientific Advisor AMRC, Sir Ronald Mason as Chairman of The Shadow Trust, Charles Marshall, Chief Executive and Prof A Goldstone, Hospital Director and a number of other distinguished individuals.

At that time, the premises and equipment were prime examples of a modern nuclear medicine setup. These were house on the 2nd floor of the Sir Jules Thorn building, Sir Jules being a significant supporter of Nuclear Medicine, funding inter alia, the first SPET cameras in the UK, data processing and staff. In the basement, the UCLH Trust had funded a first class radiopharmacy – the first major investment of the Trust in Nuclear Medicine. This was to progress with time...But as we state elsewhere, technology does not rest, and PET imaging started to make its impact. New space had to be negotiated, involving other academic departments, never an easy task. Sir Derek as Provost UCL came to the rescue, and enabled new space to be identified in the basement of The Sir Jules Thorn building.

With this decision and the outstanding support of the Trust Charity and its chair, Sir Ronald Mason, first a PET scanner and subsequently a PETCT scanner was commissioned and installed. The PETCT instrument, the 5th in the world, was to be the first PETCT scanner in the UK! The Institute was now again ready to maintain its international impact and standing. The PETCT was inaugurated by our Chancellor, the HRH Princess Royal, Princess Anne.

The two neighbouring medical schools fused in 1987, the single University College and Middlesex School of Medicine was established. In time, the designation University College London Medical School emerged and also the name University College London Hospitals. In the first wave, UCLH became a Foundation Trust Hospital. The redevelopment of UCLH at Gower Street would be a key element of the Trust's strategy.

An invitation to take part in planning the new hospital was issued by the then Chief Executive Charles Marshall, on the 11th of September 1995. By the 16th of November, 16 Task Forces were established, the date at which the Institute started planning its new premises as part of one of these. Peter Jarritt, Ian Cullum, Peter Marsden and Wendy Waddington, Dominic Lui and Caroline Townsend would also play vital roles in the planning of what was to become the newly housed Institute in the new UCLH NHS Trust Hospital. There was to be a fundamental difference though in the siting of the Institute, now planned to be housed entirely in NHS space! It is recalled that the then Dean John Pattinson supported the concept that for The Institute, both academic and NHS space, should remain integrated.

Between late 1995 and the opening of the new UCLH, 8 long years would ensue, progressively involving endless committee meetings and not always productive and or pleasant meetings with the representatives of the PFI management process. In the last two years prior the move, senior staff of the Institute would have spend between 30 and 50% of the time, entirely dedicated with the planned move. But engaging early on, and being present whenever requested, paid off – adequate space provision was fought for, and achieved, enabling a very complex infrastructure to be transferred.

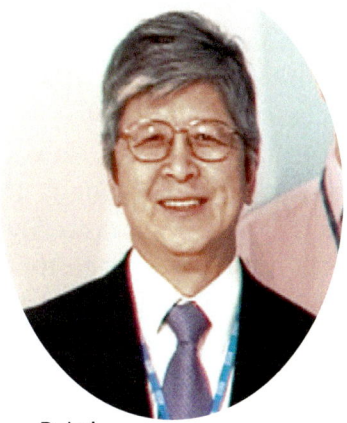

D. Lui

The requirements were significant: an entirely new IT infrastructure (I Cullum), capable of maintaining links between UCL and the Trust (complex issues arose), the design of a large GMP designated and specialist licence MHRA approved manufacturing radiopharmacy facility (D. Lui), the planning of 10 especially designed beds for radionuclide therapy, including decanting facilities for highly radioactive materials (W. Waddington), the design of a radioactive store room for most radioactive materials used throughout the Trust (W. Waddington) and the overall departmental design (Ell and all INM staff) to house patient reception and clerking and administration areas (G. MacNamara and C. Townsend), two PETCT scanners, 6 gamma cameras of which 4 has SPET capability (J Dickson and W Waddington), seminar and reporting rooms, staff and office space, etc. Most of the transfer of the technology and services was accomplished over a single extended weekend (!) without loss of a single day of some aspects of the clinical service. Below a more detailed assessment.

2005 – The Institute moves to Euston Road
Planning for the new department involved not only room layouts but also the completion of the dreaded ADBs (Activity Database) for each room, listing the environmental conditions and equipment required. The process seemed to last forever involving many heated 'discussions' with the planners. Everyone realised that this was our one chance to obtain a suitable home for the Institute and had to be taken seriously, however boring it was. Time proved this a wise decision as members of other departments not so engaged with the planning process still look at our new space with some amazement and no doubt a small degree of envy! At this stage the plan was 'everything new', with little or no movement of equipment to the new hospital.

Following planning there was a long wait while the new building slowly rose from the ground at the top of Gower Street. Small groups of staff occasionally visited to discuss specific issues but apart from this, we were not really involved. However, there was no doubt that after many false dawns (including one in the late 1970s where quite detailed plans had been made) this was really happening – the Institute was on the move. It was during this stage that the policy of 'everything new' changed into 'mostly old'; nevertheless the basic infrastructure, two gamma cameras and a PET/CT scanner were supplied directly to the new building. Even some furniture was going to make the trip. This was going to make the move more interesting!

Early in 2005 wards and departments began transferring from the Middlesex Hospital but the Institute remained. This was to have been a short term arrangement but problems with our floor in the new building meant several delays. Finally staff were able to visit our new home 'en mass' to discuss, amongst other things 'systems of work' and the 'patient journey' (words once foreign to us, but now like old friends). It was immediately clear how large and impressive the new space was; in particular the radiopharmacy seemed to have the capacity to supply most of the country. Despite all the planning, the patient reception area needed some changes. In the end this simply meant redesignation of one room and an internal window being blocked out. This was achieved with the speed and efficiency which we had come to expect and barely six months later everything was ready! Two new gamma cameras had been commissioned and another had been transferred from the Middlesex site. Unfortunately, unlike Elvis, the PET scanner was not in the building and the new radiopharmacy was not ready with ongoing problems with the air handling plant. So the decision was taken to move whilst leaving PET and radiopharmacy on the Middlesex site. Additionally, it was decided to delay moving the research group until the clinical service was running smoothly on the new site.

At the beginning of December 2005 blue crates began arriving in the department. These were filled, labelled with their destination and transferred to a neighbouring empty ward ready for transport. By this time the Middlesex H ospital had taken on the appearance of the Marie Celeste and so there was no shortage of storage areas. A full clinical service continued whilst packing progressed and it was not until the weekend before the move that the final, vital equipment was packed (this naturally included the kettle and tea bags). At this point it became apparent just how much there was to move, the ward was full! We had two days to get the department up and running on the new site, suddenly this time scale seemed rather short!

We waited confidently for Monday, after all what could go wrong, the whole process had been planned with military precision [1]. Monday morning arrived, we were all ready and …. nothing happened, no vans, no crates. The removers had been taken by surprise by the amount of equipment to be moved, by far the largest they had encountered from a single department and they had been delayed (maybe in shock). Soon though the new department whose empty rooms and corridors had seemed so large started to fill and the crates just kept on arriving. Gradually staff got to know the whereabouts of everything and crates were emptied and equipment put in place, this was no doubt aided by the lack of Gant charts and method of work statements. Many thanks are due to the removal company as amazingly during the whole process nothing was broken and only two computers were lost, later to be returned having been wrongly delivered elsewhere. A limited clinical service began within two days and following the arrival and installation of two gamma cameras from the Middlesex it was soon back to normal.

It took another two months for the research staff to transfer by which time the new PET/CT scanner was in use, leaving only radiopharmacy on the old site, the final remaining working area there. A well-worn furrow had by now been made between the Middlesex and UCLH as lots of small pieces of equipment, initially thought to be redundant, was transported for use.

After a few more months and several days when their staff seemed to work for more than 24 hours, the radiopharmacy joined the rest of the department. In the move a total of just five days of a proportion of the clinical service and no days of radiopharmacy production had been lost.

In December of 2006, a year after the move had started, the doors on the old department were closed for the last time. With it was left 37 years history, many achievements, a lot of unwanted equipment and an abundance of memories, mostly good.

Footnote: The Middlesex site was cleared during 2007 leaving only the chapel and a side facade (listed buildings) intact, ready for the building of Noho Square a proposed 'joint use' development of residential accommodation, shops and commercial space. Unfortunately plans were ruined by the financial crisis and at the time of writing the site still lays sadly empty.

1   Terry Brighton. Hell Riders – The true story of the charge of the light brigade.

Radiochemistry and Pre-clinical First Steps

Radiochemistry is integral to tracer development, not only to enable labelling of putative tracers for early pre-clinical evaluation, but also to bridge efforts in medicinal chemistry, biological evaluation, tracer selection, method development, and tracer production for early human studies. INM has historically relied on access to experimental radiotracers through national and international collaborations, and it has been a long-term strategic goal for the Institute to establish its own radiochemistry group in order to stay at the forefront of nuclear imaging. In 2008 Erik Årstad was recruited as a Senior Lecturer in Radiochemistry and generous funding was obtained from HEFCE and CBRC for construction of radiochemistry facilities and recruitment of two postdoctoral researchers. The investment formed part of a new collaborative initiative, started by the Institute of Nuclear Medicine, now involving the UCL Department of Chemistry, Division of Medicine, and UCLH, aimed to bridge expertise and accelerate translation research. Space for the facility was allocated in the Kathleen Lonsdale Building, Gower Place, and after the initial design phase in 2008 the radiochemistry lab was constructed in 2009 and commission early

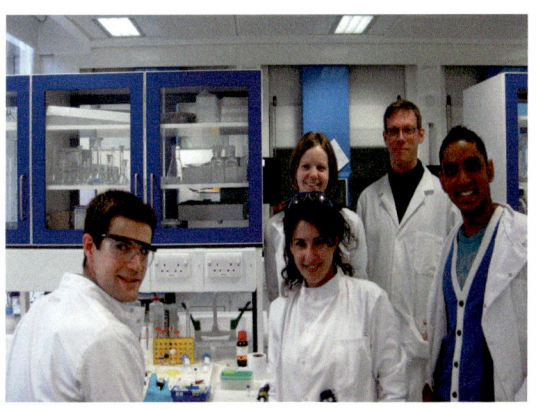

Radiochemistry lab in the Kathleen Lonsdale Building

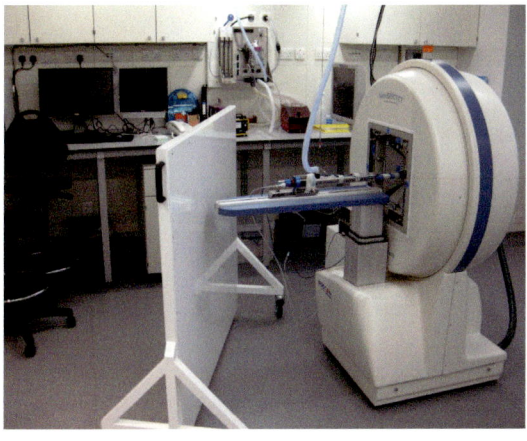

Pre-clinical imaging suite at CABI

2010. The state-of-the-art radiochemistry facility is designed for all aspects of tracer development, and is equipped with three shielded fume hoods for hands on labelling, two hot cells for scale-up and tracer production, three automated synthesis modules and analytical equipment for tracer characterisation and quality control. In parallel with this investment further funding was obtained by Mark Lythgoe at Centre for Advanced Biomedical Imaging (CABI) and Prof. Barbara Pedley at the Cancer Institute to establish a pre-clinical nuclear imaging suite equipped with a small animal SPECT/CT scanner, the scanner funded via the Comprehensive Cancer Imaging Center (CCIC) and Ell's initiative. Additional funding from the FP7 Euripides consortium enabled recruitment of two additional postdoctoral researchers in 2010, and this year the group further expanded with two PhD students recruited through internal UCL funding schemes.

The emerging radiotracer programme

The aims of the radiochemistry group are to develop radiotracers labelled with nuclides for PET and SPECT, such as ^{18}F, ^{68}Ga and ^{123}I, that will enable routine clinical applications, provide tracers for translational imaging studies, and to develop new methods and concepts that can have a profound impact on the field. One of the main limitations of current imaging methods is that no modality meets the need for cellular resolution, high sensitivity, and deep tissue penetration. In addition, chemically distinct tracers are typically used for individual imaging modalities, making image co-registration and comparison of data challenging. Imaging science would benefit from a new tracer platform technology that could report on biological processes at a systems and cellular level (multiscale imaging) to create a comprehensive picture of the molecular events. Dual optical and nuclear tracers are particularly attractive as a platform for multiscale imaging as they com-

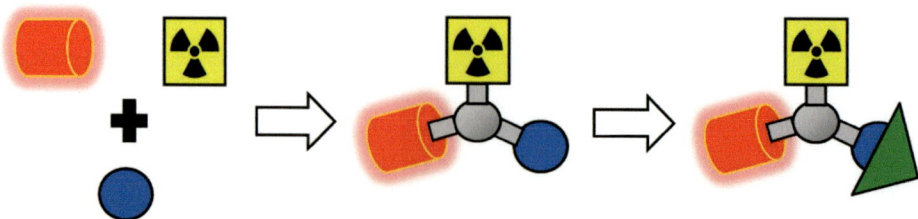

Fig. 1 Reaction of a fluorescent group (red), a radioactive element (yellow) and a group for bioconjugation (blue) to yield a dual labeling reagent. Subsequent reaction with biomolecules (green) provides dual optical and nuclear tracers

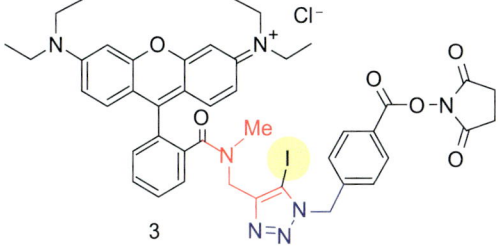

3

Dual labelling reagent used for antibody labelling

bine modalities with unrivaled sensitivity, and can bridge *in vitro* and *in vivo* preclinical imaging with human applications. In addition, high-throughput fluorescence assays can accelerate tracer development by circumventing the need to use radioactive compounds for the initial screening.

We envisaged that a three-component reaction combining a fluorescent group, a radioactive element and a group for bioconjugation could yield dual labelling reagents in a single step, providing a convenient platform for multiscale tracer development (Fig. 1). To achieve this the group recently developed a new radiochemical reaction based on previous reports that copper catalyzed cyclisation of azides and alkynes in the presence of electrophilic iodine gives 5-iodo-1,2,3-triazoles. Using a Cu(II) catalyst we were able to form a dual labelling reagent in >70% radiochemical yield using rhodamine as the fluorescent group, an active ester for bioconjugation and commercially available $[^{125}I]$NaI in water as the radioactive source. In collaboration with Prof. Barbara Pedley's group at the Cancer Institute the method was used for dual labelling of an antibody (A5B7) that binds to carcinoembryonic antigen expressed on gastrointestinal tumors. Using a combination of *in vivo* SPECT/CT, phosphor imaging *in vitro* and confocal microscopy we were able to interrogate antibody distribution in tumour bearing mice across the cellular and whole body scales. We are currently planning to use this concept to compare the behavior of murine and humanized antibodies in tumour models, which is important to assess their suitability for target radiotherapy (RIT). New dual labelling reagents are also under development to enable multiscale imaging of stem cells and cell based cancer therapies.

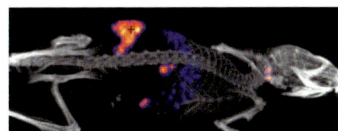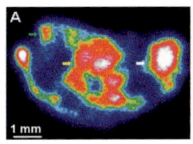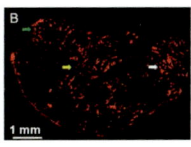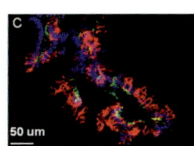

From left: SPECT/CT imaging of dual labelled A5B7 antibody in tumour bearing nude mice, phosphor imaging of tumour section, optical image (tracer in red) demonstrating co-localization of radioactivity and fluorescence, and higher magnification showing diffusion of antibodies (red) across blood vessels (blue and green)

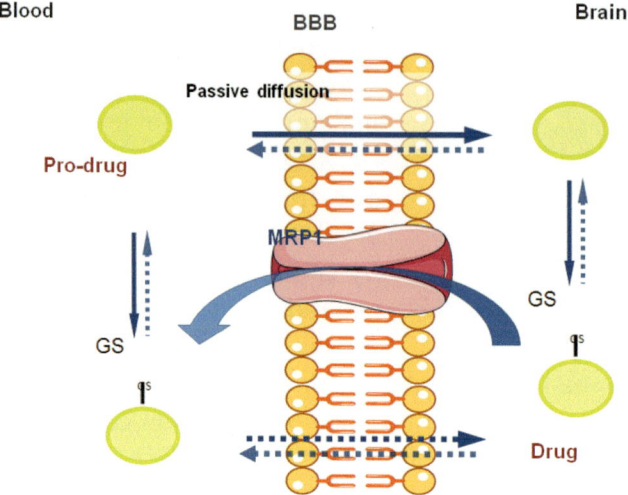

Whilst the field of nuclear Imaging has largely focused on static imaging, quantification of biological targets such as receptors and enzymes, and drug occupancy studies, PET and SPECT have the potential to also quantify dynamic biological processes. Recently, Okamura *et al.* reported a highly elegant and exiting concept for imaging of drug efflux pump function involving dynamic imaging of the efflux of a radioactive tracer from the brain. The concept, which is referred to as the metabolite extrusion method (MEM) relies on administration of a radioactive pro-drug tracer, conversion of the tracer to a metabolite (drug) that act as a substrate for drug efflux pumps, and dynamic imaging of brain clearance as a direct measured of drug efflux function. MEM overcomes many of the challenges associated with conventional imaging of efflux pumps as the initial brain uptake is high, and is attractive as it provides a dynamic measure of efflux rates than quantification of drug efflux pump expression levels. In collaboration with Prof. Matthias Koepp, IoN, and the FP7 European Euripides consortium, the group is currently developing 18F labelled MEM tracers for functional imaging of MRP1 and P-gp efflux pumps.

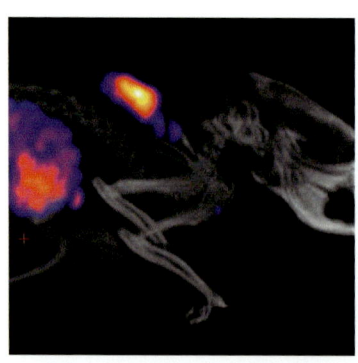

An alternative approach to image dynamic processes *in vivo* is to use state-dependent radioligands. The group is currently developing state-dependent voltage-gated sodium channel (VGSC) tracers with the view to image activated neuronal pathways in disease states. Whilst early exploratory work has focused on identifying a suitable compound class for tracer development, intriguing preliminary SPECT/CT imaging in mice has reveal what appears to be specific tracer binding in brown adipose tissue. This illustrates the value of *in vivo* imaging as a tool for tracer development as it allows identification of tracer uptake in tissues that often would be overlooked in conventional biodistribution studies.

In addition to continued development of the UCL/UCLH radiotracer development programme it is the ambition of the group to also establish production of emerging tracers for early human studies at INM, and in time establish a translational pathway to accelerate the impact of bench type research on patient care and the treatment they can be offered.

Stone JM, Erlandsson K, Årstad E, Squassante L, Teneggi V, Bressan RA, Krystal JH, Ell PJ, Pilowsky LS (2008). Relationship between ketamine-induced psychotic symptoms and NMDA receptor occupancy: a [(123)I]CNS-1261 SPET study. *Psychopharmacology* 197(3), 401-408.

Stone J.M., Erlandsson K., Årstad E., Bressan R.A., Squassante L., Teneggi V., Ell P.J., Pilowsky L.S. (2006), Ketamine displaces the novel NMDA receptor SPET probe [^{123}I]CNS-1261 in humans in vivo, *Nuclear Medicine and Biology*, 33(2), 239-43.

Stone J.M., Årstad E., Erlandsson K., Waterhouse R.N., Ell P.J., Pilowsky L.S. (2006), [^{123}I]TPCNE – A novel SPET tracer for the sigma-1 receptor: First human studies and *in vivo* haloperidol challenge, *SYNAPSE*, 60(2); 109-107.

Årstad E., Gitto R., Chimirri A., Caruso R., Constanti A., Turton D., Hume S.P., Ahmad R., Pilowsky L.S., Luthra S.K (2006). Closing in on the AMPA receptor: Synthesis and evaluation of 2-acyl-1-(p-chlorophenyl)-6-methoxy-7-[^{11}C]methoxy-1,2,3,4-tetrahydroisoquinoline as a potential PET tracer, *Bioorganic & Medicinal Chemistry*, 14 (14), 4712-4717.

Årstad E, Wester HJ, Luthra SK, Pilowsky LS, Henriksen G (2006), Towards NR2B subtype selective PET tracers: Synthesis and Evaluation of styrene-, naphthyl and 4- trifluoromethoxyphenyl N-(2-[11-C] methoxybenzyl) amidine, *Bioorganic & Medicinal Chemistry*, 14(18), 6307-6313.

Schoultz BW, Hjornevik T, Willoch F, Marton J, Noda A, Murakami Y, Miyoshi S, Nishimura S, Årstad E, Drzezga A, Matsunari I, Henriksen G (2010). Evaluation of the kappa-opioid receptor-selective tracer [(11)C]GR103545 in awake rhesus macaques. *Eur J Nucl Med Mol Imaging*. 37(6):1174-1180.

Yan R., El-Emir E., Rajkumar V., Robson M., Jathoul A.P., Pedley R.B. and Årstad E. One-pot Formation of a ^{125}I-labeled Trifunctional Reagent for Multiscale Imaging with Optical and Nuclear Techniques. *Angewandte Chemie Int Ed.*, 2011, 50, 6793 – 679

Medical physics and evolving technology: hybrid systems and solid state imaging

Introduction

Medical Physics is an important sub-group of the Institute of Nuclear Medicine's personnel, contributing to both research activity and support of clinical services. The Medical Physics group was very ably led for many years by Dr Peter Jarritt (now Clinical Director of Medical Physics and Clinical Engineering Cambridge at University Hospitals NHS Foundation Trust). He was replaced for a short period until 2003 by Dr Glyn Davies, and currently the Clinical Physics Group that supports the NHS clinical activity is led by Ms Wendy Waddington.

In 2004 Professor Brian Hutton was appointed to a newly established UCL Chair in Medical Physics in Nuclear Medicine and Molecular Imaging Science. He leads a group of scientists that undertakes research on Medical Physics relevant to Nuclear Medicine, based at INM. The group has grown to now include four research scientists and up to six PhD students, funded externally through various providers, including EC, EPSRC, CRUK, GSK, GE Healthcare and Spectrum Dynamics. The group has a range of research projects that are described briefly below, spanning single photon emission computed tomography (SPECT) system design, image reconstruction and quantitative analysis of clinical research studies, focussed on both SPECT and positron emission tomography (PET). The research activity is well reflected in the associated peer-reviewed publications which are included below which includes several reviews [3, 6, 10, 19] and book chapters [44-48]. Professor Hutton also instigated continuing education programmes for the INM with weekly seminars available for all INM staff and a London-wide Medical Physics seminar series which encourages interaction of the UCL group with other institutions. The group works closely with the Centre for Medical Image Computing at UCL and also has several international collaborative projects.

Central to most of the research work has been the introduction of novel technology at INM, providing an avenue for important research that can be translated to clinical use. The increased use of dual-modality systems is reflected in the current instrumentation at INM which includes three SPECT/CT systems and two PET/CT systems. Several projects seek to exploit the use of the additional information available on such systems and to seek solutions to unique problems that arise through use of the dual modalities. This research is set to expand further with the introduction of PET/MRI in late 2011. In addition the department was the first in the UK to introduce novel solid state technology for rapid cardiac SPECT (D-SPECT from Spectrum Dynamics) and a number of projects continue to focus on aspects of this new technology, exploiting unique features of this system. The group is also well placed to apply state-of-the-art processing techniques for analysis of studies using a range of novel tracers, especially in the clinical research setting (including amyloid imaging in patients with dementia, angiogenesis studies in patients undergoing stem cell treatment and hypoxia studies in oncology patients).

In the following sections some of the recent research projects are summarised to illustrate the activity of the group. The topics covered include projects on system design, including work on the solid state detector system, novel approaches to image reconstruction taking advantage of dual modality acquisition and improving quantification with particular emphasis on correction of partial volume effects.

Project details

System design and solid state systems

Collimator design for a novel high resolution camera: HI-CAM [4, 12, 20, 28, 29]

HI-CAM is a high-resolution Anger camera, based on state of the art detector technology, developed as part of an EU project coordinated by Prof. Carlo Fiorini from Politecnico di Milano. HI-CAM is basically a scintillation detector consisting of a CsI(Tl) crystal coupled to an array of silicon drift detectors (SDD), which act as photodetectors for read-out of the scintillation light. The SDDs thereby replace the conventional photomultiplier tubes that have been used in gamma-cameras for decades. This results in a more compact detector with better spatial resolution that is not sensitive to magnetic fields, and could therefore be used in combination with MRI.

Two prototype detectors (5x5 cm and 10x10 cm) were constructed within the project. The software for uniformity and linearity correction of the HI-CAM data as well as for geometric calibration and tomographic reconstruction of SPECT data with both parallel-hole and pinhole collimators was developed by us at the INM. The linearity and uniformity corrections are essential parts of image formation process and especially important for tomographic imaging. The reconstruction of tomographic data also requires knowledge of a number of geometric parameters. We developed a novel geometric calibration procedure for pinhole SPECT utilising two different rotation radii, in order to reduce the correlation between different parameters.

SPECT studies were made with the 10x10 cm HI-CAM detector. Two hot-rod phantoms were scanned with a parallel-hole collimator and with a pinhole collimator with 2 different focal lengths (f). The reconstructed resolution was measured from point-source studies. The results are presented in Fig. 1, showing that a tomographic resolution of 1 mm or better can be achieved. The 1-mm rods were clearly visualised with the pinhole collimator (f=110 mm). The intrinsic resolution of the camera was estimated to 0.8 mm.

We also developed a design for a brain SPECT system based on HI-CAM detectors. In order to utilise the high spatial resolution of the detectors, the system was designed with a slit-slat collimator, which is a combination of a pinhole collimator in the trans-axial direction and a parallel-hole collimator in the axial direction. A specific focus of the research was the consideration of multiplexing (projection overlap), which can increase the number of acquired counts but results in complications in the image reconstruction with artefacts being generated. A significant outcome of the work has been the recognition that mixing multiplexed and non-multiplexed data can

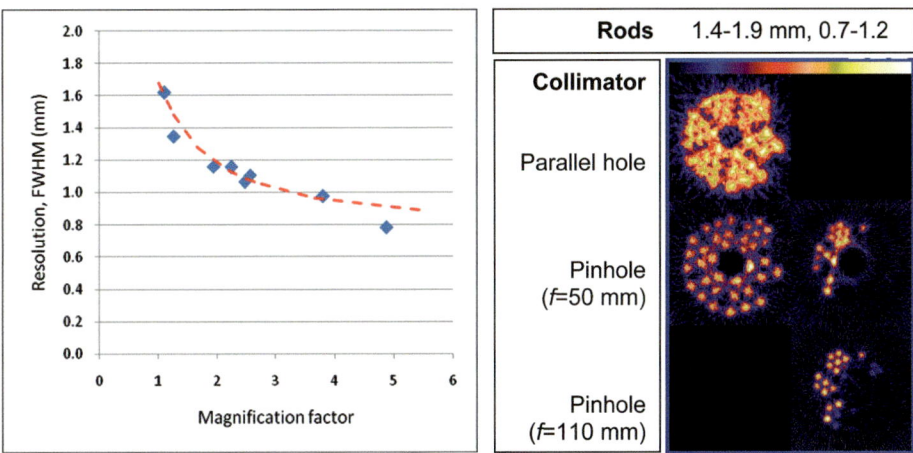

Fig. 1 Resolution measured with a pinhole collimator at different magnification factors (left), and reconstructed images for different collimators and different phantoms. (NB: The rods are only partially filled in the phantom on the right.)

result in gain in signal to noise ratio (SNR) and significant reduction (or removal) of artefacts; this has important implications for system design.

Task oriented optimisation for SPECT system design [31, 35]

In SPECT the images are blurred by the system Point Spread Function (PSF), so that a finite spatial resolution will degrade the contrast of any lesions of a size less than ~3 times the system resolution. One of the most fundamental difficulties that we want to overcome is the signal-to-noise ratio as a consequence of a trade-off between geometric efficiency and resolution of the collimator. Traditionally, the parallel hole collimator has been developed to allow only nearly parallel projections of the radionuclide distribution. Parallel hole collimator parameters can be adjusted only to improve resolution to the detriment of sensitivity and vice-versa, so it is the primary obstacle in achieving both high sensitivity and spatial resolution.

In order to obtain a tomographic image, acquired data are reconstructed using an iterative algorithm, most commonly maximum likelihood expectation maximisation (ML-EM). Iterative algorithms can incorporate a three-dimensional resolution model and so take in consideration different resolutions at different distances from the collimator. The goal of this work is to optimise collimator design with respect to the reconstruction image quality.

To be able to compare different collimator designs a method is needed that quantifies how much information is missing. Collimator designs are usually compared based on the calculation of the Linear Local Impulse Response (that quantifies the local resolution properties) and Covariance in a voxel using an iterative reconstruction algorithm and multiple noise realisations of the projection data. This methodology, however, is very time consuming. Therefore, a much faster computational method, based on approximations for the Fisher Information Matrix, has been investigated. The left of Fig. 2 shows the analytically calculated profile of covariance.

The uncertainty about the origin of the detected photons is modelled by a Point Spread Function (PSF), which, in literature, is normally assumed to be a Gaussian function, whose full width at half maximum (FWHM), is determined by the collimator's aperture. In our work, these traditional assumptions will be abandoned. In fact, it appears possible to improve resolution recovery based reconstruction by considering different shapes of PSF. We decided to use a ray-tracing algorithm to model the geometric response and the septal penetration in the collimator since no analytical treatment of this effect appears to exist in literature.

180

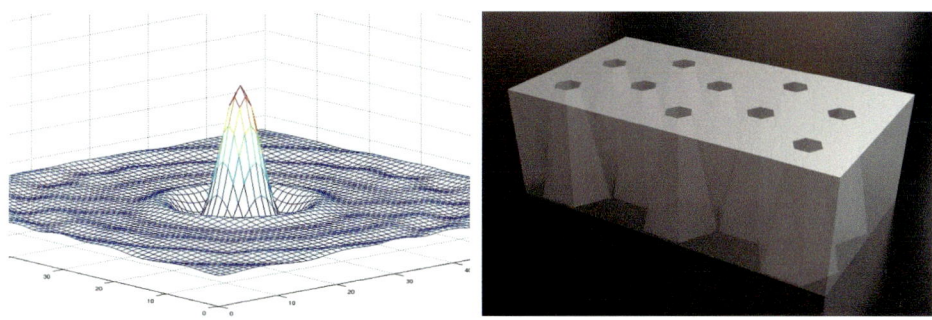

Fig. 2 Covariance profile calculated to evaluate collimator performance (left); possible collimator designed to provide non-Gaussian point spread function

Novel collimator geometries have been proposed and their performance evaluation is currently under way. The novel design does not imply necessarily parallel holes, but could involve a polygonal shape of the septa (figure on the right shows an example).

Simulation of a novel CZT based SPECT system [21, 23, 41]

Currently, the majority of clinical SPECT images are obtained using dual-head rotating Anger type gamma cameras. These consist of a scintillation detector, optically coupled to a set of photomultiplier (PM) tubes for energy and position readout, and a collimator that defines the spatial relationship between the point of gamma photon emission and the point of detection. The sensitivity of this system is largely limited by constraints in the physical collimation. This detection arrangement is physically bulky and heavy, limiting the flexibility and speed of practically achievable camera motion.

Semi-conductors offer a direct detection alternative to traditional scintillation crystal based detectors. The most extensively researched of these in the medical imaging context is cadmium zinc telluride (CZT). CZT detectors have been successfully deployed in both small animal and some clinical scale specialist SPECT imaging systems. CZT detectors are much more compact and lightweight than their conventional counterparts. They also benefit from markedly improved energy resolution and greater sensitivity. Cameras built using these detectors still require physical collimation, which continues to be the principal determinant of system sensitivity and spatial resolution.

The analytical simulator developed allows users to simulate SPECT acquisitions using gamma cameras composed of multiple pixelated CZT

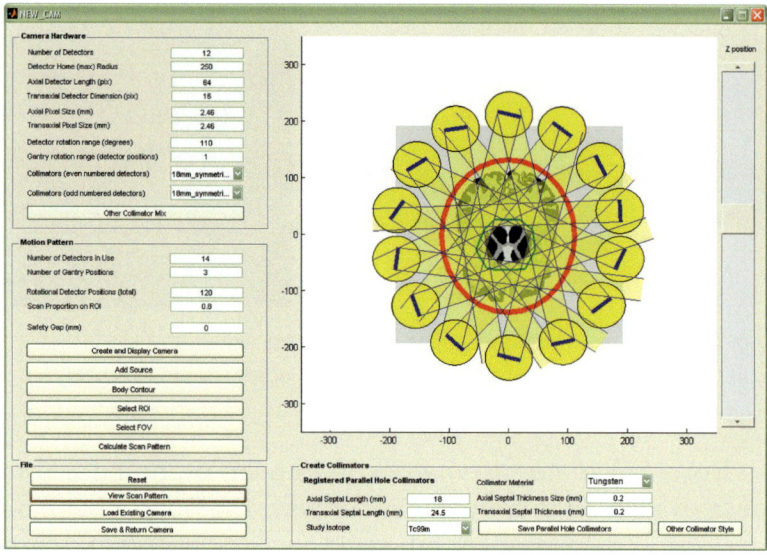

Fig. 3 Interface for simulation tool for multi-detector CZT system design

detectors equipped with parallel hole collimators registered so that each collimator hole aligns to a single detector pixel. The simulator can include or ignore attenuation effects, spatial resolution modelling and Poisson noise. It is not currently equipped to model scatter effects.

The existing D-SPECT (Spectrum Dynamics, Israel) cardiac SPECT camera at the INM represents one specific example of the set of cameras that may be simulated. It has therefore been possible to undertake validation work for the simulator using this existing physical system as a comparator. We have found excellent agreement between simulated and actual spatial resolution with the change in FWHM with distance found to be 0.875 mm/cm (R^2 = 0.98) compared to the modelled 0.872 mm/cm. We are currently investigating the simulator's tendency to overestimate sensitivity by ~20%.

We have begun exploring the optimisation of a ring gantry based system with the capacity to drive each of multiple detector heads independently to adjust radial position and angular disposition, as well as allowing rotation of the whole gantry. Early optimisation work is addressing the choice of parallel hole collimator and the trade-offs between maximising detector area, and therefore sensitivity, by using many detector heads, against achieving closer conformation to the patient, and thereby better spatial resolution, with fewer detectors.

Dual radionuclide studies on D-SPECT [8, 11]

Simultaneous cardiac SPECT imaging with the radionuclides [99mTc] and [123I] could be useful for studies of heart failure (using the radiopharmaceutical [123I]-MIBG) or fatty acid metabolism (using the radiopharmaceutical [123I]-IPPA) together with cardiac perfusion (using the radiopharmaceutical [99mTc]-MIBI). A perfusion defect in the heart could lead to misinterpretation of the [123I] data. However, the additional information provided by the [99mTc] perfusion drug can assist in interpretation of such information. One advantage of imaging two radiopharmaceuticals simultaneously is that the image data are automatically aligned to one another. Another advantage is that one scan is performed instead of two, which is of benefit to both the patient and the clinic.

In Nuclear Medicine imaging, good quality and quantitatively accurate images are required in order to obtain accurate biodistribution data. Photons which scatter in the patient and get detected in the images degrade image quality and lead to inaccurate quantification. In semiconductor detectors the effect of incomplete charge collection ('spill-down') further degrades quantitative accuracy in the images. In order to obtain quantitatively accurate images they need to be corrected for scatter and spill-down.

In this work a method for correcting images for scatter and spill-down in dual [99mTc]/[123I] cardiac imaging is being developed and investigated for a gamma camera with semiconductor detectors (D-SPECT, Spectrum Dynamics, Israel). The method involves iteratively estimating the contributions to the images. The contributions from scatter and spill-down are subtracted which results in an image free of components degrading its quality. Parameters for estimating the scatter- and spill-down contributions are estimated using experimental measurements as well as simulations.

The method is being evaluated using an experimentally measured thorax phantom with a cardiac insert containing [123I] and [99mTc] in the myocardium with two defects. The figure shows a slice of the experimentally measured [99mTc] image of the insert through the left ventricle from the insert before and after correction. These preliminary results show that there is an increased lesion-to-myocardium contrast for the 'cold-spot' (the top of the heart) in the [99mTc] image after correction compared to images without correction. The contrast increases from 0.3 to 0.6 (true contrast=1). The [123I]/[99mTc] ratio also improves in the second defect. These promising preliminary results show improved image contrast in images corrected for scatter and 'spill-down' in dual radionuclide imaging with a semiconductor cardiac SPECT scanner.

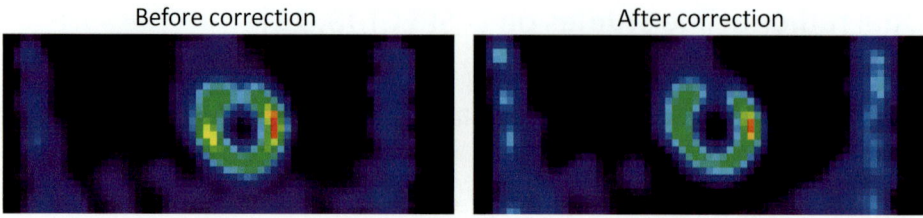

| Before correction | After correction |

Fig. 4 phantom study illustrating improvement in contrast in a physical defect in the anterior wall of the heart after correction with the proposed algorithm

Dual modality reconstruction in emission tomography

Use of anatomical priors for improved reconstruction [25, 26, 32, 36]

SPECT and PET are two main biomedical imaging techniques used for clinical neurology for purposes of visualization of biochemical and physiological processes in living tissues. The use of anatomical information from computerized tomography (CT) or magnetic resonance imaging (MRI) may show some advantages in analyzing extent and localization of radiopharmaceutical uptake, which improves diagnostic accuracy. Hybrid systems, such as SPECT/CT, PET/CT and PET/MRI, can be useful for such a task. Various statistical methods have been developed to improve the reconstruction quality of emission images. The ML-EM iterative method is a successful approach to deal with noise in the data, but it needs to be regularized to ensure a stable convergence. Anatomical data can be used to improve reconstructed activity distribution characteristics by referring to well defined anatomical boundaries.

As recent publications have shown, information theory similarity metrics, such as joint entropy and mutual information, can embed anatomical data within a Bayesian reconstruction framework with some degree of success. However, these methods can result in bias if applied solely to image intensities without taking spatial voxel dependencies into account. Encouraging results were obtained using geometrically driven techniques, such as, the Bowsher prior (BP). The incorporation of the BP in emission reconstruction is performed by local smoothing of activity values in the set which consists of the most similar neighbors on anatomy. The quadratic penalty used in the BP (QBP) tends to over-smooth the reconstructed image and degrade low contrast features. The major difficulty here is not to be too strongly biased to anatomy while reconstructing activity; some trade-off is required. It is possible to reduce the problem with use of an edge-preserving poten-

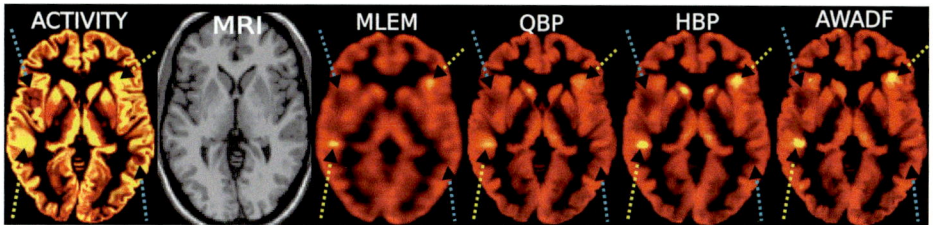

Fig. 5 Transverse section of 3D SPECT phantom with MRI and reconstructed images using ML-EM and MAP-EM algorithm with quadratic BP (QBP), Huber BP (HBP) and anatomically weighted anisotropic diffusion filtering (AWADF) method

tial function, such as the Huber function. This function is critical to the choice of the threshold parameter which precludes its wide clinical use. Post-processing of the reconstructed image after each iteration of ML-EM can be sufficient to reduce noise, although the overall resolution is degraded in favor of enhanced contrast (e.g. median filtration, anisotropic diffusion, total variation). Recently, we proposed an anatomically adaptive filtering technique to maintain resolution while retaining the important features in the data (AWADF). Work is in pregress to assess the clinical utility of the proposed algorithm.

4D reconstruction incorporating MRI for motion correction [33, 34, 39, 40]

The recent development of imaging systems that combine Emission Tomography and MRI in the same machine is enabling new biological and pathological analysis tools for clinical and pre-clinical research. Inherent co-registration and simultaneity of the acquisitions introduce a number of advantages over the separate modalities, including improved image fusion, motion correction and enhancement of the resolution of the functional image, posing new algorithmic and computational challenges.

With the advent of the fused imaging systems, the development of mathematical models that capture the hidden relation between uptake of the pharmaceutical and MR observable tissue properties is driving the new imaging paradigm where the measurement of photon counts is complemented by information from specifically designed MR sequences to enhance the resolution of pharmaceutical uptake, overcoming the resolution limits imposed by photon count statistics and motion. We have developed a novel unified probabilistic framework to merge information from the two imaging modalities, based on the existence of hidden anatomical/functional states. Combining the information from the two imaging modalities within the unified model, we inform the reconstruction of the pharmaceutical concentration in PET and SPECT about motion using fast MR sequences, obtaining time consistent estimates that account for the relation of pharmaceutical uptake with the underlying anatomy.

We are investigating an event-driven motion compensation algorithm for brain perfusion studies based on the proposed joint model, where the acquisition of a new MR image is triggered by a tracking system or by an MR navigator. The event-driven algorithm based on the joint imaging model has shown remarkable improvement of resolution in synthetic perfusion studies.

The NiftyRec reconstruction suite is the software side of our probabilistic framework. It implements algorithms for iterative Maximum Likelihood Estimation for SPECT, PET and CT. All the performance critical components are executed on GPU, accomplishing tomographic reconstructions within seconds. Fast development of new reconstruction algorithms is enabled by the modular design and the Python and Matlab scripting interfaces. NiftyRec is open source and freely distributed on Source-Forge under BSD license.

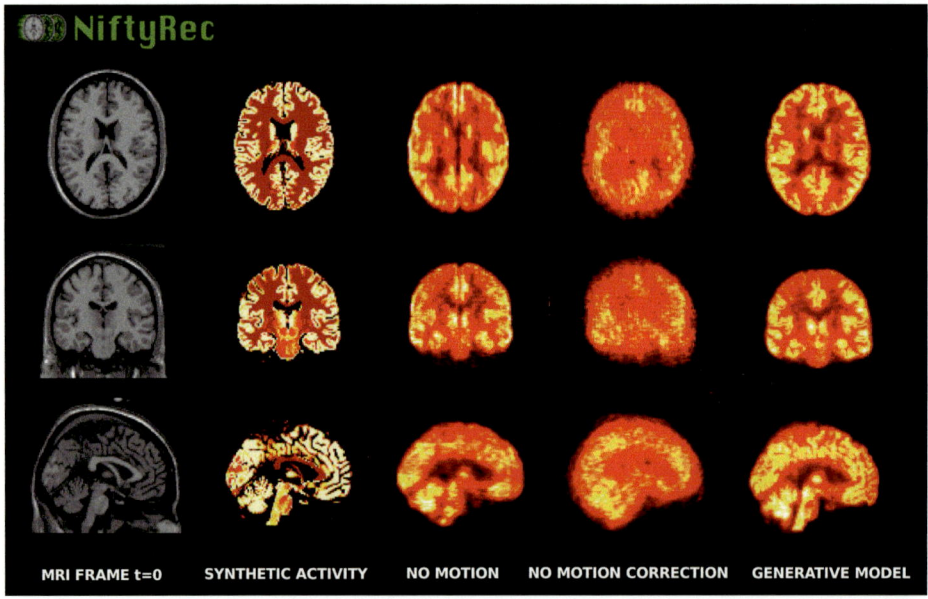

Fig. 6 Reconstruction for a brain phantom simulating uptake on an amyloid tracer; the image quality using the proposed algorithm (right) correct for motion blurring but also improves on the no-motion case (centre)

Attenuation map estimation
without transmission measurement [42]

Myocardial perfusion scintigraphy (MPS) is widely used in the diagnosis of coronary artery disease and has improved sensitivity compared to stress electrocardiography. However the sensitivity and specificity of MPS studies is limited by the variation in attenuation of different tissue types in the thorax which can lead to significant artefacts in the reconstructed images. Attenuation correction is clearly desirable since attenuation artefacts can mimic perfusion defects and hence lead to incorrect diagnosis. Attenuation correction is also essential if quantitative analysis is to be performed, e.g. comparison of images with a normal database. Currently attempts to correct MPS images for attenuation use a transmission scan (with either sealed radioactive sources or CT) which increases the scan time and the radiation dose to the patient and can be impractical in the clinical setting. It is therefore desirable to develop a technique to correct for attenuation which does not require a transmission scan. The aim of this project is to develop an image reconstruction algorithm that is optimised for MPS studies without transmission data.

The aim of this project is to develop novel algorithms for the reconstruction of myocardial perfusion scintigraphy (MPS) single photon emission computed tomography (SPECT) studies. The algorithms developed will enable MPS SPECT studies to be corrected for attenuation, in order to reduce the occurrence of artefacts, without the need to acquire a separate transmission scan in addition to the SPECT emission data. This has particular appeal for application to new instrument designs. Several different approaches to the problem will be considered including the use of measurements from multiple energy windows (e.g. scatter measurements) and differential attenuation from dual-energy radionuclides.

A rigorous analytical model of scatter has been introduced that requires the attenuation coefficients to be known as well as the activity distribution; inversely knowledge of the estimated activity distribution and the measured scatter can be used to deduce the attenuation map. The approach requires a dual estimation algorithm that first estimates activity using assumed attenuation; then estimates attenuation for the resultant activity estimate. The scatter model used has been validated using Monte Carlo simulation demonstrating that similar results are achievable independent of acquisition geometry. These results are promising although further constraints will be necessary to further improve the approach.

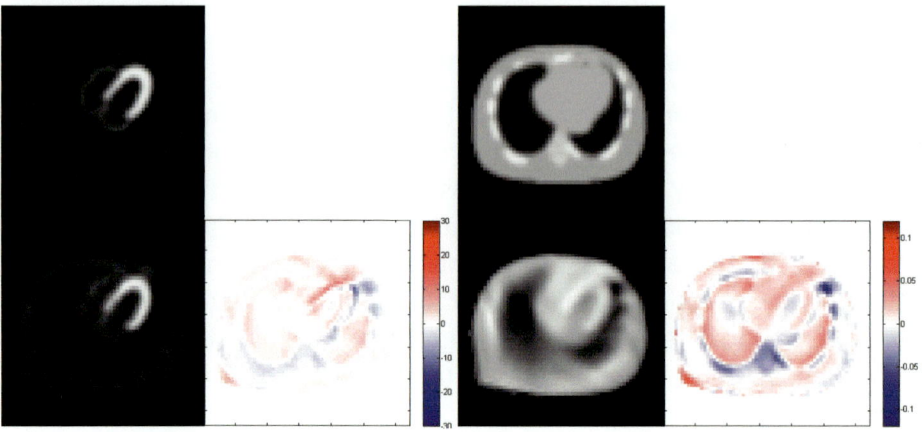

Fig. 7 Results of idealised reconstruction. top: true phantom; bottom: reconstructed emission image for pseudo-D-SPECT geometry including difference between reconstructed and true data

Quantification in emission tomography

Partial volume correction for SPECT [9, 13, 37, 38]

The partial volume effect (PVE) can be defined as the loss in apparent activity that occurs when an object partially occupies the sensitive volume of the imaging instrument (in space or time). In SPECT, PVE is caused by image blurring due to poor spatial resolution, which leads to cross-talk between different anatomical regions. Spatial or temporal variations in PVE can often be confounding factors in the image interpretation. The resolution blurring can be described by the point spread function (PSF) of the system. It is then possible to compensate for the blurring effect either during iterative reconstruction or as a post-processing operation in the reconstructed images. However, the improvement that is achievable with this type of algorithm is limited, and they can even lead to image artefacts.

A more robust approach is to utilise co-registered anatomical data from a high-resolution structural imaging modality, such as CT or MRI. The structural image is segmented into a number of anatomically distinct regions, which can be assumed to be uniform. Anatomically based partial volume correction (PVC) methods have in the past mainly been developed for PET, and operate in the image domain, assuming a position-invariant PSF. In SPECT, the resolution depends on the distance from the camera and therefore these methods are not appropriate.

We have developed a new PVC method for SPECT that operates in the projection domain and can take into account the distance dependent reso-

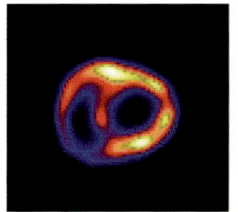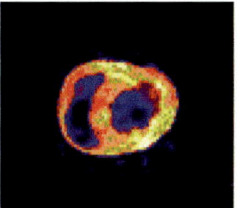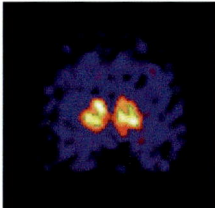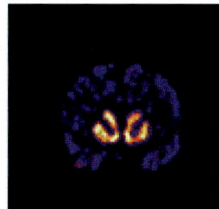

Fig. 8 Ex-vivo SPECT study of a dog heart reconstructed using OSEM with resolution modelling and OSEM with PVC (left); and a DATScan brain SPECT study on a healthy volunteer reconstructed using OSEM and OSEM with PVC (right). (NB: The cardiac SPECT/CT data were provided by Prof. Albert Sinusas, Yale University, New Haven, CT.)

lution. The correction is performed in combination with the image reconstruction, either using an analytic reconstruction algorithm, such as FBP, or an iterative algorithm, such as OSEM. We have demonstrated the performance of our PVC method with simulated and real data, and showed that it gives both qualitatively and quantitatively improved images. Fig. 1 shows examples of the method being applied to cardiac and brain SPECT data. We have also proposed, for the first time, a PVC approach that does not assume the anatomical regions to be uniform. Another type of distribution is used instead, e.g. a hyper-plane.

Partial volume correction of neurological PET data [7]

Positron emission tomography (PET) suffers from a degrading phenomenon known as the partial volume effect (PVE). The effects are due to the limited resolution of the PET scanner. Methods that correct for PVEs are known as partial volume correction (PVC) techniques and are either image-based or make use of anatomical information from other modalities such as magnetic resonance (MR) imaging. This work investigates PVC techniques for neurological applications.

PET tracers that can be used to image amyloid plaques in the brain *in-vivo* are now available. These plaques are a hallmark of Alzheimer's disease (AD), which is the most common form of dementia. In addition to increased amyloid plaque burden, AD patients often exhibit severe cerebral atrophy. Brain volume losses caused by atrophy can also induce PVEs. These PVEs become particularly important when investigating neurodegenerative diseases as apparent changes in PET signal can at least be partially attributed to PVEs.

Recently we reported an extension to existing anatomy-based PVC methods[1]. Region-based voxel-wise correction (RBV) was applied to a

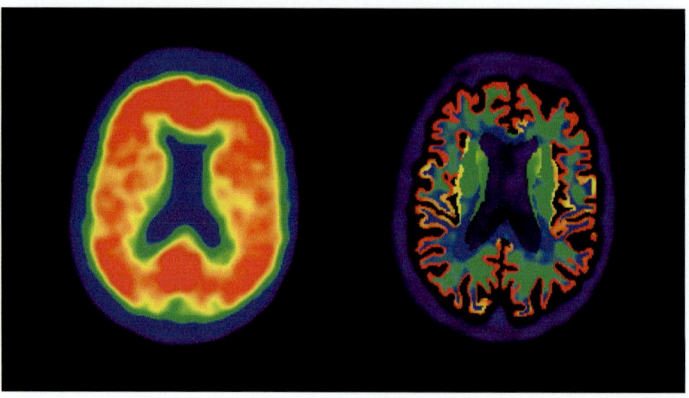

Fig. 9 Amyloid PET scan before (left) and after (right) RBV correction

clinical cohort and was shown to reduce PVE-induced bias and variance compared to commonly applied PVC technique. This was proven in phantom studies and observed in clinical data. A transaxial slice from a clinical scan can be seen in Fig. 1 below. RBV has also been used to show that previously un-reported white matter variability exists in two different amyloid tracers. This finding has implications for the application of PVC in amyloid imaging and also how scans should be normalised.

Anatomy-based PVC techniques rely on segmentations of structural images. These segmentations are not necessarily representative of the PET data. A further extension to RBV has been proposed which iteratively modifies the segmentations to find an optimal PVC in terms of the observed PET data. This novel technique reduces quantification errors due to PET-MR mismatch and has the potential to provide additional parameters in longitudinal studies.

Markov Fields and Gaussian Mixtures applied to PV correction

This work concerns the modelling of activity volumes (PET or SPECT) by a Gaussian mixture (GM) such that the underlying labels follow a Markov field (MF) distribution. This approach assumes that the activity distribution can be separated into several *classes* in which the activity has a specific behaviour, in terms on average value and variability. A Markov field Gaussian mixture (MFGM) requires the estimation of a number of parameters: mean, variance and *a posteriori* probabilities of each voxel to belong in a class conditionally to its activity value. These parameters are estimated with an expectation maximisation (EM)-like algorithm. The calculation of

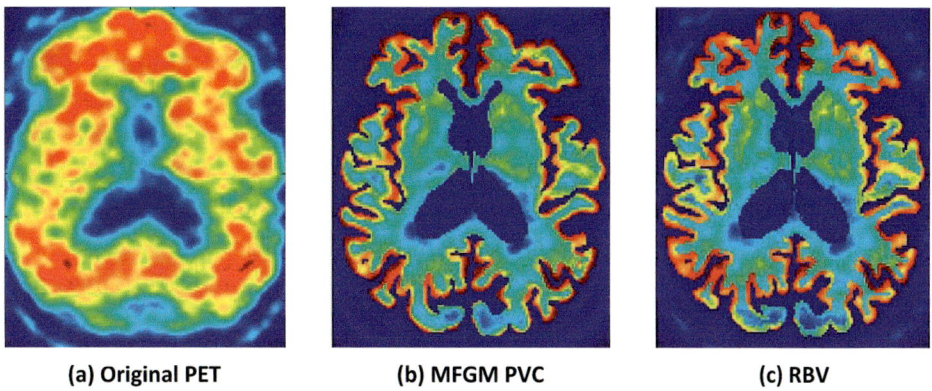

| (a) Original PET | (b) MFGM PVC | (c) RBV |

Fig. 10 Brain PET and partial volume correction using MFGM and RBV

the discrete Markov field describing the classes is challenging due to computational cost. Therefore, approximations such as *mean field* approaches are used here.

We use this model here for brain PET partial volume correction (PVC) post-processing. This task consists of restoring images with poor resolution. The MFGM is driven by an underlying co-registered MR image, in order to take advantage of its high resolution in the PVC process. The PVC problem is treated as a deconvolution inverse problem where the MRI-driven MFGM is an *a priori* distribution. The parameters of the GM are estimated jointly with the activity in a global EM algorithm. We compared our technique with a previous method developed here called *region-base voxelwise correction* (RBV). As the RBV correction assumes regions of uniform activity, our method gives better results on regions of non-uniform activity, especially if there is a feature which is not observed in the MR image. Fig. 10 shows comparative results for the two methods.

Tissue fraction correction for lung PET/CT [1]

The aim of this study is to address the issue of variation in ^{18}FDG uptake in lung tissue due to the presence of diffuse parenchymal lung disease (DPLP) or gravity-dependent tissue density variation in PET/CT (or a combination of both), and to describe a novel correction method that compensates for the variable tissue density.

The underlying assumption of our method is that the observed measurement of activity concentration in lung is considered to derive from a mixture of tracer distributed throughout the cellular component of tissue

191

and a gas component (with no activity). This is proportional to the observed density of lung tissue in CT. A CT acquired during shallow breathing is registered to PET and smoothed so as to match PET resolution. This is used to derive voxel-based tissue fraction correction factors (TF) for the individual. Our proposed technique was first applied to a phantom study (Fig. 11), as well as twelve subjects undergoing ^{18}FDG PET/CT examination where there were no observed lung abnormalities classified as "normal" lung studies. The effect of the proposed correction to the phantom study was to increase the mean activity concentration in lung to a value similar to that in the background. The mean lung value after correction was increased by a factor of 2.42 compared to the uncorrected value; however, Coefficient of Variation (CoV) remained similar.

For normal subjects, on average the corrected SUV value was increased by a factor of 2.81 compared to the original SUV, consistent with the expected density difference between lung and soft tissue. Notably the intra-subject CoV was reduced on average by 29% after correction (p<0.001). The inter-subject CoV was also significantly reduced after correction (p<0.025) with, on average, reduction by 46%, demonstrating that the correction process reduces the variability of observed SUV across and within subjects. Work is in progress to evaluate the effectiveness of the correction in determining response to disease progression and/or therapy. The proposed tissue fraction correction method is a promising technique to account for variability of density in interpreting lung PET studies.

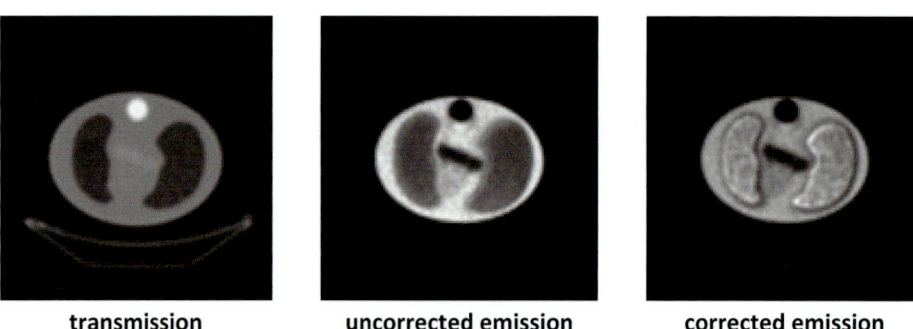

transmission	uncorrected emission	corrected emission

Fig. 11 Phantom study showing CT transmission study (left), emission study without TF correction (centre) and with correction (right)

Correction of respiratory motion artefacts in cardiac PET-CT [5, 18]

Respiratory motion during cardiac PET-CT imaging is problematic, since it results in blurring of the PET data and can induce mismatches between the PET and CT datasets, leading to attenuation-correction artefacts. The aim of this project was to obtain means of overcoming both of these issues, to allow quantitatively accurate images to be obtained.

The approach implemented was to transform a single CT such that it matched the frames of a gated PET study (Fig. 12). This enables a respiratory-matched attenuation-correction to be performed prior to motion-correction, without the need for a gated CT. This has advantages in terms of the dose associated with this type of study, as well as in reducing the presence of PET-CT mismatches, which can be problematic, even in gated studies.

The heart and diaphragm were identified through phantom studies as structures that needed to be matched during attenuation-correction to avoid artefact and hence methods of transforming their positions over the respiratory cycle were developed. The thoracic cavity (including the heart) was transformed according to rigid-registration parameters obtained from the myocardial activity, which was possible because of the high level of contrast exhibited by the myocardium in PET images. Obtaining the diaphragm motion however required additional input data, due to its poorer contrast. Therefore an approach was developed, which allowed complete diaphragm surfaces to be obtained from incomplete and noisy input data, with the use of a diaphragm shape model. This was found to be successful where information obtainable from PET images was combined with information from a single CT as input into the model fitting process.

The PET frames were then attenuation corrected with the transformed CT, reconstructed, aligned and summed, to produce motion-free images. It was found that motion blurring was reduced through alignment, although benefits were marginal in the presence of small respiratory motions. Quantitative accuracy was improved using the transformed CT for attenuation correction (compared with no CT transformation), which was attributed to both the heart and diaphragm transformations. In comparison to a gated CT, a substantial dose saving and a reduced dependence on gating techniques were achieved, indicating the potential value of the technique in routine clinical procedures.

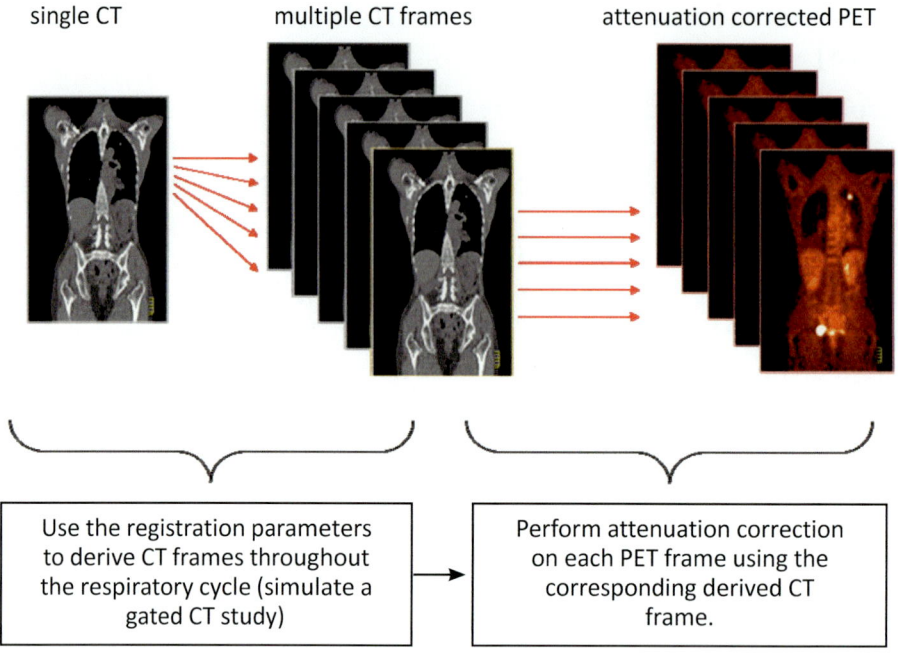

single CT   multiple CT frames   attenuation corrected PET

Use the registration parameters to derive CT frames throughout the respiratory cycle (simulate a gated CT study) → Perform attenuation correction on each PET frame using the corresponding derived CT frame.

Fig. 12 Outline of method used for correction of respiratory mismatch based on a respiratory gated PET, a single breath-hold CT and a motion model for the diaphragm

Semi-automatic analysis for lung perfusion and ventilation SPECT studies [16, 22]

The aim of the project was to develop a semi-automatic, semi-quantitative method for evaluation of lung perfusion and ventilation studies, which would help clinical decision by facilitating the interpretation of results. This should lead to a more accurate diagnosis of pulmonary embolism (PE), increasing both sensitivity and specificity of the procedure and minimizing operator's interaction.

Methodology includes performing lung perfusion and ventilation using SPECT. All data are reconstructed correcting attenuation and scatter and used to form parametric images depicting ventilation/perfusion (V/Q) mismatches which are characteristic of PE. Attenuation correction is performed through the acquisition of a scatter window to determine body and lung boundaries and fix attenuation coefficient are assigned for both, lung and soft tissue. The reconstructed SPECT data are reprojected to create 'planar like' images at any desired angle. This technique also allows contra-lateral lung to be removed and the medial view to be visualised. Normalisation of ventilation and perfusion data for subtraction is based on areas of identified 'normal' lung after hot-spots correction. Correction for respiratory motion is also considered based on dynamic SPECT acquisition. The respiratory cycle is derived from the centre of mass of acquired data.

Volumetric co-registration of perfusion and ventilation studies is performed and a 3-D parametric image generated which displays only the areas of V/Q mismatch. For anatomic reference, the abnormal areas are superimposed to a template which delineates the organ boundaries and the limits of vascular segmentation. An automatic report is generated including the presence, number, location and extension of mismatch defects and a probability of PE is calculated based on an accepted interpretation criteria. The approach has been demonstrated to improve the concordance of clinical interpretation and to reduce the number of indeterminate studies.

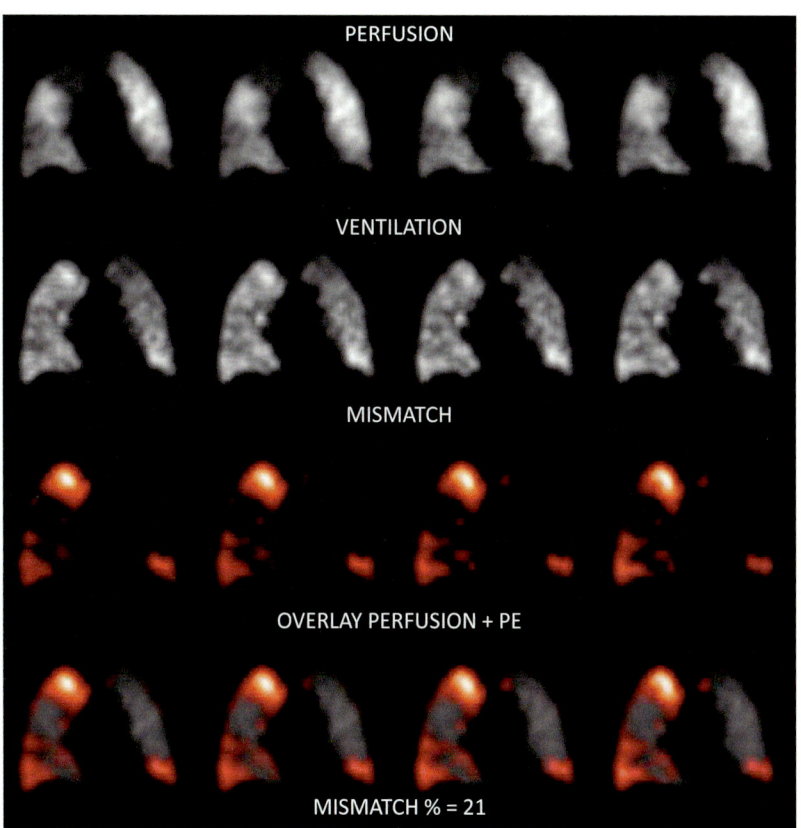

Fig. 13 Ventilation and perfusion SPECT sections with areas of mismatch highlighted

Medical Physics Research Group Staff and Students:

Group leader: Professor Brian Hutton

Primary collaborators: Professor Simon Arridge (CMIC), Dr Sebastien Ourselin (CMIC)

Scientific staff: Kjell Erlandsson, Tryphon Lambrou, Alexandre Bousse, Maria Holstensson, Daniil Kazantsev (CMIC)

PhD students: Sarah McQuaid (2005-2009), Shelan Mahmood (2006-2010), Yanni Papastavrou (p/t 2005-), Margarita Nunez (p/t 2006-2011), Benjamin Thomas (2007-2011), Sarah Cade (p/t 2008-), Niccolo Fuin (2009-), Elizabeth Howell (2010-), Stefano Pedemonte (CMIC; 2009-)

Published work in peer reviewed journals 2009–2011

1. Lambrou T, Groves A, Erlandsson K, Screaton N, Endozo R, Win T, Porter JC, Hutton BF. The importance of correction for tissue fraction effects in lung PET. *Eur J Nucl Med Mol Imaging* 2011 (in press).
2. Stute S, Carlier T, Cristina K, Noblet C, Martineau A, Hutton B, Barnden L, Buvat I. Monte Carlo simulations of clinical PET and SPECT scans: impact of the input data on the simulated images. *Phys Med Biol* 2011 (in press).
3. Hutton BF. Recent advances in iterative reconstruction for clinical SPECT/PET and CT. *Acta Oncologica* 2011; 50: 851-858.
4. Mahmood S, Erlandsson K, Cullum I, Hutton B. Experimental results from a prototype slit-slat collimator with mixed multiplexed and non-multiplexed data. *Phys Med Biol* 2011 (in press).
5. McQuaid S, Lambrou T, Hutton BF. A novel method for incorporating respiratory-matched attenuation correction in the motion correction of cardiac PET-CT studies. *Phys Med Biol* 2011; 56: 2903-2915.
6. Hutton BF, Buvat I, Beekman FJ. Review and status of SPECT scatter correction. *Phys Med Biol* 2011; 56: R85-112.
7. Thomas BA, Erlandsson K, Modat M, Thurfjell L, Ourselin S, Hutton BF. The importance of appropriate partial volume correction for PET quantification in Alzheimer's disease. *Eur J Nucl Med Mol Imaging* 2011; 38: 1104-1119.
8. Kacperski K, Erlandsson K, Hutton BF. Iterative deconvolution of simultaneous 99mTc and 201Tl projection data measured on a CdZnTe based cardiac SPECT scanner. *Phys. Med. Biol.* 2011; 56: 1397-1414.
9. Erlandsson K, Thomas B, Dickson J, Hutton BF. Partial volume correction in SPECT reconstruction with OSEM. *Nucl Instr Methods Phys Res A* 2011; 648: S85-88 (doi: 10.1016/j.nima.2010.12.106).
10. Hutton BF. New SPECT technology: potential and challenges. *Eur J Nucl Med Mol Imaging* 2010; 37: 1883-1886.
11. Ben-Haim S, Kacperski K, Hain S, Van Gramberg D, Hutton BF et al. Simultaneous dual radionuclide myocardial perfusion imaging with a solid-state dedicated cardiac camera. *Eur J Nucl Med Mol Imaging* 2010; 37: 1710-1721.
12. Mahmood S, Erlandsson K, Cullum I, Hutton BF. Potential for mixed multiplexed and non-multiplexed data to significantly improve reconstruction quality of a Multi-Slit-Slat collimator SPECT System. *Phys Med Biol* 2010; 55: 2247-2268.

13. Erlandsson K, Hutton BF. Partial volume correction in SPECT using anatomical information and iterative FBP. *Tsinghua Science & Technology* 2010; 15:50-55.

14. Dickson JC, Tossici-Bolt L, Sera T Erlandsson K, Varrone A, Tatsch K Hutton BF. The effect of reconstruction method on DaTSCAN quantification. *Eur J Nucl Med Mol Imaging* 2010; 37: 23-35.

15. Menezes LJ, Kayani I, Ben-Haim S, Hutton B, Ell PJ, Groves AM. What is the natural history of 18F-FDG uptake in arterial atheroma on PET/CT? Implications for imaging the vulnerable plaque. Atherosclerosis. 2010; 211: 136-140.

16. Núñez M, Cánepa J, Alonso O, Hutton B, Mut F. Influencia del movimiento respiratorio sobre el contraste de las lesiones en estudios de perfusión pulmonar: simulación mediante el uso de un fantoma virtual. *ALASBIMN Journal* 12 (49): July 2010. Article N° AJ49-5. http://www.alasbimnjournal.cl

17. Menezes LJ, Kotze CW, Hutton BF, Endozo R, Dickson JC, Cullum I, Yusuf SW, Ell PJ, Groves AM. Vascular inflammation imaging with 18F-DFG PET/CT: when to image? *J Nucl Med* 2009; 50: 854-857.

18. McQuaid, Lambrou T, Cunningham VJ, Bettinardi V, Gilardi MC, Hutton BF. The application of a statistical shape model to diaphragm tracking in respiratory gated PET images. *Proc IEEE* 2009; 97: 2039-2052.

19. Patton JA, Townsend DW, Hutton BF. Hybrid Imaging Technology: from dreams and vision to clinical devices. *Seminars Nucl Med* 2009; 39: 247-263.

20. Mahmood S, Erlandsson K, Hutton BF. Design of a novel slit-slat collimator system for SPECT imaging of the human brain *Phys Med Biol* 2009; 54: 3433-3449.

21. Erlandsson K, Kacperski K, van Gramberg D, Hutton BF. Evaluation of the performance characteristics of D-SPECT: a novel SPECT system designed for nuclear cardiology. *Phys Med Biol* 2009;54: 2635-2649.

22. Nunez M, Prakash V, Vila R, Mut F, Alonso O, Hutton BF. Attenuation correction for lung SPECT: evidence of need and validation of an attenuation map derived from the emission data. *Eur J Nucl Med* 2009; 36: 1076-1089.

23. Gambhir SS, Berman DS, Ziffer J, Nagler M, Dalia Dickman D, Rousso B, Sandler M. Patton J, Hutton B, Dichterman E, Ziv O, Melman H, Zilberstein Y, Ben Haim S and Ben Haim S. A Novel High Sensitivity Rapid Acquisition Single Photon Molecular Imaging Camera. *J Nucl Med* 2009; 50: 635-643.

Published conference proceedings 2009–2011

24. Bousse A, Pedemonte S, Fuin N, Kazantsev D, Erlandsson K, Ourselin S, Arridge S, Hutton BF. Log-normal distribution-based MAP-EM algorithm for edge preserving emission tomography reconstruction. Proc Fully 3D Image Reconstruction in radiology and Nuclear Medicine 2011 pp 144-147

25. Kazantsev D, Arridge S, Pedemonte S, Bousse A, Hutton BF, Ourselin S. Robust anisotropic diffusion prior with anatomical regularization for 3D SPECT reconstruction. Proc Fully 3D Image Reconstruction in radiology and Nuclear Medicine 2011 pp 237-240.

26. Kazantsev D, Pedemonte S, Bousse A, Arridge S, Hutton BF, Ourselin S. Edge preserving Bowsher prior with nonlocal weighting for 3D SPECT reconstruction. Proc International Society of Biomedical Imaging ISBI 2011 pp 1158-1161.

27. Mukherjee JM, Hutton BF, King MA. A comparison of cost functions for data-driven motion estimation in myocardial perfusion SPECT imaging. *Proc SPIE* 7962, 796209 2011 doi:10.1117/12.878393.

28. Peloso R, Busca O, Fiorini C, Abba A, Geraci A, Manenti A, Bianchi C, Poli GL, Hutton BF, Erlandsson K, Lechner P, Soltau H, Strueder L, Pedretti A, Van Mullekom P. The HICAM gamma camera. *Proc IEEE Nucl Sci Symp Med Imaging Conf 2010* pp 1957-1960.
29. Busca O, Fiorini C, Peloso R, Gola A, Abba A, Bianchi C, Poli GL, Guerra U, Hutton BF, Erlandsson K, Ottobrini L, Martelli C, Lucignani G. Applications of the HICAM gamma camera. *Proc IEEE Nucl Sci Symp Med Imaging Conf 2010* pp 2104-2107.
30. Mukherjee JM, Pretorius PH, Johnson KL, Hutton BF King MA. Comparison of data-driven and external-surrogate based motion estimation strategies in cardiac SPECT imaging. *Proc IEEE Nucl Sci Symp Med Imaging Conf 2010* pp 2987-2991.
31. Bousse A, Fuin N, Erlandsson K, Pedemonte S, Kazantsev D, Ourselin S, Arridge S, Hutton B. Point spread function optimization for parallel hole SPECT. *Proc IEEE Nucl Sci Symp Med Imaging Conf 2010* pp 2061-2065.
32. Bousse A, Pedemonte S, Kazantsev D, Ourselin S, Arridge S, Hutton B. Weighted MRI-based Bowsher priors for SPECT brian image reconstruction. *Proc IEEE Nucl Sci Symp Med Imaging Conf 2010* pp 3519-3522.
33. Pedemonte S, Bousse A, Erlandsson K, Modat M, Arridge S, Hutton BF, Ourselin S.GPU accelerated rotation-based emission tomography reconstruction. *Proc IEEE Nucl Sci Symp Med Imaging Conf 2010* pp 2657-2661.
34. Pedemonte S, Cardoso JM, Bousse A, Panagiotou C, Kazantsev D, Arridge S, Hutton B, Ourselin S. Class Conditional Joint Entropy Prior for MRI Enhanced SPECT Reconstruction. *Proc IEEE Nucl Sci Symp Med Imaging Conf 2010* pp 3292-3300.
35. Fuin N, Bousse A, Pedemonte S, Arridge S, Ourselin S, Hutton B. Collimator design in SPECT, an optimisation tool. *Proc IEEE Nucl Sci Symp Med Imaging Conf 2010* pp 3149-3154.
36. Kazantsev D, Pedemonte S, Bousse A, Panagiotou C, Arridge SR, Hutton BF, Ourselin S. ET Bayesian Reconstruction using Automatic Bandwidth Selection for Joint Entropy Optimization. *Proc IEEE Nucl Sci Symp Med Imaging Conf 2010* pp 3301-3307.
37. Erlandsson K, Thomas B, Dickson J, Hutton BF. Evaluation of an OSEM-based PVC method for SPECT with clinical data. *Proc IEEE Nucl Sci Symp Med Imaging Conf 2010* pp 2686-2690.
38. Erlandsson K, Hutton BF. Partial volume correction in SPECT using anatomical information and iterative FBP. Proc 10th *International Meeting on Fully Three-dimensional reconstruction in radiology and nuclear medicine.* 2009; pp 287-290.
39. Pedemonte S, Bousse A, Arridge S, Hutton BF, Ourselin S. 4-D Generative Model for PET/MRI Reconstruction. To be published in: G Fichtinger, A Martel and T Peters (Eds.): MICCAI 2011, Part I, LNCS 6891, pp. 581--588. Springer, Heidelberg (2011).
40. Pedemonte S, Bousse A, Arridge S, Hutton BF, Ourselin S Probabilistic Graphical Model of SPECT/MRI. MICCAI workshop of Machine Learning in Medical Imaging (MLMI). To be published: in LNCS proceedings 2011.
41. Erlandsson K, Howell E, Roth N, Hutton BF. Assessing possible use of CZT technology for application to brain SPECT. *Proc IEEE Nucl Sci Symp Med Imaging Conf 2011.*
42. Cade SC, Arridge S, Evans MJ, Hutton BF. Attenuation map estimation without transmission measurement using measured scatter data. *Proc IEEE Nucl Sci Symp Med Imaging Conf 2011.*
43. Mukherjee JM, Hutton BF, King MA. Maximum likelihood-based motion estimation in cardiac SPECT imaging. *Proc IEEE Nucl Sci Symp Med Imaging Conf 2011.*

Book Chapters 2009–2011

44. Hutton BF, Nunez M. Reconstruccion de la imagen.. In Cabrejas M (Ed) Tomografia por emision de positrones y CT 2011 (in press).
45. Hutton BF. SPECT Imaging: Basics and New Trends. In Grupen C, Buvat I, McGregor D (eds). Handbook of Particle Detection and Imaging. Springer, London 2011 (in press)
46. Hutton BF Physics applied to radiopharmacy; Imaging instruments for nuclear medicine. In Sampson's Textbook of Radiopharmacy. Theobald P (Ed). Pharmaceutical Press, London, pp61-71, 2010.
47. Hutton BF, Beekman FJ. SPECT and SPECT/CT. In Weissleder R, Ross BD, Rehemtulla A, Gambhir SS (Eds). Molecular Imaging: Principles and Practice. People's Medical Publishing House, Shelton pp40-53 2010.
48. Erlandsson K. Tracer kinetic modelling: basics and concepts. In Khalil MM (Ed) Basic Sciences of Nuclear Medicine, Springer, Berlin 2011.

Treating Disease

Radionuclide therapy is one of the pillars of Nuclear Medicine. The radionuclide therapy programme at the Institute of Nuclear Medicine started with the use of radioiodine (I-131) for treatment of the benign overactive thyroid syndromes (Grave's disease, autonomy, etc) expressed by increased thyroid hormone output - thyrotoxicosis, followed by the use of I-131 to treat malignant thyroid cancer. The management and treatment of thyrotoxicosis and of thyroid cancer was jointly carried out with the departments of Endocrinology and Radiotherapy, respectively. The treatment of these two entities comprised the bulk of the work, and remain so to date. Treating benign thyroid disease did not require any major change in practice, as patients were treated in the department of Nuclear Medicine on an outpatient basis. However, for thyroid cancer patients, designated rooms had to be identified. These had to be especially designed and lead lined, with own toilet and shower facilities, offering in-patient supervision. To this end, two rooms were set aside and designated for treating thyroid cancer in the Kathleen Ferrier and Whitbread wards of the former Middlesex Hospital.

The 1980's saw the advent of radionuclide based bone pain palliation and here the Institute was at the forefront. Strontium-89 (^{89}Sr) and Samarium-153 (^{153}Sm) were the radionuclides used (now approved in the USA and Europe) for palliation of pain from bone metastases, especially in patients with prostate and breast cancer. The Samarium-153 (^{153}Sm) labelled one of the phosphonates (EDTMP) for this purpose and data was published, showing efficacy (Resche et al European J of Cancer 33, 1583-1591, 1997, Serafini et al Journal of Clinical Oncology 16, 1574-1581, 1998, Sartor et al, Urology 63, 940-945, 2004). Although initial success with these two new ventures was encouraging, the advent of more effective means of pain control in benign and malignant conditions using non-radioactive medication somewhat reduced the interest in these treatment modalities.

Overall, there is great potential for radionuclide therapies. These have been applied widely in benign conditions, with major dissemination in the central European areas of iodine deficiency and the treatment of benign thyroid disease. In rheumatoid disease, the then available therapies were only partially successful, and often required multiple visits from patients. The Institute decided to initiate a trial of ^{153}Sm labelled to hydroxapatite, as this radiotracer could also be imaged. A project was initiated, focussing on pain palliation of large joints, especially in rheumatoid disease. The department conducted the first European survey on the use of radiation synovectomy in clinical practice (Clunie et al, European J. Nuclear Medicine 1995). To great surprise, over 3000 therapies per year were conducted in Europe, indicating a market potential for a new approach. Nevertheless, evidence based literature was almost non existent. The initial results of the Sm-153 hydroxapatite trial were encouraging, but not definitive (Clunie et al, Journal of Nuclear Medicine 36, 51-57, 1995). Despite an excellent safety profile (O'Duffy et al Rheumatology 38, 316-320, 1999), regulatory hurdles prevented this program to progress.

The 80's also saw the introduction of I-131 MIBG into clinical practice, mostly to treat malignant phaeochromocytoma, paragangliomas, neuroblastomas and carcinoids. This treatment was initially pioneered in Michigan by James Sissons, (USA), followed by Southampton and St. Bartholomew's in the UK. However, phaeochromocytomas/paragangliomas in practice was a rare condition and at The Middlesex Hospital there was not a dedicated clinic for these pathologies. Therefore, any occasional patient was sent to St Bartholomew's Hospital for treatment. However, in 1990, with a new appointment (Dr. J. Bomanji) from St. Bartholomew's, renewed interest was rekindled. The first patient with metastatic phaeochromocytoma was treated in the Whitbread ward lead lined side room. By this time the number of patients for treatment was increasing and I-131-MIBG was being produced commercially and dispensed in lead-lined containers weighing ~10 kg each, and containing 50 ml vials of 100 mCi; 3.7GBq I-131MIBG. On average, each patient received 300 mCi-11.1GBq of I-131-MIBG. Transporting these containers along with the infusion set, was not easy and this led to the requirement of a dedicated trolley for radionuclide therapy. Wendy Waddington, now Consultant Physicist, had a special interest in therapy dosimetry and took on this challenge. Wendy designed a purpose built therapy trolley, which could carry all containers along with infusion sets, meeting all the requirements of Health and Safety and radiation protection (Fig. 1). Safe operation became possible and could be adapted for other radionuclides, even including those beta emitting radionuclides for therapy. The department published its experience, which was the second largest single site experience (1) and also published guidance world-wide on thyroid blocking policy (2).

In the same decade, I-131-Lipiodol was introduced for treating hepatocellular cancer. This required placing a line into the hepatic artery feeding the tumour in the catheter laboratory, and infusing the radiolabelled Lipiodol, an extremely viscous substance, for tumour embolization. On the horizon were Y-90 SIR Spheres microspheres, which were being evaluated

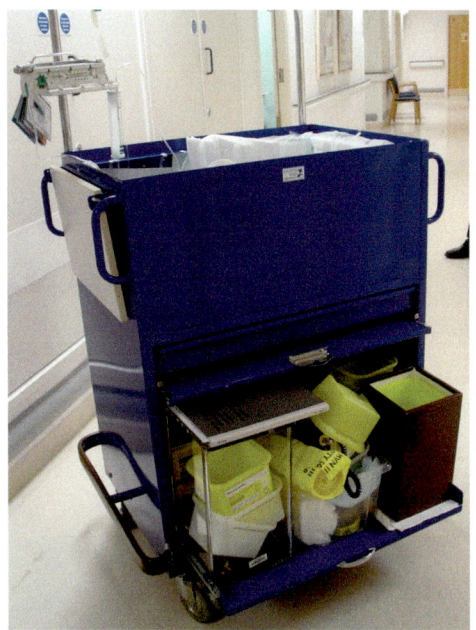
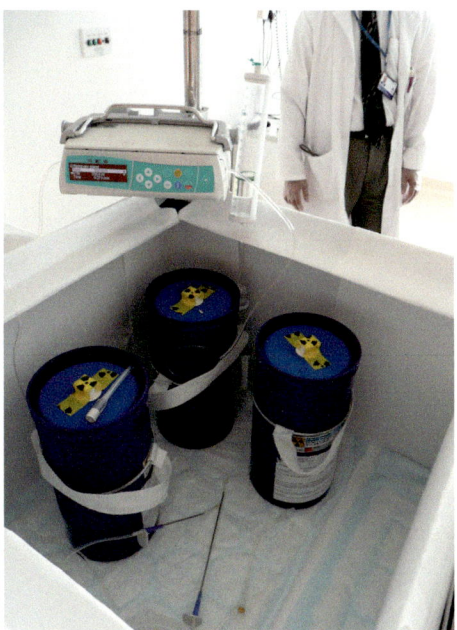

Fig. 1

in Australia to treat patients with non resectable liver cancer. This mode of treatment had achieved some success and plans were being made to introduce this therapy at the Institute, instead of I-131-Lipiodol. However, with the transfer of services in our ever changing NHS, the hepato-biliary team was relocated to the Royal Free Hospita. Hence this therapy ceased at the Institute.

The 1990's also saw the introduction of radiolabelled monoclonal antibodies for treatment. In the late 90's the Institute embarked on a Phase 1 therapy programme of using Y-90-anti-CD-45 antibody for bone marrow ablation in patients with lymphomas. At the same time, the use of Rhenium-186-HEDP was proposed for dose escalation in patients with osteosarcomas. Both therapeutic options were evaluated in the department. The antibody therapy programme required collaboration with the haematologists with Professor Steve McKinnon as the principal investigator for this study (Fig.2).

In view of this, patient were given a combination of 90Y-YAML568 (ANTI-CD45) in combination with alemtuzumab, fludarabine and melphalan, as a preparatory regimen for allogeneic stem cell transplantation in patients with haematological malignancies. On the other hand Rhenium-186-HEDP for palliative treatment of osteosarcomas was being developed in collabo-

Fig 2 PHASE I TRIAL OF
111In-YAML568 (ANTI-CD45)
LABELLED MONOCLONAL ANTI-
BODY shows increased uptake
in bone marrow and liver

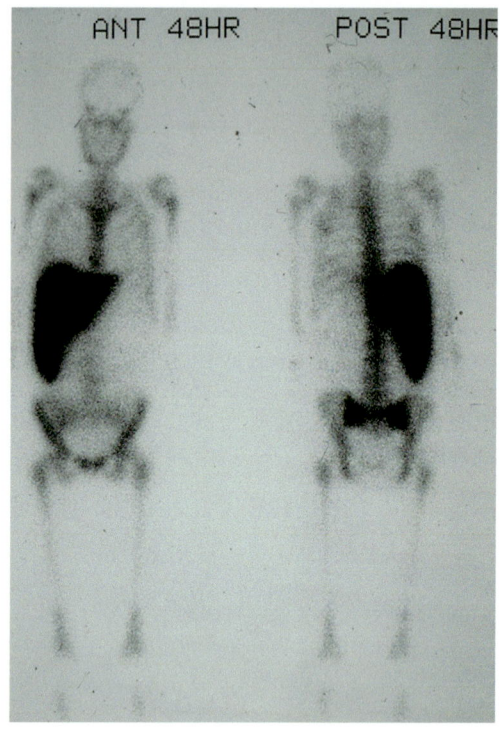

Fig 3
A) 99mTc MDP whole body bone
   scan with avid uptake in the left
   pelvic tumour
B) 186Re HEDP whole body scan
   shows uptake at the tumour site

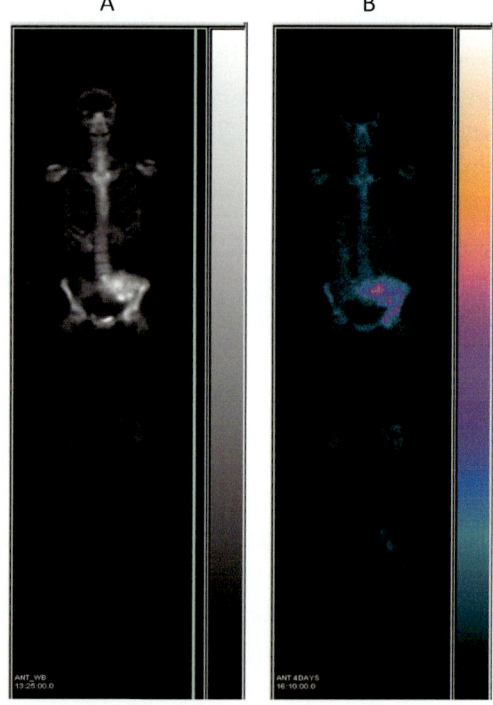

ration with the radiotherapists (Fig.3) We completed the latter study and published the first dose escalation paper for this radionuclide therapy in osteosarcomas and highlighted the potential for this approach (3, 4).

Also in the late 1999 peptide therapy came into being and initial data suggested the use of In-111-Octreotide (somatostatin type II receptor) for therapy. One patient was treated, however, it was felt that In-111 was not an appropriate radionuclide for this purpose and therefore this was not pursued further.

From a radiation delivery point of view, it was decided to pursue therapy with either Y-90-DOTATATE or Lu-177-DOTATATE. However, commercial availability was the limiting factor and the department did not have the resources to perform in-house radiolabelling of these two probes. The department of Radiotherapy continued to work closely with the department of Nuclear Medicine and in 2000 a new prospective trial (MATIN) of using high dose I-131-MIBG therapy to treat children with relapsed stage IV Neuroblastoma was proposed and started. This was a Europe wide multi-centre trial led by the oncologist/radiotherapist Mark Gaze (Fig. 4).

By this time the expanding indications for radionuclide therapy led to the then HOD Peter Ell to secure the provision of 10 purpose build led lined rooms (2 on each Floor) to be included in the design of the new UCLH building at 235 Euston Road. All members contributed to this planning but the major design and compliance work was done by Wendy Waddington. Success was achieved and the UCLH is now the only site in UK to have ten lead lined rooms for radionuclide therapy, two of which are designed for paediatric patients, two for adolescent patients and the remaining six for adult patients.

In 2004, The Institute of Nuclear Medicine moved to the new UCLH premises. The new therapy rooms are state-of-art and compliant with all the new regulations. New standard operating procedures were set up and training of nursing and medical staff in administering and handling of radioactive patients was carried out. By this time the MATIN trial came to an end. The results were encouraging and the experience is being prepared for a peer reviewed publication.

The close ties with radiotherapy also led to development of another clinical service. In 2007 the PET/CT scanner was retro-fitted with a flat radiotherapy (RT) couch top. This system is used as the sole planning modality for all upper and lower gastro-intestinal radiotherapy planning (RTP) at UCLH, and also for some head and neck, brain and lung cancer RTP. PET-CT has been described widely as improving the definition of tumour volumes, which has also been our centres experience when auditing our

205

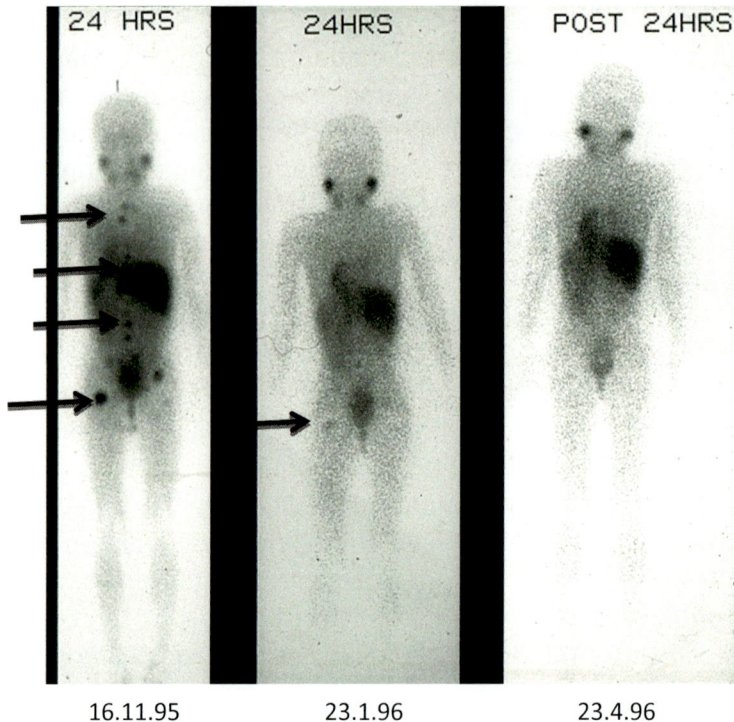

16.11.95   23.1.96   23.4.96

Fig 4 Child with stage IV neuroblastoma. Data on 16-11-95 I-123 MIBG shows bone marrow metastases (arrows). After 300mCi; 11.1 GBq of I-131 MIBG most of the metastases have resolved except one in the femur (arrow). Further treatment was given and post therapy scan on 23/4/96 shows complete resolution of disease

practice with this modality. An injection of ^{18}Fluoro-2-deoxglucose (FDG) is administered and the PET-CT scan is performed in the treatment position using standard RT protocol parameters. The CT component can therefore be directly used for dosimetric planning without the need to acquire a separate radiotherapy planning CT. The biological target volume (BTV) is delineated on the radiotherapy planning system by an experienced nuclear medicine physician using visual thresholding (Fig. 5). This volume forms the basis of the subsequent target volumes delineated by the clinical oncologist. Removing the registration anomalies with this technique enables smaller planning target volume (PTV) margins to be considered and also creates a less complex patient pathway with fewer hospital visits for multiple scans. This service is now routine and the indications are expanding to gynaecological cancers.

Patient with squamous cell carcinoma of oesophagus underwent a FDG PET scan for metabolic tumour volume assessment prior radiotherapy.

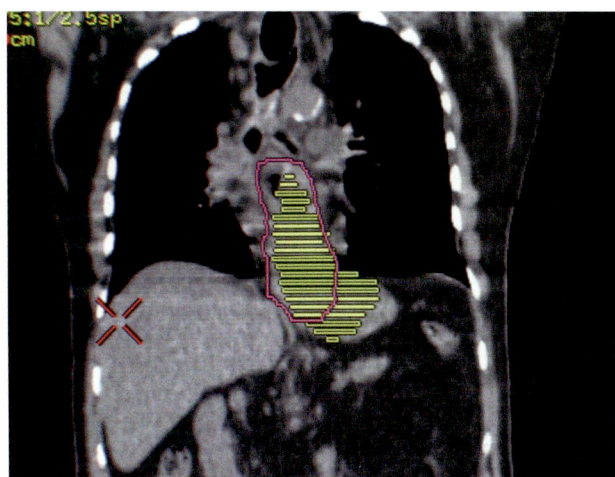

Fig. 5 BTV+GTV(CT)

Purple outline shows the biological tumour volume delineated by FDG PET scan. The yellow outline shows the volume which would have been irradiated without the benefit of FDG PET scan.

The move to the new hospital saw another major change in practice. Our pursuit to obtain either Y-90-DOTATATE or Lu-177-DOTATATE came to fruition and Lu-177-DOTATATE became available commercially. After overcoming logistic and regulatory hurdles Lu-177-DOTATATE was provided to INM for usage. Now most patients with neuroendocrine tumours have a diagnostic I-123 MIBG scan and Ga-68-DOTATATE PET scan to select patients for either I-131-MIBG therapy or Lu-177-DOTATATE.

After treating adult patients, we looked at the option of using Lu-177-DOTATATE in children with Neuroblastoma. The Dept of Nuclear Medicine and the department of Radiotherapy at UCLH published the proof of concept for this approach in 2011.

This was the first study in the world where Lu-177-DOTATATE was used for treating children (Fig. 6) with relapsed stage IV Neuroblastoma (5).

Radionuclide therapy will continue to expand at UCLH. It is now recognised as an orphan cancer service and recently a formal MDT has been introduced in line with clinical governance. It is very likely that the next decade will see an expansion of Lu-177-DOTATATE in the paediatric population and a significant expansion of Y-90 radiolabelled monoclonal antibody therapy in haematological malignancies.

Fig. 6 Child with relapsed Stage IV Neuroblastoma.
A: Anterior whole body image after first cycle of Lu-177 –DOTATATE therapy (200mCi;7.4GBq).
B: Anterior whole body image after 3rd cycle of Lu-177-DOTATATE therapy

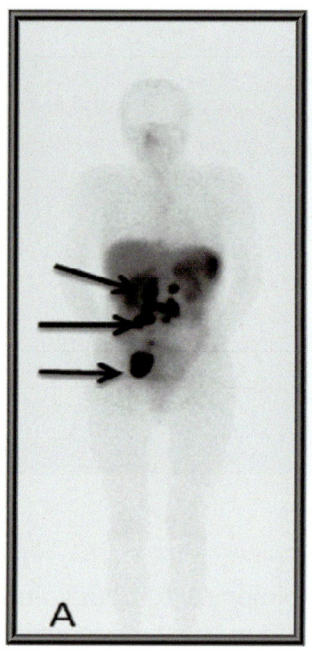
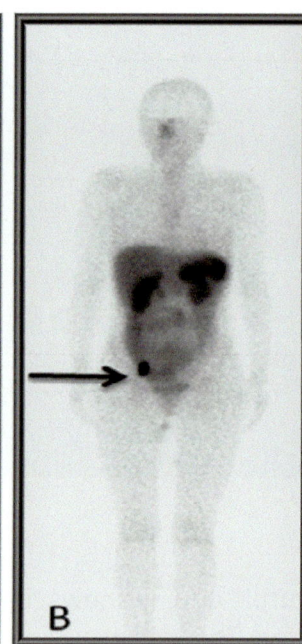

A   B

References

1. Bomanji JB, Wong W, Gaze MN, Cassoni A, Waddington W, Solano J, Ell PJ. Treatment of neuroendocrine tumours in adults with 131I-MIBG therapy. Clin Oncol (R Coll Radiol). 2003 Jun; 15(4):193-8.
2. Solanki KK, Bomanji JB, Waddington WA, Ell PJ; Thyroid blocking policy-revisited. UK Administration of Radioactive Substances Advisory Committee. Nucl Med Commun. 2004 Nov; 25(11):1071-6. No abstract available.
3. Sawyer EJ, Cassoni AM, Waddington W, Bomanji JB, Briggs TW. Rhenium-186 HEDP as a boost to external beam irradiation in osteosarcoma. Br J Radiol. 1999; 72(864): 1225-9.
4. Syed R, Bomanji J, Nagabhushan N, Kayani I, Groves A, Waddington W, Cassoni A, Ell PJ. 186Re-HEDP in the treatment of patients with inoperable osteosarcoma. J Nucl Med. 2006 Dec; 47(12):1927-35.
5. Gains JE, Bomanji JB, Fersht NL, Sullivan T, D'Souza D, Sullivan KP, Aldridge M, Waddington W, Gaze MN. 177Lu-DOTATATE Molecular Radiotherapy for Childhood Neuroblastoma. J Nucl Med. 2011 Jul; 52(7):1041-7. Epub 2011 Jun 16.

The Institute and the Comprehensive Biomedical Research Centre (CBRC)

It is only fitting to acknowledge here the important contribution the CBRC has made to the further development of the Institute. Perhaps the single most important contribution was the support given to the funding of our Radiochemistry facility, now housed within UCL Chemistry. This is described in the relevant section of this book. Further support was given by the CBRC in its first quinquennial program. We outline below the last 2 years of the outcome of our CBRC program, as part of the Imaging Theme which our staff led in the first 5 years of the CBRC.

As we write on the 17th August 2011, notice has been received that the 2nd quinquennial BRC program has received formal approval – our sincere congratulations to Professor Deenan, Director of the UCLH/UCL BRC!

Annual Report 2009/10 (Extracts from Nuclear Medicine)

A new dual accredited Consultant (nuclear medicine/radiology) has just been appointed (L Menezes). With significant expertise in cross sectional imaging and MR imaging of the heart, L Menezes will expand our R&D in oncology and the cardiovascular area. We are still the only department in the UK which offer a routine PET/CT myocardial perfusion service, with Rb82. This has shortened the patient journey in a major manner, combining CTA and Rb82 perfusion into a single investigation. Quantitative data with Rb82 perfusion has been recorded and the radiation exposure from Rb82 is a fraction of that delivered with conventional tracers (Tc99m or Tl201). In conjunction with the KCL/UCL CCIC grant, a new PhD student has also been appointed, whilst our first PhD funded in part from CBRC is now writing up the thesis (submission end of this calendar year). We have now introduced the first CZT based camera into routine practice of myocardial perfusion. This approach using conventional tracers has also sped up the standard imaging protocol, the patient journey being less than a third of the time required for a typical patient investigated with CAD prior to this novel introduction. We have provided clear solutions to the longest waiting list of NM procedures in the UK (nuclear cardiology) and provided a clear steer as to how to reduce radiation exposure (now the flavour of the month in the USA).

Novel Probes

We have continued to translate novel imaging probes into diagnostic tools. These include the somatostatin receptor ligands for neuroendocrine disease (DotaTATE and DotaNOC) and now the novel GLP-1 receptor ligand exendin for the imaging of benign and malignant insulinomas. We will by end of calendar year begin the imaging of the amyloid plaque in patients with Av-45 in patients with primary progressive aphasia (with J Schott). With the Institute of Cancer we are planning a series of trials of a novel imaging agent for the in vivo study of apoptosis. We also will apply a new probe for angiogenesis in the assessment of cardiac stem cell therapy (in collaboration with A. Mather).

Cancer Angiogenesis and Metabolic Vascular Imaging

The recruitment of this NHIR adopted study increased in 2009/10 for breast, lung and colorectal cancers. Early trends are being identified from initial data analysis. In lung cancer the metabolic vascular phenotype is showing association with mortality. In colorectal the metabolic flow relationship is intact in larger tumours but not in smaller ones. In breast cancer we have related glucose metabolism to a host of biomarkers such as angiogenesis, oestrogen and herceptin receptor status and tumour grade. This type of clinical research work will enable us to individualise patient treatment to the individual patient tumour.

Pulmonary fibrosis PET/CT Imaging

We have increased our patient recruitment of this NHIR adopted study in 2009/10. Our first (proof of concept) paper showing that FDG PET CT may be a biomarker for disease activity in interstitial lung disease, has now been published by the highest ranked imaging Journal. We have now performed work showing that PET/CT has potential to measure treatment response in interstitial lung disease. In addition we have now shown that we can get a similar disease signal using a somatostatin PET ligand analogue. This work is now gaining interest from pharmaceutical companies (see below) since the technique is translating into potential patient benefit.

Atheroma combined PET/CT3T MR Imaging

This is another NHIR adopted study. Our methodological work has seen two publications in the highest ranked Imaging journal in the last 12 months. We have used multimodality to phenotype both aneurysmal and carotid plaque disease and show interesting findings both respect to patient outcome and correlation with immune-histobiomarkers. This information has potential to risk stratify patients and thus guide patient intervention.

210

Translational studies in collaborating within and outside the Imaging Theme

We have collaborated with Imaging to combine FDG PET with CT colonography resulting in two publications in the highest ranked imaging journal. Further work is being performed with Imaging on lymphoma. We have also collaborated with Cardiology in cardiac imaging and published the first work on 64 detector PET/CT coronary angiography.

Nuclear Medicine/Physics

The following represents work in progress which has potential for future clinical impact.

Basic System Development

In conjunction with European colleagues (EC funding) we have been developing SPECT system designs that will be further developed for use in a commercial system optimised for imaging whole body and brain (KCL/UCL CCIC funded). Development of a prototype system is anticipated in 18-24 months.

Efficient reconstruction (EPSRC funded): Efforts are being made to take advantage of complex tomographic reconstruction algorithms being developed at UCL by making use of graphics processing units (GPU) typical of fast PC-based game units. A goal is to provide a comprehensive reconstruction package that incorporates state-of-the-art multimodality data.

Image Processing and Analysis

Improved partial volume correction permits more exact quantification for evaluating tracers that measure amyloid deposition (EPSRC/GE funded). This will be applied in a project to evaluate primary progressive aphasia.

A novel approach is being developed to extract transmission data from emission scatter counts for the purpose of attenuation correction; if successful this would be very widely applied.

Algorithms for processing simultaneously acquired dual radionuclide studies are being used now in human studies and evaluated for incorporation in vendor-supplied application software (industry-funded)

A technique to address the artefacts caused by PET/CT respiratory mismatch has been developed for evaluation in clinical studies but currently requires resources to continue; the imaging group at Yale University are interested in applying this work in their preclinical studies. We are also developing quantitative methods that can account for tissue fraction effects in pulmonary fibrosis studies (funded by CBRC/GSK). The work will also be extended to evaluate dual modality correction strategies in vascular imaging.

Nuclear Medicine/Radiochemistry

The radiochemistry research facility/laboratory has been constructed, equipped and validated. Within months of starting practical work, ground-breaking progress in radiochemistry has been achieved with the discovery of a new labelling reaction that provides triple functionalized radioiodinated compounds. This has allowed, for the first time, to prepare labelling reagents equipped with both fluorescent and radioactive groups for multi-scale imaging with optical and nuclear techniques. Conjugation of the new reagents to a cancer embryonic antibody (A5B7) has enabled imaging of human cancer cells in vitro. In vivo studies in animal models are due to commence within the next two weeks. UCL business has submitted a patent application for filing based on the new discovery.

The possibility of accessing dual labelled reagents and tracers in a single step has the potential to greatly accelerate tracer discovery by use of high throughput fluorescence assays for lead identification, and paves the way for unprecedented evaluation of recombinant therapies from the cellular level to whole body.

Health Care Impact

We have: introduced the imaging of neuroendocine disease with Ga-68 PET/CT probes, replacing the conventional In-111 octreotide studies; introduced ultrafast imaging protocols for CAD into routine practice, more than halving patients journeys; introduced GLP-1 receptor imaging for benign and malignant insulinomas; and offer a one stop shop for complete functional assessment of CAD, with CTA/PET/CT Rb82 studies. We will be introducing Ga-68 citrate PET/CT imaging for the investigation of infection. The worldwide impact of Tc-99m shortages had basically no impact on our service provision (in contrast to other sites in the UK and elsewhere) in view of our vision to translate PET/CT into useful alternative imaging. Finally we now offer a FDG localization service for non lesional MR patients with focal epilepsy – this is aiding diagnosis and management in 20% of all clinically difficult referred cases (Ell, Groves, Ben-Haim, Hutton, Bomanji, Dickson).

The type of translational work we are performing uses imaging to phenotype disease and investigates the possible identification of biomarkers. The imaging findings we are obtaining have important consequences with respect to the potential to guide drug discovery programs in target specific populations. Moreover we are ever identifying patient prognostic factors in populations that need more specific interventions.

Currently our work on imaging disease activity in interstitial lung disease is showing a potential role in the management of patients. This potential is now recognised by industry and we have entered collaboration with the pharmaceutical industry. Our cancer imaging is demonstrating translational benefit with identification of clear correlations of imaging findings with established cancer biomarkers (A Groves).

The Radiochemistry initiative has yet to have impact on patient benefit or care. However, discussions are ongoing with a pharmaceutical company to use nuclear imaging to optimise the treatment with one of their recombinant enzymes (E Arstad).

Patient and Public Involvement

We have conducted 2 Ethics approved research studies.

The first one, entitled: "Major Impact on Patient Journey with Novel Myocardial Perfusion Imaging and Fast D-SPECT®: Comparison with Standard Practice: First European Trial" is a validation study in 180 patients, comparing myocardial perfusion imaging on D-SPECT and conventional SPECT by visual and by quantitative analysis.

In the second study, entitled: "Major Impact on Patient Journey with Myocardial Perfusion Imaging and Fast D-SPECT: Effect of Simultaneous Dual Isotope Imaging: First World Wide Trial" we demonstrated the feasibility of simultaneous imaging of two radionuclides with D-SPECT, again significantly shortening imaging time while obtaining high quality images (S. Ben-Haim)

In addition we have assessed patients' tolerance to this novel camera; 86% of patients preferred D-SPECT for shorter imaging time and improved comfort compared to conventional camera. A. Groves is working with GSK, studying new PET ligands for the investigation pulmonary fibrosis. We are hoping this work will lead to pharmacological intervention studies.

Collaboration with Industry

A. Groves is in the process of signing a contract with the Amersham Division of GE Healthcare on an angiogenesis specific tracer.

A. Groves is submitting a grant to NIH with the PET/CT division of GE Healthcare, to investigate a novel imaging probe for hypoxia in cancer.

P. Ell has secured a grant of £ 100k with AAA (an imaging company) securing the first formal trial of Rb82 as a PET/CT agent for myocardial perfusion in comparison with conventional single photon emitters.

A grant from AVIVA (J Schott and P Ell) (equivalent to £ 100K) will allow us to start the PET/CT imaging of the amyloid plaque.

EPSRC project grant on tomographic reconstruction for which B. Hutton is PI: £ 780,962 over 3 years (commenced May 2009).

A. Groves is working with GSK, studying new PET ligands for the investigation pulmonary fibrosis. We are hoping this work will lead to pharmacological intervention studies.

We have also collaborative research work with the following companies:

GE Healthcare, Spectrum Dynamics, Nuclear Fields, GSK.

E. Arstad and he radiochemistry group has established collaboration with GE Healthcare (one grant application submitted jointly and a second about to be submitted), carried out pilot studies in collaboration with Eli Lilly, and is currently in discussion with Genzyme Therapeutics to obtain funding for tracer studies at UCL.

21 Peer Reviewed Publications (2009–2010) acknowledging CBRC

Menezes LJ, Kayani I, Bomanji J, Hutton BF, Ell PJ, Groves AM. What is the Natural History of 18F-FDG Uptake in Arterial Atheroma on PET/CT. Atherosclerosis. 2010 Jan 22. [Epub ahead of print] Pub Med PMID: 20202634.

Taylor SA, Bomanlji JB, Mezpanzure, L, Robinson C, Groves AM, Dickson JC, Greenhalgh, R Cattinin G, Obichere A, Bloom S, Ell PJ, Halligan S. Non laxative positron emission tomography CT colonography: Feasibility, performance and acceptability in patients at higher risk of colonic neoplasia. J Nucl Med. 2010 Jun; 51(6):854-61. Epub 2010 May 19. Pub Med PMID: 20484420.

Kotze CW, Yusuf SW, Menezes LJ, Hutton BF, Ell PJ, Groves AM. Vascular Imaging with FDG PET/CT: optimal FDG circulation time. J Nucl Med. 2009 Aug 18. [Epub ahead of print] Pub Med PMID: 19690039.

Kayani I, Conry BG, Groves AM, Caplan D, Win T, Bomanji J. A comparison of 68Ga-DO-TATATE and 18F-FDG PET/CT in pulmonary neuroendocrine tumors. J Nucl Med. 2009 Dec; 50(12):1927-32. Epub 2009 Nov 12. Pub Med PMID: 19910422.

Groves AM, Speechly-Dick ME, Kayani I, Pugliese F, Habib S, Menezes L, Endozo R, Pruvlovich E, McEwan J, Ell PJ. First experience cardiac PET 64-detector/CT angiography with invasive angiography validation. Eur J Nucl Med Mol Imaging. 2009 Dec; 36(12):2027-33. Epub 2009 Jul 18. Pub Med PMID: 19618180.

Menezes LJ, Groves AM, Kayani I, Dickson JC, Endozoz R, Bomanji J, Hutton B, Ell P. Assessment of LV function at rest using Rb myocardial perfusion PET; Comparison of 4 different software algorithms with simultaneous 64 detector coronary CT. Nucl Med Commun. 2009 Dec; 30(12):918-25. PubMed PMID: 19884868.

Vijayanathan S, Butt S, Gopinath G, Groves AM. Advantages and limitations of imaging the musculoskeletal system by conventional radiological, radionuclide and hybrid modalities. Semin Nucl Med. 2009 Nov; 39(6):357-68. Review. PubMed PMID: 19801216.

Kotze CW, Menezes, L, Endozo R, Groves AM, Ell, PJ Yusuf SW. Increased metabolic activity in abdominal aortic aneurysm detected by 18F- fluorodeoxyglucose (18F-FDG) positron emission tomography/computed tomography (PET/CT). Eur J Vasc Endovasc Surg. 2009 Jul; 38(1):93-9. Epub 2009 Feb 12. PubMed PMID: 19217326.

Groves AM, Win T, Screaton NJ, Berovic M, Endozo R, Booth H, Dickson JC, Ell PJ. Idiopathic Pulmonary Fibrosis and Diffuse Parenchymal Lung Disease: Implications from Initial

Experience with 18F-FDG-PET/CT. J Nucl Med. 2009 Apr; 50(4):538-45. Epub 2009 Mar 16. PubMed PMID: 19289428.

Groves AM, Wishart GC, Shastry M, Moyle P, Iddles S, Britton P, Gaskarth M, Warren RM, Ell PJ, Miles KA. Metabolic-Flow Relationships in Primary Breast Cancer: Feasibility with Combined PET/ Dynamic Contrast Enhanced CT. Eur J Nucl Med Mol Imaging. 2009 Mar; 36(3):416-21. Epub 2008 Sep 26.PMID: 18818917.

McQuaid S, Lambrou T, Cunningham VJ, Bettinardi V, Gilardi MC, Hutton BF. The application of a statistical shape model to diaphragm tracking in respiratory gated PET images. European Journal of Nuclear Medicine and Molecular Imaging 2009; 36:416-421 Proc IEEE 2009; 97: 2039-2052. PubMed PMID:

Patton JA, Townsend DW, Hutton BF. Hybrid Imaging Technology: from dreams andVision to clinical devices. Semin Nucl Med. 2009 Jul; 39(4):247-63. Review. PubMed PMID: 19497402.

Mahmood S, Erlandsson K, Hutton BF. Design of a novel slit-slat collimator system for SPECT imaging of the human brain. Phys Med Biol. 2009 Jun 7; 54(11):3433-49. Epub 2009 May 13. PubMed PMID: 19436098.

Erlandsson K, Kacperski K, van Gramberg D, Hutton BF. Performance Evaluation of D-SPECT: a novel SPECT system designed for nuclear cardiology. Phys Med Biol. 2009 May 7; 54(9):2635-49. Epub 2009 Apr 8. PubMed PMID: 19351981.

Nunez M, Prakash V, Vila R, Mut F, Alonso O, Hutton BF. Attenuation correctionfor lung SPECT: evidence of need and validation of an attenuation map derived fromthe emission data. Eur J Nucl Med Mol Imaging. 2009 Jul; 36(7):1076-89. Epub 2009 Feb 24. PubMed PMID: 19238381.

Gambhir SS, Berman DS, Ziffer J, Nagler M, Dalia Dickman D, Rousso B, Sandler M. Patton J, Hutton B, Dichterman E, Ziv O, Melman H, Zilberstein Y, BenHaim S and Ben Haim S. A Novel High Sensitivity Rapid Acquisition Single PhotonMolecular Imaging Camera. J Nucl Med. 2009 Apr; 50(4):635-43. PubMed PMID: 19339672.

Ben-Haim SS, Kacperski K, Hain S, van Gramberg D, Hutton B, Erlandsson K, Sharir T, Roth N, Waddington WA, Berman DS and Ell PJ. Simultaneous dual-radionuclide myocardial perfusion imaging with a solid-state dedicated cardiac camera. Eur J Nucl Med Mol Imaging. 2010 Apr 11. PubMed PMID: 20383705.

Menezes LJ, Kotze CW, Hutton BF, Endozo R, Dickson JC, Cullum I, YusufSW, Ell PJ, Groves AM. Vascular inflammation imaging with 18F-DFG PET/CT:when to image? J Nucl Med. 2009 Jun; 50(6):854-7. Epub 2009 May 14. PubMed PMID: 19443587.

Erlandsson K, Hutton BF. Partial volume correction in SPECT using anatomicalinformation and iterative FBP. Proc 10th International Meeting on Fully Three-DimensionalReconstruction in Radiology and Nuclear Medicine. 2009; pp 287-290. PubMed PMID:

Torres Martin de Rosales R, Arstad E, Blower PJ. Nuclear Imaging of Molecular Processes in Cancer. Target Oncol. 2009 Sep; 4(3):183-97. Epub 2009 Sep 25. Review. PubMed PMID: 19779864.

Dickson JC, Tossici-Bolt L, SeraT, Erlandssson K, Varrone A, Tatsch K and Hutton B. The impact of reconstruction method on the quantification of DaTScan images. Eur J Nucl Med Mol Imaging. 2010 Jan; 37(1):23-35. Epub. PubMed PMID: 19618181.

PETMR and
The Charity University College London Hospitals

In early 2011, the UCLH Charity under the chair of Lord Crispin supported UCLH with a major grant, allowing for an infrastructure to be build and for the purchase of the first fully integrated 3T PETMR in the UK. Managed by the Institute of Nuclear Medicine, the instrument will be able to start clinical work in time for the opening of the new MacMillan Cancer Center in April 2012. So the Charity continues to support major initiatives of UCLH Trust Hospitals, as it supported the Institute of Nuclear Medicine with the funding of the first PETCT scanner in the UK in 2002!

PETMR: a UK first: a disruptive technology and a paradigm change in imaging

MR in cancer

A Google search opens up 28,100,000 entries. The relevance of MR in cancer is beyond dispute. The FDA (USA) supports MR in breast cancer staging since 1991 and numerous guidelines are available for MR in several cancers (head and neck, breast, prostate, brain, etc). From Cancer Research UK, a few years ago: MR is particularly good for some types of brain tumour, primary bone tumours, soft tissue sarcomas and for tumours affecting the spinal cord, deep seated lesions, etc.

PETCT in cancer

PETCT is now established in the staging, re-staging and therapy response assessment in many cancer types. We now perform some 3700+ PETCT studies per annum, 85% of these in cancer. Many patients are referred more than once, for response assessment and prognostication. The DH has recognised the role of PETCT in oncology, with a funded 5 year PETCT program based on mobile scanners providing services outside the London area.

Why PETMR

Many new probes, both for MR and PET are in current development. These will address specific biological signals, relevant to the understanding of the underlying pathology and the evaluation of novel forms of treatment. Most should be used in a combined manner, each imaging modality investigating one specific probe. This implies multiple visits to separate sites and separate scanners. The combined power of PETMR will offer unique multiplexing capacity – from a single patient visit, multiple biological parameters could be recorded simultaneously!

Combining the power of PET with the power of MR, we achieve, in a single setting, unique patient and population benefits:

- 50% Reduction in Radiation Exposure (as compared to PETCT) in all referrals
- Major New Clinical Indication: The Dementias and the worried well
- Paradigm Change in Imaging Cancer: Phenotyping Disease via Multi-modality Imaging in most cancers
- Specific indications for (inter alia) Brain Tumours, Head and Neck Cancer, Breast Cancer, Soft Tissue Sarcomas, Colon Cancer, Prostate Cancer, Paediatric Cancer
- Evolving new Imaging Paradigm, as a **one stop single** test with PET **and** MR will dramatically increase the diagnostic power: RT planning, response monitoring in lymphoma, tumour grade assessment in neuro-oncology, and others
- Multimodality Molecular Imaging of the Cardiovascular System: imaging atheroma, inflammation, apoptosis, neo-vessel formation, proliferation, etc

As outlined above, the opportunity is major, opening up entirely new avenues for diagnosis, disease monitoring and response assessment:

A. Major population benefit is achieved with a combined PETMR approach – a reduction of at least 50% of the radiation exposure to all patients referred to a PETCT, often even a greater reduction, since patients come to a PETCT after having had a CT exposure! This becomes very relevant in circumstances where patients are offered repeated CT and or PETCT exposures – some of our lymphoma patients have been referred for disease monitoring with PETCT, five and more times over. Similar observation can be made for other types of cancer, such as colorectal, head and neck, etc. In all of these above listed cancers, UCLH has a major stake and PETMR can play a significant if not unique role. Many if not most of referrals submitted hitherto to a separate CT, MR or PETCT instrument, would be referred directly to a single PETMR investigation. A fusion of the anatomy and discriminatory power of MR with the metabolic information offered by PET, will offer a step change in the staging and disease monitoring of these patients. Multiple separate investigations will be reduced to a one stop imaging referral. New imaging paradigms will be tested and applied, investigating the role of cell signalling, apoptosis, angiogenesis, proliferation, perfusion, hypoxia, receptor status. This has at present not been possible since patient journey and flow and the inherent separation of the imaging technologies have prevented this multiplexing approach. PETMR is the solution in this exciting world of molecular imaging.

B. The Early Diagnosis of the Dementias and the assessment of the worried well. With an aging population, the prevalence of Alzheimer dementia represents a major health burden. At age 60, it is 2%, and it doubles every 5 years to reach approximately 20% at age 80! Whilst the standard present imaging modality for Alzheimer type dementia is MR, the technology is far from perfect. PET now offers at least 3 probes, able to visualise the deposition of the amyloid plaque. In early studies, PET imaging can detect amyloid up to 10 years before first clinical symptoms manifest. Adults with only mild cognitive impairment and a positive PET scan, are 13 times more likely to develop full blown Alzheimer dementia. A PETMR approach is likely to offer the solution to the early diagnosis of this terrifying condition, avoiding invasive procedures such as CSF taps, but also opens up the window of opportunity for disease modifying approaches. Major industries and academic centres are actively engaged in developing a specific treatment.

C. Multimodality Imaging of the Cardiovascular System.
Whilst some of the clinical potential of PETMR in the heart remains a challenge, inroads are being made. Some academic centres are focusing on MR for the investigation of the vulnerable atheroma plaque. Our own group has published on this topic with PET (Atherosclerosis 2009). The JUPITER trial (Lancet 2009) has shown that patients with normal cholesterol levels but elevated C reactive protein can their risk for an event halved if treated with aggressive statins. Can PETMR further identify the populations at risk, since long term treatment with statins carries an unknown risk. Inflammation (imaged by PETMR) will decline more rapidly after stating therapy than plaque load, giving early indices of treatment success and more importantly, a possible tool to titrate the amount of stating given to an individual. A PETMR approach will attempt to char-

acterize the plaque in terms of its macrophage load, apoptosis and metalloproteinase expression, fibrin deposition, etc. Clinical cell tracking is possible with supraparamagnetic iron oxide nanoparticles (SPIO's) and stem cell tracking has been achieved with radiolabelled probes, so far investigated in separate settings and instruments. PETMR offers a unique single approach. Myocardial integrin expression can be investigated with PETMR using specific probes looking into angiogenesis. Industry is committed to the development of these probes, to be used with PETMR.

2011 Platform

Radiochemistry Laboratory (CBRC Funded)
Pre-Clinical SPETCT (CCIC Funded)
Large Radiopharmacy (UCLH Funded)
Major Equipment base:
16 + 64 Slice PETCT (Charity UCLH Funded): UK First
3T PETMT (Charity UCLH Funded): UK First
Solid State Camera (Industry funded): UK First
16 Slice SPETCT (CRUK Funded)
16 Slice PETCT (UCLH Funded)
DEXA Densitometer (first scanner was UK first – INM Funded)
Ga-68 Radionuclide Generator for In-House Peptide Labelling
Rb-82 Generator for In-House Low Dose Rapid PET Perfusion Studies
10 Radionuclide Therapy Beds (UCLH Funded)

UCL/UCLH Radiochemistry Operational since March 2010

- Equipped with 3 shielded fume hoods, 2 hot cells and 3 synthesis modules
- Suitable for tracer development, automation and scale-up (PET and SPECT)

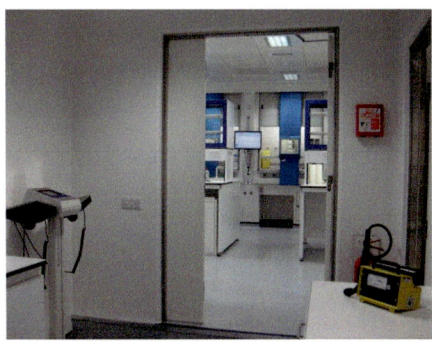 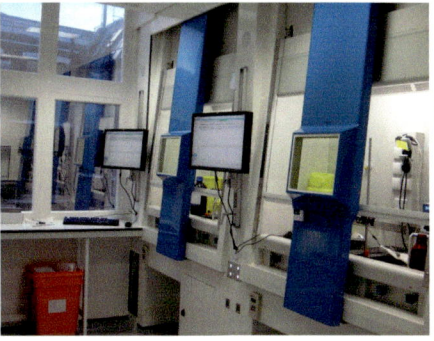

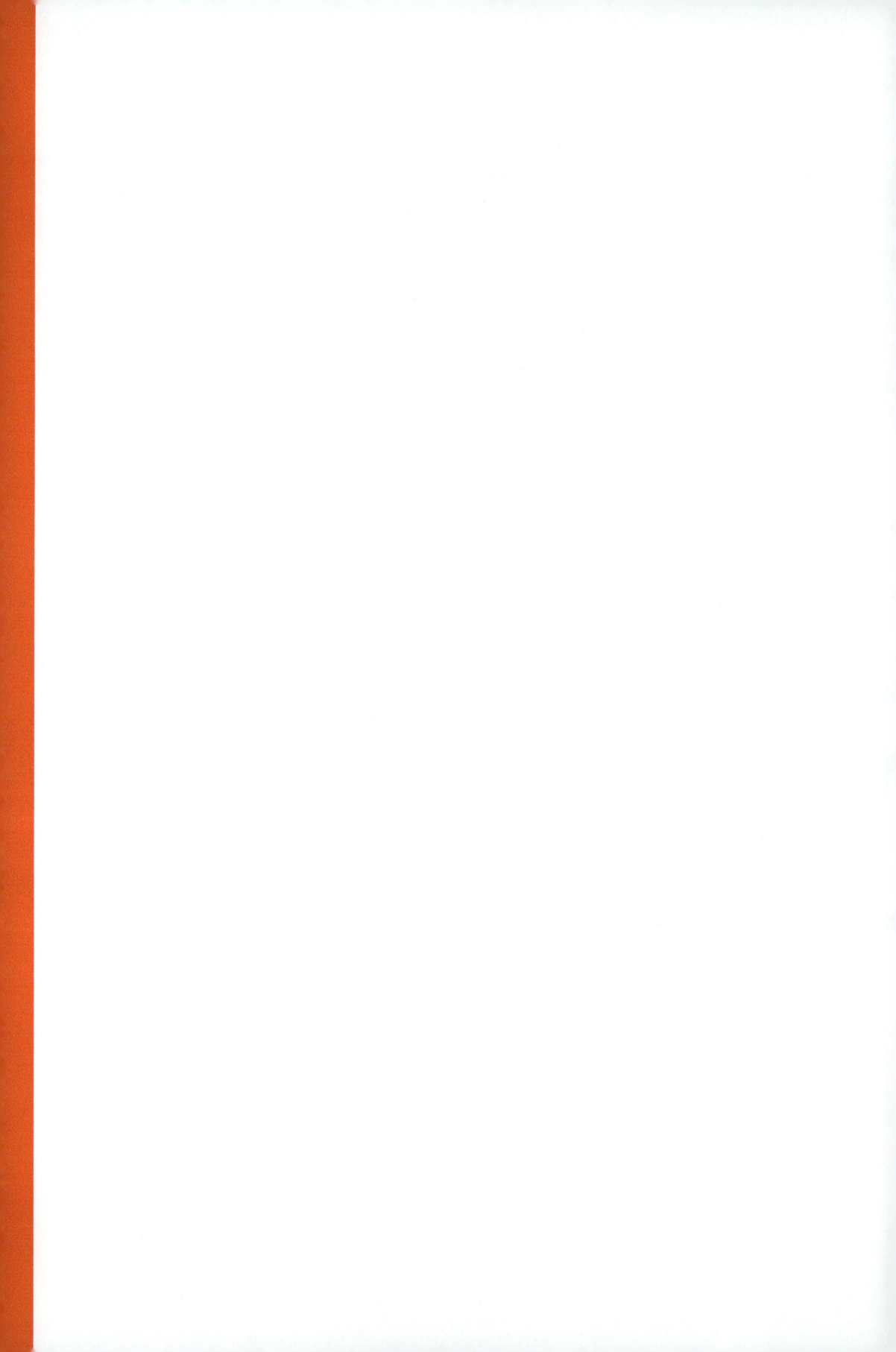

Conclusion

Several decades ago the program Atoms for Peace was launched. No one would have predicted where atoms for medicine would have led us to. Five Nobel laureates have been intimately involved in the biological use of radioactive tracers in man.

The WHO defines Nuclear Medicine as embracing all applications of radioactive materials in diagnosis, treatment or research, with the exception of the use of sealed sources in Radiotherapy. This then defines our field of endeavour. Today, Nuclear Medicine is a safe methodology, applied in all ages, from children to the elderly. A significant impact in health care and patients lives is made.

For therapy purposes, we use nuclides such as Yt-90, Sr-89, Re-186, Sm153, Ra-222, and of course, I-131. Progress is expected with the use of Bi-123 and At-211. Novel magic bullets, protein, antibody receptor and peptide based, are in use. In diagnostics, we make daily use of nuclides such as Tc-99m, I-123, Tl-201, F-18, Rb82. Exciting applications have emerged with the use of Ga-68, I-124 and Cu-64. Novel ligands are in development for the targeting of cellular proliferation, hypoxia, apoptosis, neo-vessell formation, and the deposition of amyloid, tau and atheroma.

In 1991, the British National Society Audit team wrote: "The department and its staff to be commended for the high level of care, clinical expertise, original research and the teaching skills for which the Institute has earned an international reputation". "We single the commitment to care as their overall impression". More recent audit in 2003 and 2011 has further documented the above, with high level of governance, compliance with standards, and patient care.

A patient letter received August 7th, 2011 states:

> Tank you for your letter dated as typed 26 July 2011, which I received yesterday. Naturally, I am very pleased about the result of my recent coronary angiogram.
>
> I should like to take this opportunity to express my gratitude to the staff of the Deparment of Nuclear Medicine for the care and consideration shown to me during the course of the procedure. The apparatus involved (to say nothing of the name of the department!) might well have proved intimidatin, but the tratment I received was very reassuring. I am most grateful

The future is bright

PETCT Started Multimodality Imaging at UCLH/UCL and UK
In 2002

Multisignalling Probes will Extend Molecular Imaging

PETMR Extends Multimodality Imaging at UCLH/UCL and UK
In 2012

References: 1986–2011

1986

447. Task groups and the European Societies of Nuclear Medicine. Ell PJ. Editorial Nuclear Medicine Communications, 7, 81-82, 1986.
448. Cerebral consequences of cardiopulmonary bypass. Smith PLC, Newman SP, Ell PJ, Treasure T, Joseph P, Schneidau A and Harrison MJG. The Lancet, I, 823-825, 1986.
449. Does it help to know the left ventricular ejection fraction? Ell PJ and Underwood SR. The Lancet, I, 909, 1986.
450. Clinical aspects of detection and imaging of brain tumours. Ell PJ. In Nuclear Medicine in Clinical Oncology. E.C. Winkler, Springer-Verlag, 55-60, 1986.
451. Experimental studies of 99mTc HMPAO with an rCBF model. Costa DC, Jones BE, Steiner TJ, Aspey BS, Ell PJ, Cullum ID and Jewkes RF. Nuclear Medicine Communications, 7, 282, 1986.
452. Clinical studies using a new regional cerebral blood flow agent 99mTc-hexamethyl-propyleneamine oxime (HMPAO). Hocknell JML, Cullum ID, Smith PLC, Costa DC and Ell PJ. Nuclear Medicine Communications, 7, 295, 1986.
453. Radionuclide venography - how accurate an examination. Watkin GT and Ell PJ. Nuclear Medicine Communications, 7, 322, 1986.
454. A quantitative study of biliary dyskinesia using 99mTc-EHIDA. Jarritt PH, Pagtakhan E and Ell PJ. Nuclear Medicine Communications, 7, 280, 1986.
455. Nuclear medicine practice, cost benefit and risk assessment: an introduction. Ell PJ. CEIR Forum on the Microdosimetry of Radiopharmaceuticals International Journal of Radiation Biology, 50, 556-558, 1986.
456. Stress induced right ventricular dysfunction: an indication of reversible right ventricular ischaemia. Underwood SR, Campos Costa D, Walton S, Laming PJ, Ell PJ, Emanuel RW and Swanton RH. In: Nuklearmedizin, 119-123, 1986. Proceedings, Ed. Britton, Schmidt, and Ell, Schattauer Verlag, Stuttgart.
457. Quantitative analysis of stress induced phase changes in the detection of coronary artery disease. Underwood SR, Walton S, Laming PJ, Ell PJ, Emanuel RW and Swanton RH. In: Nuklearmedizin, 77-79, 1986. Proceedings, Ed. Britton, Schmidt and Ell, Schattauer Verlag, Stuttgart.
458. Determination of the accuracy of ventricular volume measurement by single photon emission tomography. Laming PJ, Underwood SR, Walton S and Ell PJ. In: Nuklearmedizin, 15-17, 1986. Proceedings, Britton, Schmidt and Ell, Schattauer Verlag, Stuttgart.
459. 99mTc compound assists imaging of CBF. Ell PJ and Costa DC. Diagnostic Imaging, 8, 6, 112-117, 1986.
460. The in vivo distribution of 99Tcm-HMPAO in normal man. Costa DC, Ell PJ, Cullum ID and Jarritt PH. Nuclear Medicine Communications 7, 647-658, 1986.

1987

461. Radionuclide imaging of the central nervous system. Ell PJ. RAD, 18-19, 1987.
462. Cerebral blood flow. Ell PJ. Editorial, Nuclear Medicine Communications, 8, 7, 1987.
463. Stress induced right ventricular dysfunction: an indication of reversible right ventricular ischaemia. Underwood SR, Costa DC, Walton S, Laming PJ, Ell PJ, Emanuel RW and Swanton RH. European Journal of Nuclear Medicine, 12, 529-532, 1987.
464. 99Tcm-HMPAO brain uptake: sensitivity to physiological and pharmacological intervention in vivo. Costa DC, Lui D and Ell PJ. Nuclear Medicine Communications 8, 239, 1987.
465. The value of radionuclide oesophageal transit (OT). de Gara CJ, Wakeling H, Langford J, Jarritt PH, Hobsley M and Ell PJ. Nuclear Medicine Communications 8, 247, 1987.
466. Cerebral blood flow and arterial CO2 during cardiopulmonary bypass. Venn G, Sherry K, Treasure T, Newman S, Harrison M, Klinger L and Ell PJ. Nuclear Medicine Comunications 8, 295, 1987.
467. Neuropsychological sequelae of bypass 12 months after coronary artery surgery. Venn GE, Sherry K, Treasure T, Newman S, Harrison M and Ell PJ. British Heart Journal, 57, 565, 1987.
468. Functional imaging of the brain. Ell PJ, Jarritt PH, Costa DC, Cullum ID and Lui D. Seminars in Nuclear Medicine, 17, 3, 214-229, 1987.
469. Bone imaging and skeletal radiology in dysbaric osteonecrosis. Williams ES, Khreisat S, Ell PJ and King JD. Clinical Radiology, 38, 589-592, 1987.
470. Cerebral blood flow imaging in migraine. Costa DC, Davies PTG, Jones BE, Steiner TJ, Ell PJ and Clifford Rose F. In Advances in Headache Research, 75-80, Ed. F. Clifford Rose. Pub. John Libbey & Co. Ltd. 1987.
471. Cerebral blood flow. Editorial. Ell PJ. Nuclear Medicine Communications, 8, 453-455, 1987.
472. High resolution images of regional cerebral blood flow. Costa DC, Cullum ID, Jarritt PH and Ell PJ. Nuclear Medicine Communications, 8, 573-580, 1987.
473. Imaging cerebral damage in HIV infection. Ell PJ, Costa DC and Harrison M. The Lancet, II, 569-570, 1987.
474. Acute neuropsychological consequences of coronary artery bypass surgery. Newman S, Smith P, Treasure T, Joseph P, Ell PJ and Harrison M. Current Psychological Research and Reviews, 6, 2, 115-124, 1987.
475. Relative and absolute 99mTc-DMSA uptake measurements in normal and obstructed kidneys. Zananiri MC, Jarritt PH, Sarfarazi M and Ell PJ. Nuclear Medicine Communications, 8, 11, 869-880, 1987.

1988

476. New instrumentation, new tracers. The answer to clinical brain SPET. In PET/SPECT 1987. Ell PJ. Proceedings ACNP/SNM Symposium, Washington, 238-252, 1988 ACNP Publication 1988-7.

478. 99mTc-d, l-HMPAO and 201Tl-DDC show different intracellular distribution in rat brain. Costa DC, Lui D, Sinha AK, Jarritt PH and Ell PJ. Nuklearmedizin, Suppl. 24: 762-765; 1988.

479. Tracer options for single photon emission tomography of the brain. Ell PJ, Cullum ID, Lui D, Costa DC and Jarritt PH. In Impact of Functional Imaging in Neurology and Psychiatry, Current Problems in Neurology, 5, 54-70, Ed. by Wade, J. et al. John Willey, 1988.

480. 99mTc-HMPAO labelled white cell imaging - a new technique for the dynamic assessment of inflammatory bowel disesase. Heagerty AHM, Costa DC, Cairns SR, Ell PJ and McNeil NI. Gut, 28, A1389-A1390, 1987.

481. Determinants of cerebral blood flow during cardiopulmonary bypass. Venn GE, Sherry K, Treasure T, Newman S, Harrison M, Klinger L and Ell PJ. British Heart Journal, 59, 1, 103-104, 1988.

482. Single photon emission tomography: a practical methodology. Ell PJ. British Journal of Radiology, 61, 428-429, 1988.

483. Simultaneous dual radionuclide labelled white cells: 111In-oxine vs. 99mTc-HMPAO. A comparative study. Lui D, Costa DC, Jarritt PH and Ell PJ. Nuklearmedizin, 483-486, Ed. by Csernay, L, and Schmidt, H.A.E. Schattauer Verlag, 1988.

484. Unusual hypersensitivity to MDP: report of 2 cases. Costa DC, Eustace M, Lui D and Ell PJ. Nuclear Medicine Communications 9, 4, 322, 1988.

485. Preliminary data on 99mTc-HMPAO studies of patients with dementia (Alzheimer type and HIV) and Parkinson's disease. Costa DC, Ell PJ, Burns A, Philpot M and Levy R. Journal of Cerebral Blood Flow and Metabolism, 8, S109-S115, 1988.

486. Cerebral blood flow during cardiopulmonary bypass. Venn GE, Sherry K, Klinger L, Newman S, Treasure T, Harrison M and Ell PJ. European Journal of Cardiothoracic Surgery, 2, 360-363, 1988.

487. The differential sensitivity of radionuclide ventriculography for the selection of anterior and inferior infarction. Underwood SR, Walton S, Laming PJ, Ell PJ, Emanuel RW and Swanton RH. British Heart Journal, 60, 5, 411-416, 1988.

488. 99TcmECD: an alternative choice in 99Tcm cerebral blood flow studies. Ell PJ, Costa DC and Williams ES. British Journal of Radiology, 61, 659, 1988.

489. HMPAO - fundamental and clinical research. Biersack H, Büll U and Ell PJ. Nuclear Medicine, 27, 108-117, 1988.

490. White cells radiolabelled with 111In and 99mTc- a study of relative sensitivity and in vivo viability. Costa DC, Lui D and Ell PJ. Nuclear Medicine Communications, 9, 725-731, 1988.

1989

491. Impairment of cerebral function following cardiac and other major surgery. Treasure T, Smith P, Newman S, Schneidau A, Joseph PH, Ell PJ and Harrison M. European Journal of Cardiothoracic Surgery, 3, 216-221, 1989.

492. Quantitative phase analysis in the assessment of coronary artery disease. Underwood SR, Walton S, Laming PJ, Ell PJ, Emanuel RW and Swanton RH. British Heart Journal, 61, 14-22, 1989.

493. The investigation of Alzheimer's disease with single photon emission tomography. Burns A, Philpot M, Costa DC, Ell PJ and Levy R. Journal of Neurology, Neurosurgery and Psychiatry, 52, 248-253, 1989.

494. 99mTc-Pentavalent DMSA imaging detects metastases of poorly differentiated carcinoma of the thyroid. Costa DC, Glynne-Jones R, Falzon H, Lui D, Ryder JP and Ell PJ. Clinical Nuclear Medicine, 14, 218-221, 1989.

495. Changing patterns in patient referral: 1980-1987. Ell PJ and Lui D. Invited Paper to 1st issue of Medicina Nuclearis, 1, 35-41, 1989.

496. Biodistribution, dosimetry and clinical evaluation of 99mTc-ethyl-cisteinate dimer (ECD) in normal subjects and in patients with chronic cerebral infarction. Holman BL, Hellman RS, Goldsmith SJ, Mena IG, Leveille J, Oberadi PG, Moretti JL, Delaloye AB, Hill THC, Rigo P, van Heertum RL, Ell PJ, Buell U, De Roo MC and Morgan RA. Journal of Nuclear Medicine, 30, 6, 1018-1024, 1989.

497. X-ray dual photon absorptiometry - a new method for the measurement of bone density. Cullum I, Ell PJ and Ryder J. British Journal of Radiology, 62, 587-592, 1989.

498. Temporal lobe epilepsy - role of routine functional brain imaging. Costa DC and Ell PJ. The Lancet, I., 959, 1989.

499. Prognosis in stroke. Costa DC and Ell PJ. The Lancet, I., 218, 1989.

500. 99Tcm HMPAO washout from brain. Ell PJ and Costa DC. The Lancet, I, 665-666, 1989.

501. Brain blood flow imaging by SPET. Ell PJ. RAD, 15, 17-18, 1989.

502. Preliminary data obtained using a new densitometry methodology. Hall ML, Cullum I, Ryder J and Ell PJ. Nuclear Medicine Communications, 10, 5, 372 1989.

503. One year follow-up of dementia of Alzheimer type (DAT) patients: clinical and rCBF/SPET correlations. Costa DC, Philpot M, Burns A, Ell PJ and Levy R. Journal of Nuclear Medicine, 30, 5, 895, 1989.

504. Epithelial membrane antigen (EMA): a target antigen for radiolabelled monoclonal antibodies (MABs) in colorectal cancer imaging? Davidson B, Young H, Waddington W, Clarke G, Short M, Boulos P, Styles J, Dean C and Ell PJ. Journal of Nuclear Medicine, 30, 5, 800, 1989.

505. Intracellular localisation of 99Tcm-d, l-HMPAO and 201Tl-DDC in rat brain. Costa DC, Lui D, Sinha AK, Jarritt PH and Ell PJ. Nuclear Medicine Communications 10, 459-466, 1989.

506. 99Tcm-HMPAO SPET and cerebral blood flow: a study of CO_2 reactivity. Choksey MS, Costa DC, Iannotti F, Ell PJ and Crockard HA. Nuclear Medicine Communications 10, 609-618, 1989.

507. Nuclear medicine in AIDS. Ell PJ. British Journal of Radiology, 62, 878, 1989.

508. Tc-99m-d, l-HMPAO uptake mechanism in cultured astrocytes. Costa DC, Hubank M, Sinha AK, Lui D and Ell PJ. The Journal of Nuclear Medicine and Allied Sciences, 33, 3, 279, 1989.

509. Modern imaging procedures for ventricular function and myocardial perfusion and their clinical significance. Ell PJ. European Journal of Nuclear Medicine, 15, 8, 533, 1989.

510. New trends and facilities in nuclear medicine. Ell PJ. European Journal of Nuclear Medicine, 15, 8, 589, 1989.

511. SPET studies of the human brain. Ell PJ. European Journal of Nuclear Medicine, 15, 8, 432, 1989.

512. 99mTc-HIG: a new agent for the identification and localisation of active inflammatory bowel disease and intra-abdominal sepsis. Ell PJ. European Journal of Nuclear Medicine, 15, 8, 562, 1989.

513. Subcellular localization of 99mTc-HMPAO and 201Tl-DDC in rat brain - preliminary results. Costa DC, Lui D, Sinha AK, Jarritt PH, Ell PJ and Ekins RP. In Blood Flow in the Brain ed. W.J. Angerson et al., Clarendon Press, Oxford, chap. 5, 44-49, 1989.

1990

514. Skeletal scintigraphy in carcinoma of the breast - ten year retrospective study of 389 patients. Ahmed A, Glynne-Jones R and Ell PJ. Nuclear Medicine Communications, 11, 421-426, 1990.

515. 99mTc-d, l-HMPAO uptake mechanism in astrocytes in culture. Costa DC, Hubank M, Sinha A and Ell PJ. In Technetium and Rhenium in Chemistry and Nuclear Medicine ed. M. Nicolini, G. Bandoli, and U. Mazzi, Cortina International, Verona, Raven Press, New York; pp 773-776, 1990.

516. 99mTc-human immunoglobulin (HIG) - first results of a new agent for the localization of infection and inflammation. Buscombe JR, Lui D, Ensing G, Jong R and Ell PJ. European Journal of Nuclear Medicine, 16, 649-655, 1990.

517. A comparison of SPET and CT in the investigation of chronic low back pain. Buscombe JR, Summers B, Edgar M, Hogg P and Ell PJ. Nuclear Medicine Communications, 11, 199, 1990.

518. First study of the efficacy of 99Tcm-HIG as a new agent for the investigation of infection and inflammation. Buscombe JR, Lui D and Ell PJ. Nuclear Medicine Communications, 11, 210, 1990.

519. Dobutamine thallium myocardial perfusion imaging: an alterntive form of stress. Pennell DJ, Underwood SR, Ell PJ, Swanton RH and Walker JM. Nuclear Medicine Communications, 11, 190, 1990.

520. Dobutamine magnetic resonance imaging in ischaemic heart disease; a new technique. Pennell DJ, Underwood SR, Ell PJ, Swanton RH, Walker JM and Longmore DB. European Journal of Nuclear Medicine, 16:420, 1990.

521. MRI of reversible myocardial ischaemia during dobutamine stress. Pennell DJ, Underwood SR, Manzara CC, Mohiaddin RH, Poole-Wilson PA, Ell PJ, Swanton RH, Walker JM and Longmore DB. Proceedings European Congress of NMR, 4, 1990.

522. The assessment of aortic flow and acceleration during dobutamine stess by magnetic rsonance imaging. Pennell DJ, Underwood SR, Manzara CC, Mohiaddin RH, Firmin DN, Poole-Wilson PA, Ell PJ, Swanton RH, Walker JM and Longmore DB. European Heart Journal (Abstr. Suppl), 11: 26, 1990.

523. Detection of reversible myocardial ischaemia with magnetic resonance imaging during dobutamine infusion. Pennell DJ, Underwood SR, Manzara CC, Mohiaddin RH, Poole-Wilson PA, Ell PJ, Swanton RH, Walker JM and Longmore DB. Radiology 177 (P): 101, 1990.

524. Magnetic resonance imaging of reversible myocardial ischaemia using intravenous dipridamole. Pennell DJ, Underwood SR, Ell PJ, Swanton RH, Walker JM and Longmore DB. Journal of Magnetic Resonance Imaging, 8 (suppl 1): 69, 1990.

525. Magnetic resonance imaging of reversible myocardial ischaemia during dobutamine stress. Pennell DJ, Underwood SR, Manzara CC, Mohiaddin RH, Poole-Wilson PA, Ell PJ, Swanton RH, Walker JM and Longmore DB. Journal of Magnetic Resonance Imaging, 8 (suppl 1): 451, 1990

526. Dipyridamole magnetic resonance imaging: a comparison with 201thallium emission tomography. Pennell DJ, Underwood SR, Ell PJ, Swanton RH, Walker JM and Longmore DB. British Heart Journal, 64, 362-369, 1990.

527. In-vivo characterisation of 3-iodo-6-methoxybenzamide 123I in humans. Costa DC, Verhoeff NPLG, Cullum I, Ell PJ, Syed GHS, Barrett J, Pallazidou E, Toome B and van Royen E. European Journal of Nuclear Medicine, 16, 813-817, 1990.

528. Effect of disease activity on bone density on rheumatoid arthritis. Hall ML, Ell PJ and Spector TD. British Journal of Rheumatology, 29, 21, 1990.

529. An assessment of the effect of oral corticosteroids on bone mineral density in systemic lupus erythematosis: a preliminary study with dual energy X-ray absorptiometry. Dhillon VB, Davies MC, Hall ML, Ell PJ, Jacobs HS, Snaith ML and Isenberg DA. Annals of Rheumatic Diseases, 49:624-626, 1990.

530. Single photon emission computed tomography (SPET) of the brain. Ell PJ. Journal of Neurosciences Methods, 34, 207-217, 1990.

531. Editorial. Ell PJ. European Journal of Nuclear Medicine, 16, 1, 1990.

532. Highlights of the European Association of Nuclear Medicine Congress, Amsterdam, 1990. Ell PJ. European Journal of Nuclear Medicine, 16, 873-890, 1990.

533. The range of bone density in normal British women. Hall M, Heavens J, Cullum I and Ell PJ. British Journal of Radiology, 63, 266-269, 1990.

534. Brain perfusion patterns in human immunodeficiency virus (HIV) positive patients. Hall ML, Miller R, Costa DC, Shields J and Ell PJ. Nuclear Medicine Communications, 11, 210, 1990.

535. Dominant versus non-dominant femoral density. Hall ML, Heavens J and Ell PJ. In: Current Research in Osteoporosis and Bone Mineral Measurement - page 55 of 1990 Bath Osteoporosis Conference Proceedings Ed. Ring EFI. British Institute of Radiology, 1990.

536. Amenorrhoea: a risk factor for osteoporosis. Davies MC, Hall ML, Ell PJ and Jacobs HS. In: Current Research in Osteoporosis and Bone Mineral Measurement - page 65

of the 1990 Bath Osteoporosis Conference Proceedings, Ed. Ring EFI. British Institute of Radiology, 1990.

537. Diagnosis of inflammation and infection: a new approach. Houston EA, Nockles J and Ell PJ. Nuclear Medicine Communications, 11, 245, 1990.

538. Nanocolloid imaging in the distinction of bone and bone marrow metastatic spread. Huggett SM, Nimalaraj T, Costa DC and Ell PJ. Nuclear Medicine Communications, 11, 230, 1990.

539. Alveolar targeting of inhaled 99Tcm-DTPA with a new delivery system - the APE nebulizer. Miller RF, Jarritt PH, Lui D, Kidery J, de Jong R and Ell PJ. Nuclear Medicine Communications, 11, 182, 1990.

540. Use of 99Tcm-MIBI in conjunction with monophasic action potential in the detection of myocardial ischaemia. John RM, Costa DC, Taggart P, Sutton P, Ell PJ and Swanton RH. Nuclear Medicine Communications, 11, 185, 1990.

541. Assessment of regional myocardial ischaemia by a combination of nuclear imaging (99mTc-methoxyisobutylisonitrile) and monophasic action potential recordings. John RM, Sutton P, Taggart P, Costa DC, Ell PJ and Swanton RH. British Heart Journal, 64, 10, 1990.

542. Effect of ischaemia on the relation between monophasic action potential duration and cycle length in the human left ventricle. John RM, Taggart P, Sutton P, Ell PJ and Swanton RH. British Heart Journal, 64, 76, 1990.

543. Advantages and limitations of 99Tcm-DMSA scans in routine clinical work. MacSweeney AF, Lythgoe M, Costa DC and Ell PJ. Nuclear Medicine Communications, 11, 230, 1990.

544. Myocardial perfusion SPET imaging with 99mTc-MIBI in the detection and localisation of coronary artery disease: a comparison with 201Tl. Mittal RB, Ahmed A, Costa DC and Ell PJ. Medicina Nuclearis, 2, 179-186, 1990.

545. Symptomatic bradycardia complicating the use of intravenous dipyridamole for thallium-201 myocardial perfusion imaging. Pennell DJ, Underwood SR and Ell PJ. International Journal of Cardiology, 27, 272-274, 1990.

546. Dipyridamole thallium myocardial perfusion imaging: differential coronary flow or ischaemia? Pennell DJ, Underwood SR, Ell PJ, Swanton RH, Walker JM and Longmore DB. Nuclear Medicine Communications, 11, 189-190, 1990.

547. Thallium myocardial perfusion imaging using dobutamine; an alternative to dipyridamole. Pennell DJ, Underwood SR, Ell PJ, Swanton RH and Walker JM. Nuclear Medicine Communications, 11, 190, 1990.

548. Dobutamine magnetic resonance imaging in patients with coronary artery disease. Pennell DJ, Underwood SR, Ell PJ, Swanton RH, Walker JM and Longmore DB. British Heart Journal, 69, 100, 1990.

549. The investigation of osteoradionecrosis of the mandible by 99mTc-methylenediphosphonate radionuclide bone scans. Hutchinson IL, Cullum ID, Langford JA, Jarritt PH, Ell PJ and Harris M. British Journal of Oral and Maxillofacial Surgery, 28, 143-149, 1990.

550. Neurocamara: Una Gammacamara de 3 detectores para gamagrafia cerebral. Costa DC, Townsend CE, Jarritt PH and Ell PJ. Revista Esp. Med. Nuclear, Supl III, 33-37, 1990.

551. PET reflections. Ell PJ. Editorial. Eur. J. Nucl. Med., 17, 1, 1990.

1991

552. The action of dipyridamole for thallium myocardial perfusion imaging: differential coronary artery flow or ischaemia? A comparative assessment with magnetic resonance imaging. Pennell DJ, Underwood SR, Ell PJ, Swanton RH, Walker JM and Longmore DB. Radioactive Isotopes in Clinical Medicine and Research, 56-62, 1991.
553. 99mTc HMPAO SPET studies in traumatic intracerebral haematoma. Choksey MS, Costa DC, Iannotti F, Ell PJ and Crockard HA. The Journal of Neurology, Neurosurgery and Psychiatry, 54, 6-11, 1991.
554. Variation between femurs as measured by dual energy X-ray absorptiometry (DEXA). Hall ML, Heavens J and Ell PJ. European Journal of Nuclear Medicine 18, 38-49, 1991.
555. Nanocolloid imaging in early bone or marrow metastatic spread. Huggett SM, Nimalaraj T, Costa DC and Ell PJ. Journal of Nuclear Medicine and Technology, 19, 33-35, 1991.
556. The APE nebulizer - a new delivery system for the alveolar targeting of particulate technetium-99mDTPA. Miller RF, Jarritt PH, Lui D, Kidery J, Temple SJG and Ell PJ. European Journal of Nuclear Medicine, 18, 164-170, 1991.
557. The use of cerebral activation procedure with single photon emission tomography. A review. Ring HA, George M, Costa DC and Ell PJ. European Journal of Nuclear Medicine, 18, 133-142, 1991.
558. Nuclear medicine and medical literature. Editorial. Ell PJ. European Journal of Nuclear Medicine, 18, 713-714, 1991.
559. Dobutamine 201Thallium myocardial perfusion tomography. Pennell DJ, Underwood SR, Swanton RH, Walker JM and Ell PJ. Journal of American College of Cardiology, 18, 1471-1479, 1991.
560. First demonstration of human parietal lobe activation using SPET. Ring HA, George MS, Costa DC, Kouris K and Ell PJ. Nuclear Medicine Communications, 12, 273, 1991.
561. Post gastrectomy osteoporosis. Tovey FI, Hall ML, Ell PJ and Hobsley M. British Journal of Surgery, 78, 1335-1337, 1991.
562. Neuroreceptor imaging. Ell PJ. Nuclear Medicine Communications, 12, 829-830, 1991.
563. Single photon emission tomography in Alzheimer's disease. A longitudinal study of changes in relative regional cerebral blood flow. Philpot MP, Costa DC, Burns A, Levy R and Ell PJ. Journal of Neurology, Neurosurgery and Psychiatry, 6, 767-774, 1991.
564. Central D2 dopaminergic receptor status in treatment responsive and treatment resistant schizophrenic patients as measured by I-123 IBZM single photon emission tomography (SPET). Pilowsky LS, Costa DC, Kerwin R, Murray RM and Ell PJ. Schizophrenia Research, 4, 3, 410, 1991.
565. How far investigations for occult metastases in breast cancer aid the clinician. Glynne-Jones R, Young T, Ahmed A, Ell PJ and Berry RJ. Clinical Oncology 3, 65-72, 1991.
566. Nuclear medicine and receptor studies. Ell PJ. Wiener Klinische Wochenschrift. Editorial, 15, 437, 1991.
567. Imaging the endocrine glands. Ell PJ. British Journal of Hospital Medicine, 46, 331-334, 1991
568. Bone Scanning in Cancer. Ell PJ. Current Opinion in Radiology, 3, 791-796, 1991.

569. Qualitative vs Bullseye quantitative analysis of myocardial perfusion SPET maps with Tcc-99m MIBI. Mahmood S, John RM, Costa DC, Jarritt PH and Ell PJ. Nuclear Medicine Communications, 12, 266-267, 1991.

570. Tc-99m HMPAO SPET abnormalities in infantile autism. George MS, Costa DC, Kouris K, Ring H and Ell PJ. Nuclear Medicine Communications, 12, 275, 1991.

571. Bone marrow scintigraphy with Tc-99m HMPAO labelled white blood cells. Nockles J, Carthy TB, Lui D, Costa DC and Ell PJ. Nuclear Medicine Communications, 12, 306, 1991.

572. Tc-99m HMPAO and In-111 oxime labelled white blood cells (WBC) in the investigation of infective chest disease. Buscombe JR, Miller RF, Hounslow N, Costa DC and Ell PJ. Nuclear Medicine Communications, 12, 318-319, 1991.

573. Brain tumour uptake of Iodo-alpha-methyl-tyrosine. Ell PJ. Journal of Nuclear Medicine, 32, 2193, 1991.

574. The evaluation of a new three detector tomographic gamma camera (IGE Neurocam) in a clinical environment. Townsend CE, Costa DC, Jarritt PH, Kidery J and Ell PJ. In: Nuclear Medicine: The State of the Art in Europe. Ed. HAE Schmidt & JB van der Schoot, Schattauer Verlag, 11-13, 1991.

575. Benzodiazepine receptor density in human brain measured in vivo with 123I-Iomazenil SPECT. Verhoeff NPLG, von Royen EA, Ell PJ, Costa DC and Hasler PH. In: Nuclear Medicine: The State of the Art in Europe. Ed. HAE Schmidt & JB van der Schoot, Schattauer Verlag, 203-206, 1991.

576. Dopamine D2-receptor imaging with dynamic I-123 SPET in patients with schizophrenia or HIV Encephalopathy Nuclear Medicine. Verhoeff NPLG, Costa DC, Ell PJ et al. In: Nuclear Medicine: The State of the Art in Europe. Ed. HAE Schmidt & JB van der Schoot, Schattauer Verlag, 207-212, 1991.

577. Radionuclide bone marrow imaging with 99Tcm-HMPAO labelled white blood cells (WBC). Costa DC, Lui D, Lythgoe M and Ell PJ. In: Nuclear Medicine: The State of the Art in Europe. Ed. HAE Schmidt & JB van der Schoot, Schattauer Verlag, 318-320, 1991.

578. Thallium scintigraphy. Underwood SR, Tweddel A, Hutton I, Ell PJ and Walton ST. The Lancet, 338, 1405-1406, 1991.

579. Endocardial monphasic action potential recordings for the detection of myocardial ischemia in man: A study using atrial pacing stress and myocardial perfusion sctingraphy. John RM, Taggart PI, Sutton PM, Costa DC, Ell PJ and Swanton RH. American Heart Journal, 122, 1559-1609, 1991.

580. Brain perfusion patterns with 99Tcm-HMPAO/SPET in patients with Gilles de la Tourette Syndrome - short report. Hall M, Costa DC, Shields J, Heavens M, Robertson M and Ell PJ. In: Nuclear Medicine Ed. Schmidt & Schoot, 243-245, Schattauer-Verlag, 1991.

581. Dobutamine thallium myocardial perfusion tomography. Pennell DJ, Underwood SR and Ell PJ. British Heart Journal, 66: 88-89, 1991.

582. Dobutamine thallium myocardial perfusion tomography. Pennell DJ, Underwood SR, Swanton RH, Walker JM and Ell PJ. European Heart Journal (Abstr. Suppl), 12: 16, 1991.

583. Use of dobutamine in thallium myocardial perfusion tomography: Useful alternative to dipyridamole. Pennell DJ, Underwood SR, Swanton RH, Walker JM and Ell PJ. Radiology, 181 (P), 289, 1991.

584. MR velocity mapping of aortic acceleration during dobutamine induced myocardial ischaemia. Pennell DJ, Underwood SR, Manzara CC, Firming DN, Ell PJ, Swanton RH, Walker JM and Longmore DB. Journal of Magnetic Resonance Imaging 9 (suppl 1): 242, 1991.

585. Magnetic resonance assessment of aortic flow during dobutamine stress predicts extent of myocardial ischaemia. Pennell DJ, Underwood SR, Manzara CC, Firmin DN, Ell PJ, Swanton RH, Walker JM and Longmore DB. British Heart Journal, 105, 1991.

586. Dopamine D2 receptor binding in drug naive schizophrenics. Gray NS, Pedro BM, Pilowsky L, Costa DC, Verhoeff NPLG, Ell PJ and Kerwin RW. Neuropsychiatry. Journal of Psychopharmacology. British Association of Psychopharmacology. Abstract Book, p177.

587. A 123 I-IBZM single photon emission tomography study of in vivo dopamine receptor occupancy in typical antipsychotic responders and non responders. Pilowsky L, Costa DC, Ell PJ, Verhoeff N and Kerwin RW. British Journal of Pharmacology, 107, 68P.

588. A single photon emission tomography study of in-vivo dopamine receptor occupancy for typical antipsychotics and the atypical drug clozapine in schizophrenia. Pilowsky L, Costa DC, Ell PJ, Verhoeff N and Kerwin RW. British Journal of Pharmacology, 107, 69P.

1992

589. The interrelation between the monophasic action potential duration, cycle length and ischaemia in the human left ventricle. John RM, Taggart PI, Sutton PM, Ell PJ and Swanton H. European Heart Journal, 13, 310-315, 1992.

590. Challenges for nuclear medicine in the 90's. Ell PJ. Nuclear Medicine Communications, 13, 65-75, 1992.

591. Clinical audit: Does 67Ga-citrate (67Ga) scintigraphy in AIDS patients provide clinically useful information? Wassie E, Buscombe JR, Miller RF and Ell PJ. Nuclear Medicine Communications, 13, 209, 1992.

592. Safety of combined dipyridamole-exercise 201Tl myocardial perfusion scintigraphy. Hall ML, Mahmood S and Ell PJ. Nuclear Medicine Communications, 13, 217, 1992.

593. Physical comparison of two three-headed SPET systems with emphasis on brain studies. Clarke G, Kouris K, Jarritt PH, Townsend CE, Costa DC and Ell PJ. Nuclear Medicine Communications, 13, 220, 1992

594. rCBF/SPET in patients with myalgic encephalomyelitis. Douli V, Brostoff J, Costa DC, Kouris K and Ell PJ. Nuclear Medicine Communications, 13, 222, 1992.

595. Regional cerebral blood flow during verbal memory challenge - a split-dose single photon emission tomography (SPET) study. Busatto G, Kerwin RW, Costa DC, David AS, Pilowsky L and Ell PJ. Nuclear Medicine Communications, 13, 4, 28, 1992

596. Fast skeletal SPET in the assessment of chest metastases in young patients with primary bone tumours. Buscombe JR, Townsend, CE, Clarke G, Kouris K and Ell PJ. Nuclear Medicine Communications, 13, 248, 1992.

597. Myocardial perfusion of patients with left bundle branch block: a comparison between dynamic exercise and vasodilator pharmacological stress. Marinho NVS, Costa DC and Ell PJ. Nuclear Medicine Communications, 13, 302, 1992.

598. Nuclear Medicine. Ell PJ. Postgraduate Medical Journal, 68: 82-105, 1992.

599. Physical assessment of GE/CGR Neurocam and comparison with a single rotating gamma camera. Kouris K Jarritt PH, Costa DC and Ell PJ. European Journal of Nuclear Medicine, 19, 163-242, 1992.

600. SPECT in epilepsy. Markus HS, Kouris K, Costa DC and Ell PJ. Neurology, 42, 1127-1128, 1992.

601. Post viral fatigue syndrome. Costa DC, Brostoff J, Douli V and Ell PJ. British Medical Journal, 304, 1567-1992.

602. Hepatobiliary scintigraphy in the diagnosis of AIDS-related sclerosing cholangitis. Buscombe JR, Miller RF and Ell PJ. Nuclear Medicine Communications, 13, 154-160, 1992.

603. Diagnosing Alzheimer's disease. Butler RE, Costa DC, Ell PJ and Katona CLE. British Medical Journal, 304, 574-575, 1992.

604. Mapping cerebral blood flow. Editorial. Ell PJ. Journal of Nuclear Medicine, 33, 1843-1845, 1992.

605. Clozapine, single photon emission tomography, and the D2 dopamine receptor blockade hypothesis in schizophrenia. Pilowsky LS, Costa DC, Ell PJ, Murray RM, Verhoeff NPLG and Kerwin RW. The Lancet, 340: 199-202, 1992.

606. Elevated frontal cerebral blood flow in Gilles de la Tourette syndrome (GTS): A 99Tcm-HMPAO SPECT study. George MS, Trimble MR, Costa DC, Robertson MM, Ring HA and Ell PJ. Psychiatry Research, Neuroimaging 45, 143-151, 1992.

607. Demonstration of human motor cortex activating using SPECT. George MS, Ring HA, Costa DC, Kouris K and Ell PJ. Journal of Neural Transmission, 87, 231-236, 1992.

608. Functional brain imaging - SPECT and PET. Ell PJ and Costa DC. Current Opinion in Neurology and Neurosurgery, 5, 863-869, 1992.

609. Magnetic resonance imaging during dobutamine stress in coronary artery disease. Pennell DJ, Underwood SR, Manzara CC, Ell PJ, Swanton RH, Walker JM and Longmore DB. American Journal of Cardiology, 70, 34-40, 1992.

610. Vasodilator myocardial perfusion imaging: demonstration of local electrophysiological changes of ischaemia. John RM, Taggart PI, Sutton PM, Costa DC, Ell PJ and Swanton H. British Heart Journal, 68, 21-30, 1992.

611. The use of thallium-201 lung/heart ratios. Mahmood S, Buscombe JR and Ell PJ. European Journal of Nuclear Medicine, 19, 807-814, 1992.

612. Clinical high resolution skeletal SPET in 8 minutes utilizing a multi-detector gamma camera. Buscombe JR, Townsend CE, Kouris K, Clarke G, Jarritt PH, Mahmood S and Ell PJ. British Journal of Radiology, 65 (Congress Suppl), 34, 1992.

613. Cerebral blood flow abnormalities in adults with infantile autism. George MS, Costa DC, Kouris K, Ring HA and Ell PJ. The Journal of Nervous and Mental Disease, 180, 413-417, 1992.

614. Effect of vigabatrin on striatal dopamine receptors: Evidence in humans for interactions of GABA and dopamine systems. Ring HA, Trimble MR, Costa DC, George MS, Verhoeff P and Ell PJ. Journal of Neurology, Neurosurgery and Psychiatry, 55, 758-761, 1992.

615. Direct effect of dobutamine on action potential duration in ischaemic compared with normal areas in the human ventricle. John RM, Taggart PI, Sutton PM, Ell PJ and Swanton H. Journal of American College of Cardiology, 20, 896-903, 1992.

616. Recent advances with SPET: from instrumentation to clinical practice. Ell PJ. Revista Espanola di Medicina Nuclear, 11, 44-50, 1992.

617. Assessment of myocardial viability with 201Tl SPET and reinjection technique: a quantitative approach. Mahmmod S, Buscombe JR, Hall ML, Jarritt PH, Costa DC and Ell PJ. Nuclear Medicine Communications, 13, 783-789, 1992.

618. The role of blood flow SPET in the investigation of epilepsy - a comparison with other methods. Schmitz B, Jackson G, Costa DC, Ring H, Moriarty J, Conelly A, Duncan J, Trimble M and Ell PJ. Epilepsy, 1, (Suppl. A), 10, 1992.

619. Hippocampus-Beurteilung mittels HMPAO-SPECT: Vergleich mit MRI und MR-Spektroskopie. Schmitz B, Costa DC, Ring H, Moriarty J, Conelly A, Duncan J, Trimble M and Ell PJ. Epilepsie-Blätter, 5, 29, 1992.

620. Temporal lobe activation during memory challenge: a SPET study. Busatto G, Kerwin RW, Costa DC, David AS, Pilowsky LS and Ell PJ. Schizophrenia Research 6 (2) (Special issue) VIth Biennial European Workshop on Schizophrenia, Badgastein, Austria, January 26-31, 148-149, 1992.

621. Thallium myocardial perfusion tomography using dobutamine stress. Pennell DJ, Underwood SR, Swanton RH, Walker MJ and Ell PJ. Postgraduate Medical Journal, 68 (Suppl. 2), S12-S13, 1992.

622. Regional cerebral blood flow during verbal memory challenge - split-dose single photon emission tomography (SPET) study. Busatto G, Kerwin RW, Costa DC, David AS, Pilowsky LS and Ell PJ. Nuclear Medicine Communications, 13, 28, 1992.

1993

623. Nuclear Medicine in Europe. Ell PJ. Nuclear Medicine Communications, 14, 239, 1993.

624. Simultaneous low level dynamic exercise and adenosine infusion in the assessment of myocardial perfusion. Mahmood S, Yepes-Mora S, Costa DC, Buscombe JR and Ell PJ. Nuclear Medicine Communications, 14, 239, 1993.

625. Effect of lung scintigraphy report on clinician's use of anticoagulants. Kaboli P, Buscombe JR and Ell PJ. Nuclear Medicine Communications, 14, 278, 1993.

626. Ceretec® brain perfusion SPET: a reference normal file. Costa DC, Kaboli P, Douli V and Ell PJ. Nuclear Medicine Communications, 14, 269, 1993.

627. D2 dopamine receptor abnormalities in schizophrenia: a 123I-IBZM SPET study. Pilowsky LS, Costa DC, Ell PJ, Verhoeff NPLG, Murray RM and Kerwin RW. Nuclear Medicine Communications, 14, 268, 1993.

628. D2 dopamine receptor blockade and response to anti-psychotic treatment: a 123I-IBZM SPET sudy. Pilowsky LS, Costa DC, Ell PJ, Verhoeff NPLG, Murray RM and Kerwin RW. Nuclear Medicine Communications, 14, 267, 1993.

629. Regional cerebral blood flow (rCBF) in schizophrenia during verbal memory activation: a 99Tcm-HMPAO split-dose single photon emission tomographic study. Busatto GF, Costa DC, Ell PJ, Pilowsky LS, David AS and Kerwin RW. Nuclear Medicine Communications, 14, 267, 1993.

630. A study of Gilles de la Tourette syndrome using HMPAO SPET. Moriarty J, Costa DC, Schmitz B, Trimble MR, Robertson MM and Ell PJ. Nuclear Medicine Communications, 14, 266-267, 1993.

631. Safety of dobutamine for thallium imaging in asthma. Pennell DJ, Underwood SR and Ell PJ. Nuclar Medicine Communications, 14, 265, 1993.

632. Comparison in the efficacy of gallium and radiolabelled immunoglobulin in identifying infection in HIV positive patients. Buscombe JR, Miller RF, Oyen WJG, Classens RAM, Corstens FHM and Ell PJ. British Journal of Radiology, 66, 55-56, 1993.

633. The future of nuclear medicine: a perspective from Europe. Ell PJ. Journal of Nuclear Medicine, 33, 169-170, 1993.

634. Antipsychotic medication, D2 dopamine receptor blockade and clinical response-a 123I-IBZM SPET (single photon emission tomography) study. Pilowsky LS, Costa DC, Ell PJ, Verhoeff NPLG, Murray RM and Kerwin RW. Psychological Medicine.23, 791-797, 1993

635. Thallium myocardial perfusion tomography using intravenous dypiridamole combined with maximal dynamic exercise. Pennell DJ, Mavrogeni S, Anagnostopoulos C, Ell PJ and Underwood SR. Nuclear Medicine Communications, 14, 939-945, 1993.

636. Safety of Dobutamine stress thallium myocardial perfusion tomography in patients with asthma. Pennell DJ, Underwood SR and Ell PJ. American Journal of Cardiology, 71, 1346-1350, 1993.

637. Biodistribution and tumour localisation of 131I SWA11 recognising the cluster W4 antigen in patents with small cell lung cancer. Ledermann JA, Marston NJ, Stahel EA, Waitel, R, Buscombe JR and Ell PJ. British Journal of Cancer, 68, 119-121, 1993.

638. High sensitivity of optimized interictal HMPAO SPECT in focal epilepsies. Schmitz B, Jackson G, Costa DC, Ring H, Moriarty J, Connell A, Duncan J, Trimble M and Ell PJ. Epilepsia, 34, (2), 111-112, 1993.

639. Hippocampal blood flow in epilepsy: comparison with MRI, MR spectroscopy and T-2 relaxometry. Schmitz B, Jackson G, Costa DC, Ring H, Moriarty J, Connelly A, Ducan J, Trimble M, Gadian D and Ell PJ. Epilepsia, 34 (2), 195, 1993.

640. Indium-111 labelled polyclonal human immunoglobulin: Identifying focal infection in patients positive for human immunodeficiency virus. Buscombe JR, Oyen Wim JG, Grant A, Roland AMJ, Jos van der Meer, Corstens FHM, Ell PJ and Miller RF. Journal of Nuclear Medicine, 34, 1621-1625, 1993.

641. D2 receptor abnormalities in schizophrenia. A 123 I-IBZM single photon emission study of drug naive schizophrenic patients. Pilowsky L, Costa DC, Ell PJ, Verhoeff NPLG, Murray RM and Kerwin RW. Journal of Cerebral Blood Flow and Metabolism, 13, S512, 1993.

642. Latent inhibition in drug naive schizophrenics. Gray NS, Pilowsky LS, Costa DC, Verhoeff NPLG, Ell PJ and Kerwin RW. Schizophrenia Research, 9, 176, 1993.

643. Temporal lobe activation derive verbal memory challenge: A single photon emission tomography study. Busatto GF, Kerwin RW, Costa DC, David AS, Pilowsky LS and Ell PJ. Schizophrenia Research, 6(2), 148, 1992.

644. Left lateralised asymmetry of striatal D2 receptor binding in antipsychotic free schizophrenic patients: a 123I-IBZM SPET study. Pilowsky LS, Costa DC, Verhoeff NPLG, Ell PJ and Kerwin RW. Schizophrenia Research, 9, 200, 1993.

645. D2 Dopamine receptor occupancy and response to typical and atypical antipsychotics. Kerwin RW, Pilowsky LS, Costa DC, Ell PJ, Murray RM and Verhoeff NPLG. Schizophrenia Research 9, 200, 1993.

646. Activation studies of medial temporal and frontal lobes in schizophrenia: a study using 99mTc-HMPAO SPET. Busatto G, Costa DC, Ell PJ, Pilowsky LS and Kerwin RW. Schizophrenia Research 9 (2-3): 195, 1993.

647. Dopamine D2 receptor binding in the basal ganglia in patients with schizophrenia: relationship to stereotypy. Pedro BM, Gray NS, Pilowsky L, Costa DC, Hemsley DR, Gray JA, Verhoeff NPLG, Ell PJ and Kerwin R. Schizophrenia Research, 9, 186, 1993.

648. Reporting ventilation perfusion lung scintigraphy: impact on subsequent use of anticoagulant therapy. Kaboli P, Buscombe JR and Ell PJ. Postgraduate Medical Journal, 69, 851-855, 1993.

649. Medial temporal and frontal lobe activity during memory activation in schizophrenia. Busatto G, Costa DC, Ell PJ, Pilowsky L, David AS and Kerwin RW. Journal of Cerebral Blood Flow and Metabolism, 13, S513, 1993.

650. A clinical high resolution single photon emission tomography using a triple-headed gamma camera. Buscombe JR, Townsend CE, Kouris K, Clarke G, Mahmood S, Jarritt PH and Ell PJ. British Journal of Radiology, 66, 817-822, 1993.

651. Tc-99m HMPAO single photon emission tomography in late life depression: a pilot study of regional cerebral blood flow at rest and during a verbal fluency task. Philpot M, Banerjee S, Needham-Bennett H, Costa DC and Ell PJ. Journal of Affective Disorders, 28, 233-240, 1993.

652. Role of radionuclide venography in the detection of proximal deep vein thrombosis: a prospective comparative study. Mohamadiyeh MKh, Shaban AA, El-Desouki M, Malabarey T and Ell PJ. Nuclear Medicine Communications, 14, 1014-1022, 1993.

653. If I were a patient. Ell PJ. Journal of Royal College of Physicians of London, 27, 478, 1993.

654. Dopamine D2 receptor occupancy in vivo and response to the new anti psychotic risperidone: A case study. Busatto, GF, Pilowsky LS, Kerwin RW, Ell PJ, Costa DC and Verhoeff NPLG. British Journal of Psychiatry, 163, 833-834, 1993

655. Stereotype, schizophrenia and dopamine D2 receptor binding in the basal ganglia. Pedro BM, Pilowsky LS, Costa DC, Hemsley DR, Ell PJ, Verhoeff NPLG, Kerwin RW and Gray NS. Psychological Medicine. Psychological Medicine, 24, 423-429, 1993.

656. Regional cerebral blood flow in schizophrenia: A 99mTc HMPAO single photon emission tomography (SPET) study during verbal memory activation. Busatto GF, Costa DC, Ell PJ, Pilowsky LS, David AS and Kerwin RW. Psychological Medicine, 24, 463-472, 1993.

1994

657. Bradycardia progressing to cardiac arrest during adenosine thallium myocardial perfusion imaging in occult sino-atrial disease. Pennell DJ, Mahmood S, Ell PJ and Underwood SR. European Journal of Nuclear Medicine, 21, 170-172, 1994.

658. The diagnosis and assessment of an adult with anomalous origin of the left coronary artery from the pulmonary artery. Cowie MR, Mahmood S and Ell PJ. European Journal of Nuclear Medicine, 21, 1017-1019, 1994.

659. Cyclical etidronate therapy and postgastrectomy osteoporosis. Tovey FI, Hall ML, Ell PJ and Hobsley M. British J of Surgery, 81, 468-469, 1994.

660. Whole body imaging of thallium-201 after six different stress regimes. Pennell DJ and Ell PJ. Journal of Nuclear Medicine, 35, 425-428, 1994.

661. D2 dopamine receptor binding in the basal ganglia of anti-psychotic free schizophrenic patients. A 123 I-IBZM single photon emission computerized tomography study. Pilowsky L, Costa DC, Ell PJ, Verhoeff NPLG, Murray RM and Kerwin RW. British Journal of Psychiatry, 164, 16-26, 1994.

662. Science citation index and impact factors. Ell PJ. Nuclear Medicine Communications, 15, 205, 1994.

663. Planar 99mTc-DMSA renal scintigraphy and interobserver variability. Gacinovic S, Costa DC, Buscombe JR and Ell PJ. Nuclear Medicine Communications, 15, 203-204, 1994.

664. Tomographic imaging of 99mTc-DMSA post renal transplant. Buscombe JR, Gacinovic S, Hilson AJ and Ell PJ. Nuclear Medicine Communications, 15, 196, 1994.

665. Recognition of mental state terms: clinical findings in children with autism, and a functional neuroimaging study of normal adults. Baron-Cohen S, Ring M, Moriarty J, Schmitz B, Costa DC and Ell PJ. British Journal of Psychiatry, 165, 640-649, 1994.

666. Thallium-201 myocardial perfusion SPET: Adenosine alone or combined with dynamic exercise. Mahmood S, Gupta NK, Gunning M, Bomanji J, Jarritt PH and Ell PJ. Nuclear Medicine Communications, 15, 586-592, 1994.

667. Clinical experience with a multidetector SPET system (Toshiba GCA-9300A). Mahmood S, Buscombe JR, Kouris K, Clarke GA, Townsend CE, Jarritt PH, Costa DC and Ell PJ. Nuclear Medicine Communications, 15, 643-652, 1994.

668. Striatal dopamine receptor binding in epileptic psychoses. Ring HA, Trimble MR, Costa DC, Moriarty J, Verhoeff NPLG and Ell PJ. Biological Psychiatry, 35, 375-380, 1994.

669. Diagnostic accuracy of adenosine technetium-99m methoxy isobutyl isonitrile myocardial tomography in patients with coronary artery disease: comparison with exercise. Cuocolo A, Soricelli A, Pace I, Nicolai E, Castelli L, Nappi A, Imbriaco M, Morisco C, Ell PJ and Salvatore M. Journal of Nuclear Biology and Medicine, 38, 191, 1994.

670. Radiation synovectomy in chronic knee synovitis Samarium-153 hydroxyapatite particles. Clunie G, Lui D, Edwards JCW and Ell PJ. Journal of Nuclear Medicine, 35, 378, 1994.

671. The results of a multi-center clinical trial of indium-111 pooled human IgG in AIDS patients with lung infection. Buscombe JR, Khalkhali I, Datz F, Meatherall J, Raub D, Miller RF, Ell PJ, Oyen WJG and Corstens FHM. Journal of Nuclear Medicine, 35, 240P, 1994.

672. 67Ga scintigraphy in HIV antibody positive patients; a review of its clinical usefulness. Wassie E, Buscombe JR, Miller RF and Ell PJ. The British Journal of Radiology, 67, 349-352, 1994.

673. Adenosine technetium-99m-methoxy isobutyl isonitrile myocardial tomography in patients with coronary artery disease: comparison with exercise. Cuocolo A, Soricelli A, Pace L, Nicolai E, Castelli L, Nappi A, Imbriaco M, Morisco C, Ell PJ and Salvatore M. Journal of Nuclear Medicine, 35, 1110-1115; 1994.

674. Can Ga-67 citrate diagnose atypical mycobacterial disease in patients with AIDS? Buscombe JR, Buttery P, Miller RF and Ell PJ. European Journal of Nuclear Medicine, 10, S130, 1994.

675. Determinants of knee synovitis relapse following intra-articular Samarium-153 particulate hydroxyapatite radiation synovectomy. Clunie G, Lui D, Edwards JCW and Ell PJ. European Journal of Nuclear Medicine, 10, S115, 1994.

676. Dynamic whole-volume 123I-Iomazenil SPECT- Applications to schizophrenia research. Busatto GF, Costa DC, Pilowsky LS, Lingford-Hughes A, Ell PJ and Kerwin RW. European Journal of Nuclear Medicine, 10, S109, 1994.

677. Dopamine D2 receptor blockade and extrapyramidal side-effects with the novel antipsychotics remoxipride and risperidone - a 123I-IBZM SPECT study. Busatto GF, Pilowsky LS, Costa DC, Ell PJ, Verhoeff NPLG and Kerwin RW. European Journal of Nuclear Medicine, 10, S14, 1994.

678. D2 Dopamine receptor binding in the basal ganglia of antipsychotic free schizophrenic patients: a 123I-IBZM SPET study. Pilowsky LS, Costa DC, Ell PJ, Verhoeff NPLG, Murray RM and Kerwin RW. Journal of Psychiatry, 164, 16-26, 1994.

1995

679. Dopamine D2 receptor blockade in vivo with the novel antipsychotics risperidone and remoxipride - an 123I-IBZM single photon emission tomography study. Busatto GF, Pilowsky LS, Costa DC, Ell PJ, Verhoeff NPLG and Kerwin RW. Psychopharmacology, 117, 55-61, 1995.

680. In-vivo imaging of GABA A receptors using dynamic whole volume 123I-Iomazenil single photon emission tomography (SPET). Busatto G, Pilowsky LS, Costa DC, Ell PJ, Lingford-Hughes A and Kerwin RW. European Journal of Nuclear Medicine, 22, 12-16, 1995.

681. Nuclear Medicine. Ell PJ. Editorial. Quarterly Journal of Medicine, 88, 1-2, 1995.

682. Clinical Brain radionuclide imaging studies. Messa C, Fazio F, Costa DC and Ell PJ. Seminars in Nuclear Medicine, 2, 111-143, 1995.

683. Samarium-153 particulate hydroxyapatite radiation synovectomy: biodistribution data for chronic knee synovitis. Clunie G, Lui D, Cullum I, Edwards JOCW and Ell PJ. Journal of Nuclear Medicine, 36, 51-57, 1995.

684. Does three dimensional display of SPECT data improve the acccuracy of technetium-99m DMSA imaging of the kidney? Buscombe JR, Wilson AJ, Hall ML, Townsend D, Clarke G and Ell PJ. Journal of Nuclear Medicine Technology, 23, 1-6, 1995.

685. Dopamine receptor availability in Tourette's Syndrome. George MS, Robertson MM, Costa DC, Ell PJ, Trimble MR, Pilowsky L and Verhoeff NPLG. Psychiatry Research: Neuroimaging, 55, 193-203, 1995.

686. Highlights of the 6th World Congress of Nuclear Medicine and Biology. Ell PJ. European Journal of Nuclear Medicine, 22, 159-176, 1995.

687. Nuclear Medicine in Cardiology. A position paper for an open debate. Ell PJ, Bourguignon MH, Pauwels EKJ, Martin-Comin J, De Roo M and Dige-Petersen H. European Journal of Nuclear Medicine, 22, 189-192, 1995.

688. Combined rest thallium-201 / stress Tc-99m Tetrofosmin SPECT: a study of feasibility and diagnostic accuracy of a 90 minute protocol. Mahmood S, Gunning M, Bomanji JB, Gupta NK, Costa DC, Jarritt PH and Ell PJ. Journal of Nuclear Medicine, 36, 932-935, 1995.

689. Localization of infection in HIV antibody positive patients with fever: comparison of the efficacy of Ga-67 citrate and radiolabeled human IgG. Buscombe JR, Oyen WJG, Corstens FHM, Ell PJ and Miller RF. Clinical Nuclear Medicine, 20, 334-339, 1995.

690. High resolution renal SPECT in eight minutes using a multi-detector gamma camera. Buscombe JR, Townsend CE, Kouris K, Clarke G, Mahmood S, Jarritt PH and Ell PJ. Clinical Nuclear Medicine 20, 13-17, 1995.

691. Adenosine 201Tl SPET imaging in patients undergoing major non-vascular abdominal surgery. Mumtaz H, Bomanji J, Gupta NK, Zaidi F, Costa DC, Taylor I and Ell PJ. Nuclear Medicine Communications, 16, 209, 1995.

692. Evaluation of 99Tcm-L,L-etylenedicysteine (99Tcm-L,L-EC) in patients with chronic renal failure. Prvulovich E, Bomanji J, Waddington W, Rudrasingham P and Ell PJ. Nuclear Medicine Communications, 16, 213, 1995.

693. GABAA receptor density and clinical dimensions of schizophrenia: a 123I-Iomazenil SPET investigation. Busatto GF, Pilowsky LS, Costa DC, Ell PJ, David AS and Kerwin RW. Nuclear Medicine Communications, 16, 216, 1995.

694. Regional cerebral blood flow in obsessive-compulsive disorder measured by 99Tcm-HMPAO uptake and SPET: differential correlates with obsessive-compulsive and anxious-avoidant features. Lucey JV, Busatto G, Costa DC, Blanes T, Takei N, Pilowsky LS, Ell PJ, Marks M and Kerwin RW. Nuclear Medicine Communications, 16, 217, 1995.

695. Role of 201Tl brain SPET in the detection of intracerebral lymphoma in HIV-positive patients. Costa DC, Gacinovic S, Miller RF, Harrison MJG and Ell PJ. Nuclear Medicine Communications, 16, 218, 1995.

696. Bolus injection of D-ribose in the identification of thallium redistribution: quantitative analysis. Gunning MG, Clunie G, Bradley J, Gupta NK and Ell PJ. Nuclear Medicine Communications, 16, 224, 1995.

697. A survey of European radiation synovectomy practice 1991-93 by postal questionnaire. Clunie GPR and Ell PJ. Nuclear Medicine Communications, 16, 230, 1995.

698. Identification of focal infection in HIV-infected patients: the role of imaging with the monoclonal antibody BW 250/183. Prvulovich E, Miller RF, Costa DC, Severn A, Corbett E, Bomanji J, Becker W and Ell PJ. Nuclear Medicine Communications, 16, 247, 1995.

699. The pathophysiology of hibernating myocardium studied by PET during hyperinsulinemic-euglycemic clamp. Marinho NVS, Keogh BE, Costa DC, Ell PJ, Lammertsma AA and Camici PG. Journal of Nuclear Cardiology, 2, S3, 1995.

700. Adenosine technetium-99m tetrofosmin cardiac tomography in patients with coronary artery disease: comparison with exercise. Cuocolo A, Pace L, Nicolai E, Nappi A, Squame F, Sullo P, Ell PJ and Salvatore M. Journal of Nuclear Cardiology, 2, S74, 1995.

701. 99Tcm-L, L-ethylenedicysteine (99Tcm-L,L-EC) scintigraphy in patients with renal disorders. Gupta NK, Bomanji JB, Waddington W, Lui D, Costa DC, Verbruggen AM and Ell PJ. European Journal of Nuclear Medicine, 22: 617-624, 1995.

702. Nuclear medicine: radiologists must love it or leave it (letter). Ell PJ. Clinical Radiology, 50, 507, 1995.

703. Immunoscintigraphy with a 99Tcm labelled antigranulocyte monoclonal antibody in patients with human immunodeficiency virus infection and AIDS. Prvulovich EM, Miller RF, Costa DC, Severn A, Corbett E, Bomanji J, Becker WS and Ell PJ. Nuclear Medicine Communications, 16, 838-845, 1995.

704. Nuclear medicine and AIDS. Ell PJ and Lucignani G. Journal of Nuclear Medicine and Biology, 39, 1-2, 1995.

705. Brain perfusion abnormalities in Gilles de la Tourette's syndrome. Moriarty J, Costa DC, Schmitz B, Trimble MR, Ell PJ and Robertson MM. British Journal of Psychiatry, 167, 249-254, 1995.

706. Patterns of Ga-67 citrate accumulation in human immunodeficiency virus positive patients with and without mycobacterium avium intracellulare infection. Buscombe JR, Buttery P, Ell PJ and Miller RF. Clinical Radiology, 50, 483-488, 1995.

707. Assessment of magnetic resonance velocity mapping of global ventricular function during dobutamine infusion in coronary artery disease. Pennell DJ, Firmin DN, Burger P, Yang GZ, Manzara CC, Ell PJ, Swanton RH, Walker JM, Underwood SR and Longmore DB. British Heart Journal, 74, 163-170, 1995.

708. Nuclear Medicine in Europe. De Roo M and Ell PJ. European Journal of Nuclear Medicine, 22, 719-720, 1995.

709. Regional cerebral blood flow in obsessive compulsive disorder measured by 99m Tc-HMPAO uptake and single photon emission tomography. Lucey JV, Costa DC, Busatto GF, Pilowsky LS, Marks IM, Ell PJ and Kerwin RW. Journal of Nuclear Medicine, 36, 20P, 1995.

710. Reduced regional I-123-iomazenil binding correlates with severity of psychotic symptoms in schizophrenia: a single photon emission tomography (SPECT) study. Busatto GF, Costa DC, Pilowsky LS, David AS, Lucey JV, Ell PJ and Kerwin RW. Journal of Nuclear Medicine, 36, 20P, 1995.

711. Role of Tl-201-brain SPET in the diferential diagnosis of intracerebral space occupying lesions in HIV+ve patients. Costa DC, Gacinovic S, Severn A, Sweeney B, Miller RF, Harrison MJG and Ell PJ. Journal of Nuclear Medicine, 36, 192P, 1995.

712. Bolus injection of D-ribose in the identification of thallium redistribution following combined adenosine/dynamic exercise stress. Gunning MG, Clunie G, Bradley J, Gupta NK and Ell PJ. European Journal of Nuclear Medicine, 22, 496, 1995.

713. Identification of focal infection in human immunodeficiency virus infected patients - the role of imaging with monoclonal antibody BW 250/183. Prvulovich E, Miller RF, Costa DC, Severn A, Corbett E, Bomanji J, Becker W and Ell PJ. European Journal of Nuclear Medicine, 22, 737, 1995.

714. Gated-99mTc-Tetrofosmin compared with cine magnetic resonance imaging in the assessment of left ventricular wall motion characteristics. Gunning MG, Anag-

nostopoulos C, Davies G, Forbat SM, Ell PJ and Underwood SR. European Journal of Nuclear Medicine, 22, 755, 1995.

715. Relapse of synovitis in patients treated with intra-articular samarium-153 particulate hydroxyapatite for chronic synovitis. Clunie G, Lui D, Edwards JCW, Cullum I and Ell PJ. European Journal of Nuclear Medicine, 22, 808, 1995.

716. European radiation synovectomy practice 1991-3. Clunie GPR and Ell PJ. European Journal of Nuclear Medicine, 22, 829, 1995.

717. Evaluation of 99m-Tc-L,L.-etylenedicysteine (99mTc-L,L,-EC) in patients with chronic renal failure. Prvulovich E, Bomanji J, Waddington W, Jarritt PH, Rudrasingham P and Ell PJ. European Journal of Nuclear Medicine, 22, 854, 1995.

718. Third generation bone densitometry. The impact of fan beam technology. Ell PJ, Bouyoucef SE and Cullum I. European Journal of Nuclear Medicine, 22, 875, 1995.

719. Effect of adenosine on cerebral blood flow as evaluated by single photon emission comptuted tomography in normal subjects and in patients with occlusive carotid disease. Soricelli A, Postiglione A, Cuocolo A, De Chiara S, Ruocco A, Brunetti A, Salvatore M and Ell PJ. Stroke, 26, 1572-1576, 1995.

720. Regional cerebral blood flow in obsessive-compulsive disordered patients at rest. Differential correlates with obsessive-compulsive and anxious-avoidant dimensions. Lucey JV, Costa DC, Blanes T, Busatto GF, Pilowsky LS, Takei N, Marks IM, Ell PJ and Kerwin RW. British Journal of Psychiatry, 167, 629-634, 1995.

721. Optimised interictal HMPAO-SPECT in the evaluation of partial epilepsies. Schmitz EB, Costa DC, Jackson GD, Moriarty J, Duncan JS, Trimble MR and Ell PJ. Epilepsia Research, 21, 159-167, 1995.

722. Schizophrenic auditory hallucinations are associated with increased regional cerebral blood flow during verbal memory activation in a study using single photon emission computed tomography. Busatto GF, David AS, Costa DC, Ell PJ, Pilowsky LS, Lucey JV and Kerwin RW. Psychiatry Research: Neuroimaging, 61, 255-264, 1995.

1996

723. Targeting disseminated melanoma with radiolabelled methylene blue: comparative bio-distribution studies in man and animals. Link EM, Costa DC, Lui D, Ell PJ, Blower PJ and Spittle MF. Acta Oncologica, 3, 331-341, 1996.

724. Pathophysiology of chronic left ventricular disfunction: new insights from the measurement of absolute myocardial blood flow and glucose utilization. Marinho NVS, Keogh BE, Costa DC, Lammerstma AA, Ell PJ and Camici PG. Circulation, 93, 737-744, 1996.

725. Dopamine D2 receptor occupancy in vivo by the novel atypical antipsychotic olanzapine - a 123I IBZM single photon emission tomography (SPET) study. Pilowsky LS, Busatto GF, Taylor M, Costa DC, Sharma T, Sigmundsson T, Ell PJ, Nohria and Kerwin RW. Psychopharmacology, 124, 148-153, 1996.

726. Adenosine coronary vasodilation quantitative Tc-99m methoxy isobutyl isonitrile myocardial tomography in the identification and localization of coronary artery dis-

ease. Nicolai E, Cuocolo A, Pace L, Nappi A, Sullo P, Cardei S, Argenziano L, Squame F, Ell PJ and Salvatore M. Journal of Nuclear Cardiology, 3, 9-17, 1996.

727. The role of 18F-FDG SPET in detection of hibernating myocardium: Comparison with rest-redistribution 201Thallium SPET. Prvulovich E, Bomanji J, Holdright D, Costa DC and Ell PJ. Heart, 75, (suppl. 1), 72, 1996.

728. Identification of hibernating myocardium: a comparison of Tl-201, Tc-99m Tetrofosmin, and Dobutamine cine magnetic resonance imaging. Gunning MG, Knight CJ, Anagnostopoulos C, Chua TP, Burman E, Pennell DJ, Pepper J, Ell PJ, Fox K and Underwood SR. Heart, 75, (suppl. 1), 72, 1996.

729. Efficacy and safety of 153Sm-EDTMP in alleviating the pain of bone metastases in patients with prostate carcinoma. Reid, RH, Hoskin P, Ell PJ, Coleman, R, Quick D and the 153Sm-EDTMP Phase 3 Study Group. Nuclear Medicine Communication, 17, 258, 1996.

730. A comparison of attenuation-corrected and non-attenuation-corrected 201Tl studies for the detection of coronary artery disease. Prvulovich E, Lonn AHR, Bomanji J, Jarritt PH and Ell PJ. Nuclear Medicine Communication, 17, 276-277, 1996.

731. Adenosine stress test in patients with coronary artery disease: comparison between technetium-99m tetrofosmin cardiac tomography and echocardiography. Cuocolo A, Sullo P, Nicolai E, Nappi A, Pace L, Gisonni P, Cardei S, Ell PJ and Salvatore M. Journal of Nuclear Medicine, 37, 5, 178P, 1996.

732. Technetium-99m tetrofosmin myocardial tomography in patients with coronary artery disease: comparison between adenosine and exercise stress testing. Cuocolo A, Soricelli A, Nicolai E, Pace L, Nappi A, Squame F, Sullo P, Cardei S, Ell PJ and Salvatore M. Journal of Nuclear Cardiology, 3, 194-203, 1996.

733. Gallium imaging in the diagnosis of pericardial lymphoma in a patient with acquired immunodeficiency syndrome. Prvulovich MD, Costa DC, Bomanji J, Clarke GA, Townsend CE, Miller RE and Ell PJ. Journal of Nuclear Medicine, 37, 995-996, 1996.

734. Slow bolus injection of ribose in the identification of thallium-201 redistribution following combined adenosine/dynamic exercise stress. Gunning MG, Clunie G, Bradley J, Gupta NK, Bomanji JB and Ell PJ. European Heart Journal, 17, 1438-1443, 1996.

735. Performance assessment of a fourth generation fan-beam x-ray densitometer. Bouyoucef SE, Cullum ID and Ell PJ. British Journal of Radiology, 69, 522-531, 1996.

736. 20 years of the European Journal of Nuclear Medicine. Ell PJ. European Journal of Nuclear Medicine, 23, 1025-1026, 1996.

737. HMPAO SPECT in non epileptic seizures. Preliminary results. Varma AR, Moriarty J, Costa DC, Gacinovic S, Schmitz EB, Ell PJ and Trimble MR. Acta Neurologica Scandinavica, 94, 88-92, 1996.

738. Clinical outcome following samarium-153 particulate hydroxyapatite radiation synovectomy. Clunie G, Lui D, Cullum I, Ell PJ and Edwards J. Scandanavian J. Rheumatology, 25, 360-366, 1996.

739. Contrast media nephrotoxicity and the role of the radionuclide renal scan. Dhawan RT, Foo M, Bomanji JB, Setna FJ and Ell PJ. Journal of Nuclear Medicine, 37, 1828-1830, 1996.

740. Myocardial perfusion scintigraphy in patients undergoing major non-vascular abdominal surgery. Mumtaz H, Bomanji JB, Gupta NK, Davidson T, Costa DC, Taylor I and Ell PJ. Annals Royal College of Surgeons of England, 78, 420-425, 1996.

741. Inter-observer agreement in the reporting of Tc-99m DMSA renal studies. Gacinovic S, Buscombe J, Costa DC, Hilson A, Bomanji J and Ell PJ. Nuclear Medicine Communications, 17, 596-602, 1996.
742. Brain blood flow in anxiety disorders: obsessive compulsive disorder, panic disorder with agorophobia, and post traumatic stress disorder on 99mTc-HMPAO single photon emission tomography. Lucey JV, Costa DC, Adshead G, Deahl M, Gacinovic S, Travis M, Pilowsky LS, Ell PJ, Marks IM and Kerwin RW. British Journal of Psychiatry, 171, 346-351, 1996.

1997

743. HMPAO SPET does not distinguish obsessive-compulsive and Tic syndromes in families multiply affected with Gilles de la Tourette's syndrome. Moriarty J, Eapen V, Costa DC, Gacinovic S, Trimble M, Ell PJ and Robertson MM. Psychological Medicine, 27, 737-740, 1997.
744. Gated 99m-Tc-Tetrofosmin SPECT and cine MRI to assess left ventricular contraction. Gunning MG, Anagnostopoulos C, Davies G, Forbat SM, Ell PJ and Underwood SR. Journal of Nuclear Medicine, 38, 438-442, 1997.
745. Correlation between reduced in vivo benzodiazepine receptor binding and severity of psychotic symptoms in schizophrenia. Busatto GF, Pilowsky LS, Costa DC, Ell PJ, David AS, Lucey JV and Kerwin RW. American Journal of Psychiatry, 154, 56-63, 1997.
746. Effect of attenuation correction on myocardial 201Thallium distribution in patients with low likelihood for coronary artery disease. Prvulovich EM, Lonn AHR, Bomanji JB, Jarritt PH and Ell PJ. European Journal of Nuclear Medicine, 24, 266-275, 1997.
747. Transmission imaging for attenuation correction of myocardial 201Thallium images in obese patients. Prvulovich EM, Lonn AHR, Bomanji JB, Jarritt PH and Ell PJ. Nuclear Medicine Communications, 18, 207-218, 1997.
748. Clinical evaluation of Technetium-99m-L,L-Ethylenedicysteine in patients with chronic renal failure. Prvulovich EM, Bomanji JB, Waddington WA, Rudrasingham P, Verbruggen A and Ell PJ. Journal of Nuclear Medicine, 38, 1-6, 1997.
749. In vivo effects on striatal dopamine D2 receptor binding by the novel atypical antipsychotic drug sertindole- a 123I IBZM single photon emission tomography (SPET) study. Pilowsky LS, O'Connell P, Davies N, Busatto GF, Costa DC, Murray RM, Ell PJ and Kerwin RW. Psychopharmacology, 130, 152-158, 1997.
750. Tc-99m Furifosmin (Q-12) myocardial perfusion SPECT in detection of coronary artery disease. Mahmoud S, Bomanji J, Ayub M, Aleem, M Sheikh SA and Ell PJ. Journal of Nuclear Cardiology, 4, S45, 1997.
751. Transmission scanning for attenuation correction in obese patients. Prvulovich E, Lonn AHR, Bomanji JB, Jarritt PH and Ell PJ. Journal of Nuclear Cardiology, 1, S104, 1997.
752. Improved 201Tl uniformity with attenuation correction in patients with low risk for CAD. Prvulovich E, Lonn AHR, Bomanji JB, Jarritt PH and Ell PJ. Journal of Nuclear Cardiology, 1, S108, 1997.

753. Economics of myocardial perfusion imaging - Empire study. Underwood SR, Godman B, Salyani S, Ogle J, Sechtem U and Ell PJ. Journal of Nuclear Cardiology, 4, 598, 1997.

754. The contribution of brain receptor imaging to understanding schizophrenia. Pilowsky LS, Costa DC, Busatto GF, Mulligan RL, Acton PD, Gacinovic S, Travis MJ, Bigliani V, Stephenson C, Ell PJ and Kerwin RW. British Journal of Radiology, 70, 47, 1997.

755. Reduced levels of the GABA benzodiazepine receptor in alcohol dependency - An 123 I-Iomazenil SPET study. Lingford-Hughes AR, Acton PD, Gacinovic S, Busatto GF, Costa DC, Boddington S, Marshall JE, Ell PJ, Kerwin RW and Pilowsky LS. Journal of Nuclear Medicine, 38, 107P, 1997.

756. Clozapine shows selective occupancy of extra-ST dopamine D2/D2-like receptors - A 123I epidepride SPET preliminary findings. Pilowsky LS, Mulligan RS, Acton PD, Gacinovic S, Busatto GF, Kessler RM, Ell PJ, Travis MJ, Bigliani V, Stephenson C, Costa DC and Kerwin RW. Journal of Nuclear Medicine, 38, 94P, 1997.

757. Nuclear Medicine: Provision of a Clinical Service. Ell PJ, Coakley A, Clarke S and Lewington V. Journal of the Royal College of Physicians, 31, 384-388, 1997.

758. Limbic selectivity of clozapine. Pilowsky LS, Acton P, Mulligan RS, Ell PJ, Costa DC and Kerwin RW. The Lancet, 350, 490-491, 1997.

759. A dose-controlled study of 153Sm-EDTMP in the treatment of patients with painful bone metastases. Resche I, Chatal JF, Pecking A, Ell PJ, Duchesne G, Fogelman I, Houston S, Fauser A, Fischer M and Wilkins D. European Journal of Cancer, 33, 1583-1591, 1997.

760. Tc-99m MDP patterns in patients with painful shoulder lesions. Clunie G, Bomanji J and Ell PJ. Journal of Nuclear Medicine, 38, 1491-1495, 1997.

761. Undergraduate Teaching of Radiology and Nuclear Medicine. Ell PJ. European Journal of Nuclear Medicine, 24, 1081-1082, 1997.

762. Psychiatric profiles and patterns of cerebral blood flow in focal epilepsy: interaction between depression, obsessionality and perfusion related to the laterality of the epilepsy. Schmitz EB, Moriarty J, Costa DC, Ring HA, Ell PJ and Trimble MR. Journal of Neurology, Neurosurgery and Psychiatry, 62, 458-463, 1997.

763. Multivariate cluster analysis of dynamic 123I-IBZM SPET dopamine D2 receptor images in schizophrenia. Acton PD, Pilowsky LS, Costa DC and Ell PJ. European Journal of Nuclear Medicine, 24, 111-118, 1997.

764. Registration of dynamic dopamine D2 receptor images using principal component analysis. Acton PD, Pilowsky LS, Suckling J, Brammer MJ and Ell PJ. European Journal of Nuclear Medicine, 24, 1405-1412, 1997.

765. Initial evaluation of 123I-5-I-R91150, a selective 5-HT2a ligand for single photon emission tomography (SPET) in healthy human subjects. European Journal of Nuclear Medicine, 24, 119-125, 1997.

766. Caudate regional cerebral blood flow in obsessive-compulsive disorder, panic disorder and healthy controls on single photon emission computerised tomography. Lucey JV, Costa DC, Busatto G, Pilowsky LS, Marks IM, Ell PJ and Kerwin RW. Psychiatric Research: Neuroimaging, 14, 74, 1, 25-33, 1997.

767. Serotonin 5-HT2a occupancy in vivo and response to the new antipsychotics olanzapine and sertindole. Travis MJ, Busatto GF, Pilowsky LS, Kerwin W, Mulligan RS, Gacinovic S, Costa DC, Ell PJ, Mertens J and Terriere D. British Journal of Psychiatry, 171, 290-291, 1997.

768. Wisconsin card-sorting errors and cerebral blood flow in obsessive compulsive disorder (OCD). Lucey JV, Costa DC, Busatto G, Pilowsky LS, Ell PJ, Marks IM and Kerwin RW. British Journal of Medical Psychology, 70, 403-411, 1997.

1998

769. Palliation of pain associated with metastatic bone cancer using 153Sm-EDTMP: A double blind placebo-controlled clinical trial. Serafini A, Rubens RD, Chatal JF, Quick DP, Grund FM, Ell PJ, Betrand A, Ahmann FR, Orihuela E, Reid RH, Lerski RA, Collier BD, McKillop JH, Purnell GL, Pecking AP, Thomas FD and Harrison KA. Journal of Clinical Oncology, 16, 1574-1581, 1998.
770. Recurrent follicular carcinoma-oxyphilic cell type (Hurthle cell carcinoma) of the thyroid, imaging with iodine-131 and technetium-99m tetrofosmin before and after radiotherapy. Bomanji JB, Gacinovic S, Gaze MN, Costa DC and Ell PJ. The British Journal of Radiology, 71, 87-89, 1998.
771. Foot pain: specific indications for scintigraphy. Duffy EO, Clunic G, Gacinovic S, Edwards JC, Bomanji J and Ell PJ. British Journal of Rheumatology, 37, 1998.
772. Progress with Nuclear Medicine audit in the UK. Ell PJ. Nuclear Medicine Communications, 19, 95-96, 1998.
773. Cognitive functioning and GABAA/Benzodiazepine receptor binding in schizophrenia: A 123I-Iomazenil SPET study. Ball S, Busatto GF, David AS, Jones SH, Hemsley DR, Pilowsky LS, Costa DC, Ell PJ and Kerwin RW. Biological Psychiatry, 43, 107-117, 1998.
774. Preliminary results: D1/D2-like receptor binding in temporal cortex and striatum in sertindole and olanzapine treated patients. Bigliani V, Mulligan RS, Acton PF, Stephenson C, Gacinovic S, Ell PJ, Kerwin RW and Pilowsky LS. Journal of Nuclear Medicine, 39, 82P, 1998.
775. Broad-spectrum typical antipsychotics and in vivo 5-HT2A receptor occupancy in schizophrenic patients: SPET findings. Travis MJ, Busatto GF, Pilowsky LS, Mulligan RS, Gacinovic S, Acton PD, Costa DC, Ell PJ and Kerwin RW. Journal of Nuclear Medicine, 39, 83P, 1998.
776. Reduced levels of the GABA-benzodiazepine receptor in alcohol dependency in the absence of grey matter atrophy. Lingford-Hughes AR, Acton PD, Gacinovic S, Suckling JO, Busatto GF, Boddington S, Bullmore E, Woodruff PW, Costa DC, Pilowsky LS, Marshall EJ, Ell PJ and Kerwin RW. British Journal of Psychiatry, 173, 116-122, 1998.
777. Early detection of melanoma metastases with radioiodinated methylene blue. Link EM, Blower PJ, Costa DC, Lane D, Lui D, Brown RSD, Ell PJ and Spittle MF. European Journal of Nuclear Medicine, 25, 1322-1329, 1998.
778. Magnetic resonance imaging, Thallium-201 SPET scanning and laboratory analyses for discrimination of cerebral lymphoma and toxoplasmosis in AIDS. Miller RF, Hall-Craggs MA, Costa DC, Brink NS, Scaravilli F, Lucas SB, Wilkinson ID, Ell PJ, Kendall BE and Harrison MJG. Sex Trans. Inf, 74, 258-264, 1998.

779. 5-HT2A receptor blockade in patients with schizophrenia treated with risperidone or clozapine. A SPET study using the novel 5-HT2A ligand 123I-5-I-R-91150. Travis MJ, Busatto GF, Pilowsky LS, Mulligan R, Acton PD, Gacinovic S, Mertens J, Terriere D, Costa DC, Ell PJ and Kerwin RW. British Journal of Psychiatry, 173, 236-241, 1998.

780. I-131 MIBG therapy of a patient with carcinoid liver metastases. Prvulovich E, Stein RC, Bomanji JB, Lederman JA, Taylor I and Ell PJ. Journal of Nuclear Medicine, 39, 1743-1745, 1998.

781. Technetium-99m human immunoglobulin imaging in patients with sub-acromial impingement on adhesive capsulitis. Clunie G, Bomanji J, Renton P, Edwards JCW and Ell PJ. Clinical Rheumatology, 17, 419-421, 1998.

782. The Profession and the Industry. Ell PJ. European Journal of Nuclear Medicine, 25, 1472-1474, 1998.

783. Sentinel lymph node biopsy in breast cancer. Keshtgar M and Ell PJ. The Lancet, 352, 1471-1472, 1998.

784. Neurology and Psychiatry. CME in Nuclear Medicine. Ell PJ, Costa DC and McKillop JH. Journal of the Royal College of Physicians, 32, 529-536, 1998.

785. Comparison of thallium-201, technetium-99m-tetrofosmin and dobutamine magnetic resonance imaging for identifying hibernating myocardium. Gunning MG, Anagnostopoulos C, Knight CJ, Pepper K, Burman ED, Davies G, Fox KM, Pennell DJ, Ell PJ and Underwood SR. Circulation, 98(18), 1869-1874, 1998.

1999

786. Nuclear Medicine and the challenge of the 21st century. Ell PJ. In "Radioactive Isotopes in Clinical Medicine and Research XXIII". Ed. by Bergman H, Kohn H, Sinzinger H. Published by Birkhauser, 3-18, 1999.

787. Sentinel lymph node: detection and imaging. Keshtgar M and Ell PJ. European Journal of Nuclear Medicine, 26, 57-68, 1999.

788. The practice of medical and surgical synovectomy: a UK survey. O'Duffy EK and Ell PJ. British Journal of Rheumatology. Nuclear Medicine Communications, 1, 21-24, 1999.

789. Economics of Myocardial Perfusion Imaging in Europe. The Empire Study. Underwood SR, Godman B, Salyani S, Ogle J and Ell PJ. European Heart Journal, 20(2), 157-166, 1999.

790. Changes in articular synovial lining volume measured by magnetic resonance in a randomised, double-blind, controlled trial of intra-articular samarium-153 particulate hydroxyapatite for chronic knee synovitis. Clunie GPR, Wilkinson ID, Lui D, Hall-Craggs MA, Paley MN, Edwards JCW and Ell PJ. Rheumatology 38, 113-117, 1999.

791. The sentinel node and lymphoscintigraphy in breast cancer. Ell PJ and Keshtgar M. Nuclear Medicine Communications, 41, 303-305, 1999.

792. Scientific poster presentations at the EANM Annual Congress. Bischof Delaloye A and Ell PJ. European Journal of Nuclear Medicine, 26, 1, 1999.

793. Needle-free vehicle for administration of radionuclide for sentinel node biopsy. Keshtgar MRS and Ell PJ. Lancet, 355, 1410-1411, 1999.
794. Costs of Health Care: A lopsided debate. Ell PJ and Deszy J. European Journal of Nuclear Medicine, 26, 435-436, 1999.
795. Automatic segmentation of dynamic neuroreceptor SPECT images using fuzzy clustering. Acton PD, Pilowsky LS and Ell PJ. European Journal of Nuclear Medicine, 26, 581-590, 1999.
796. The cost implications of sentinel node biopsy in breast cancer management. Keshtgar MRS, Howard Jones E, Davidson T, Waddington WA, Saunders C, Baum M, Taylor I and Ell PJ. Journal of Nuclear Medicine, 40, 139P, 1999.
797. A randomised comparison of MIBI and Tetrofosmin for myocardial perfusion imaging with and without a fatty meal before imaging. Kapur A, Latus KA, Davies G, Jarritt PH, Young MC, Roussakis G, Pennell DJ, Ell PJ and Underwood SR. Journal of Nuclear Medicine, 40, 85P, 1999.
798. The ROBUST study: a randomised comparison of three tracers for myocardial perfusion scintigraphy. Kapur A, Latus KA, Davies G, Jarritt PH, Young MC, Roussakis G, Pennell DJ, Ell PJ and Underwood SR. Journal of Nuclear Medicine, 40, 85P, 1999.
799. Breast carcinoma and Nuclear Medicine. Ell PJ. Radiology Now, 16, 1, 7-9, 1999.
800. Preparation of [123I]epidepride from trialkylstannyl precursors in the presence of chloramine-T - some cautionary observations. Mulligan RS, Osman S, Pilowsky LS, Ell PJ and Pike VW. J. Lab. Cpds. Radiopharm, 1999, S6.
801. Radioiodination of SB 207710 as a prospective radioligand for imaging 5-HT4 receptors in vivo - autoradiography of [125I]SB 207710 against human brain tissue. Mulligan RS, Halldin C, Hall H, Pilowsky LS, Ell PJ, Farde L and Pike VW. J. Lab. Cpds. Radiopharm, 1999, M29.
802. [123I]5-iodo-R91150, a radioligand for 5-HT2A receptors - radiochemical stability and metabolism. Mulligan RS, Osman S, Travis MJ, Eersel JLH, Pilowsky LS, Ell PJ and Pike VW. J. Lab. Cpds. Radiopharm, 1999, Q24.
803. Langer's axillary arc in association with sentinel lymph node. Keshtgar MRS, Saunders C, Ell PJ and Baum M. The Breast, 8, 152-153, 1999.
804. In vivo occupancy of striatal and temporal cortical D2/D3 dopamine receptors by typical antipsychotic drugs. Bigliani V, Mulligan RS, Acton PD, Visvikis D, Ell PJ, Stephenson C, Kerwin RW and Pilowsky L. The British Journal of Psychiatry, 175, 231-238, 1999.
805. Double-blind glucocorticoid controlled trial of Samarium-153 particulate hydroxyapatite radiation synovectomy for chronic knee synovitis. O'Duffy EK, Clunie GPR, Lui D, Edwards JCW and Ell PJ. Annals of the Rheumatic Diseases, 58, 554-558, 1999.
806. Bright future for Nuclear Medicine. Ell PJ. The Lancet, 354, 616, 1999.
807. False negative rates in sentinel node in breast cancer. Keshtgar MRS and Ell PJ. The Lancet, 354, 773, 1999.
808. Chromosomal analysis of peripheral lymphocytes of patients before and after radiation synovectomy with samarium-153 particulate hydroxyapatite. O'Duffy EK, Oliver FJ, Chatters SJ, Walker H, Lloyd DC, Edwards JCW and Ell PJ. Rheumatology, 38, 316-320, 1999.
809. Nuclear Medicine in Neurology and Psychiatry. Costa DC, Pilowsky L and Ell PJ. The Lancet, 354, 1007-1111, 1999.

810. Acipimox does not augment Tl-201 redistribution in the fasting state. Gunning MG, Clunie G, Yepes-Mora S, Eastick S, Underwood SR, Bomanji J and Ell PJ. Journal of Nuclear Cardiology, 6, 586-592, 1999.

2000

811. Nuclear Medicine: an exciting past and a stimulating future. Ell PJ. European Journal of Nuclear Medicine, 27, 55-57, 2000.

812. In vivo serotonin 5-HT2A receptor occupancy and Quetiapine. Jones HM, Travis MJ, Mulligan R, Visvikis D, Gacinovic S, Ell PJ, Kerwin RW and Pilowsky LS. American Journal of Psychiatry, 157, 1148, 2000.

813. Impact of European Societies. Ell PJ. Seminars in Nuclear Medicine, 3, 225-230, 2000.

814. Radiation safety of the sentinel lymph node in breast cancer. Waddington WA, Keshtgar MRS, Taylor I, Lakhani SR, Short MD and Ell PJ. European Journal of Nuclear Medicine, 27, 377-391, 2000.

815. Impact Factors or Common Sense. Ell PJ. Clinical Radiology, 55, 413, 2000.

816. Striatal and temporal cortical D2/D3 receptor occupancy by olanzapine and sertindole in vivo: a [123I] epidepride single photon emission tomography (SPET) study. Bigliani V, Mulligan RS, Acton PD, Ohlsen RI, Pike VW, Ell PJ, Gacinovic S, Kerwin RW and Pilowsky LS. Psychopharmacology, 150, 132-140, 2000.

817. Medicina Nuclear: O Futuro. Ell PJ. Revista Esp. Medicina Nuclear, 19, 82-84, 2000.

818. Striatal and extra-striatal D2/D3 dopamine receptor occupancy by quetiapine in vivo [123I]epidepride SPET study. Stephenson CME, Bigliani V, Jones HM, Mulligan RS, Acton PD, Visvikis D, Ell PJ, Kerwin RW and Pilowsky LS. British Journal of Psychiatry, 177, 408-415, 2000.

819. Nuclear medicine in the next decade. Ell PJ. European Journal of Nuclear Medicine, 27, 1277-1279, 2000.

820. Influence of arm positioning on tomographic thallium-201 myocardial perfusion imaging and the effect of attenuation correction. Prvulovich E, Jarritt PH, Lonn AHR, Vorontsova E, Bomanji JB and Ell PJ. European Journal of Nuclear Medicine, 27, 1349-1355, 2000.

821. Levels of GABA-benzodiazepine receptors in female abstinent alcohol dependent subjects: preliminary findings from a 123I-iomazenil single photon emission tomography study. Lingford-Hughes AR, Acton PD, Gacinovic S, Boddington SJA, Costa DC, Pilowsky LS, Ell PJ, Marshall EJ and Kerwin RW. Alcoholism: Clinical and Experimental Research, 24, 1449-1455, 2000.

2001

822. Positron emission tomography in colorectal cancer. Arulampalam THA, Costa DC, Loizidou M, Visvikis D, Ell PJ and Taylor I. British Journal of Surgery, 88, 176-189, 2001.

823. Functional imaging as an aid to decision making in metastatic paraganglioma. Bomanji J, Hyder SW, Gaze MN, Gacinovic S, Costa DC, Coulter C and Ell PJ. British Journal of Radiology, 74, 266-269, 2001.

824. The clinical role of positron emission tomography. Bomanji JB, Costa DC and Ell PJ. The Lancet Oncology, 3, 157-164, 2001.

825. Functional imaging of malignant paragangliomas and carcinoid tumours. Le Rest C, Bomanji JB, Costa DC, Townsend CE, Visvikis D and Ell PJ. European Journal of Nuclear Medicine, 38, 478-482. 2001.

826. Dopamine D2 receptor blockade in Schizophrenia. Bressan RA, Jones HM, Ell PJ and Pilowsky LS. American Journal of Psychiatry, 158, 6, 2001.

827. The sentinel node in anal carcinoma. Keshtgar MRS, Amin A, Taylor I and Ell PJ. European Journal of Surgical Oncology, 27, 113-122, 2001.

828. Influence of OSEM and segmented attenuation correction in the calculation of standardised uptake values for 18FDG-PET. Visvikis D, Le Rest C, Costa DC, Bomanji JB, Gacinovic S and Ell PJ. European Journal of Nuclear Medicine, 28, 1326-1335, 2001.

829. A revolution in surgical oncology: sentinel lymph node biopsy. Ell PJ. Imaging, 13, 197-205, 2001.

830. The role of fluorodeoxyglucose positron emission tomography scanning in the diagnosis of paraneoplastic neurological disorders. Rees J, Hain, Johnson N, Hughes, Costa DC, Ell PJ, Keir and Rudge. Brain. 124, 2223-2231, 2001.

831. The impact of FDG-PET on the management algorithm for recurrent colorectal cancer. Arulampalam, THA, Costa DC, Visvikis D, Boulos B, Taylor I and Ell PJ. European Journal of Nuclear Medicine. 28, 12, 1758-1765, 2001.

832. Optimal nuclear medicine support in sentinel node detection. Waddington WA, Keshtgar MRS and Ell PJ. Annals of Surgical Oncology, 8, 9-12, 2001.

833. The clinical application of positron emission tomography to colorectal cancer management. Arulampalam THA, Costa DC, Bomanji JB and Ell PJ. The Quarterly Journal of Nuclear Medicine, 45, 3, 215-230, 2001.

834. The effect of polyethylene glycol 400 on gastrointestinal transit: Implications for the formulation of poorly-water soluble drugs. Basit AW, Newton JM, Short MD, Waddington WA, Ell PJ and Lacey LF. Pharmaceutical Research, 18, 8, 1146-1150, 2001.

835. In vivo 5HT2a receptor blockade by quetiapine-An R91150 single photon emission tomography study. Jones H, Travis MJ, Mulligan RS, Visvikis D, Gacinovic S, Ell PJ, Kerwin RW and Pilowsky LS. Psychopharmacology, 157, 1, 60-66, 2001.

836. OSEM and segmented attenuation correction in the calculation of SUV's for FDG PET. Visvikis D, Townsend CE, Taylor L, Costa DC, Bomanji JB, Le Rest C and Ell PJ. Journal of Nuclear Medicine, 42, 5, 103p, 2001.

837. Typical antipsychotic drugs – D2 receptor occupancy and depressive symptoms in schizophrenia. Bressan RA, Costa DC, Jones HM, Ell PJ and Pilowsky LS. Schizophrenia Research, 56, 31-36, 2001.

838. Keynote Lecture (Special Issue): The role of PET in oncology. Ell, P.J. Cancer Imaging, 2, Special Issue 2, 54-55(2), 2001.

2002

839. Clinical role of sentinel-lymph node biopsy in breast cancer. Keshtgar MRS and Ell PJ. Lancet Oncology, 3, 105-110, 2002.

840. The Future of Nuclear Medicine. Ell PJ, Hoejgaard C and Becker W. The Lancet, 359, 629-630, 2002.

841. Welcome to the European Journal of Nuclear Medicine and Molecular Imaging. Gambhir SS and Ell PJ. European Journal of Nuclear Medicine and Molecular Imaging, 29, 1, 1-2, 2002.

842. The role of dynamic imaging in sentinel lymph node biopsy in breast cancer. Lee AC, Keshtgar MRS, Waddington WA and Ell PJ. European Journal of Cancer, 38, 6, 784-787, 2002.

843. Glucose utilisation and cell proliferation in colorectal cancer. Visvikis D, Francis DL, Costa DC, Mulligan RS, Townsend CE, Arulampalam THA, Islam MS, Taylor I and Ell PJ. European Journal of Nuclear Medicine and Molecular Imaging, 29, 2, 280, 2002.

844. 18FDG and 18FLT in colorectal carcinoma: preliminary results of a comparative study. Visvikis D, Francis DL, Costa DC, Mulligan RS, Townsend CE, Islam S and Ell PJ. Nuclear Medicine Communications, 23, 4, 386, 2002.

845. Is there a role for sentinel node biopsy and 18F-FDG PET in the preoperative staging the clinically NO neck in early oral squamous cell carcinoma? Hyde NC, Prvulovich EM, Visvikis D, Waddington WA, Keshtgar MRS and Ell PJ. Journal of Nuclear Medicine, 43, 158, 2002.

846. PET/CT: A new road map. Ell PJ and von Schulthess GK. European Journal of Nuclear Medicine, 29, 719-720, 2002.

847. Nuclear Medicine in primary breast cancer imaging. Gopalan D, Bomanji JB, Costa DC and Ell PJ. Clinical Radiology, 7, 565-574, 2002.

848. The comparative values of bone marrow aspirate and trephine for obtaining bone scan-targeted metastases from hormone-refractory prostate cancer. Brown RSD, Dogan A, Ell PJ, Payne HA, Masters JRW and Harland SJ. Prostate Cancer and Prostatic Diseases, 5, 2, 144-151, 2002.

849. Fluorodeoxyglucose positron emission tomography in clinical oncology: The Referrers perspective. Gopalan D, Griffiths D, Townsend CE, Prvulovich EM, Bomanji JB, Costa DC and Ell PJ. Nuclear Medicine Communications, 23, 1041-1046, 2002.

850. Colonic delivery of 4-aminosalicylic acid using amylose-ethylcellulose coated hydroxyproplymethyl cellulose capsules. Tuleu C, Basit AW, Waddington WA, Ell PJ and Newton JM. Alimentary Pharmacology and Therapeutics, 16, 1771-1779, 2002.

851. A comparison of three radionuclide myocardial perfusion tracers in clinical practice: the ROBUST study. Kapur A, Latus KA, Davies G, Dhawan RT, Eastick S, Jarritt PH, Roussakis G, Young MC, Anagnostopoulos C, Bomanji JB, Costa DC, Pennell DJ, Prvulovich EM, Ell PJ and Underwood SR. European Journal of Nuclear Medicine 29, 1608-1616, 2002.

852. Influence of polyethylene glycol 400 on the gastrointestinal absorption of ranitidine. Basit AW, Podczeck F, Newton JM, Waddington WA, Ell PJ and Lacey LF. Pharmaceutical Research, 19(9), 2002.

853. Exercise trained following myocardial infarction improves myocardial perfusion assessed by thallium-201 scintigraphy. Gunning MG, Walker J, Eastick S, Bomanji JB, Ell PJ and Walker JM. International Journal of Cardiology, 84, 233-239, 2002.

854. Challenging cases and diagnostic dilemmas: case 2. Pitfalls of positron emission tomography for assessing residual mediastinal mass after chemotherapy for Hodgkin's disease. Bomanji JB, Syed R, Brock C, Jankowska P, Dogan A, Costa DC, Ell PJ and Lee SM. Journal of Clinical Oncology, 20(15), 3347-3349, 2002.

2003

855. Optimizing limbic selective D2/D3 receptor occupancy by risperidone: A [^{123}I] – epidepride SPET study. Bressan RA, Erlandsson K, Jones HM, Mulligan RS, Ell PJ, and Pilowsky LS. Journal of Clinical Psychopharmacology, 23 (1), 5-14, 2003.

856. CT based attenuation correction in the calculation of SUVs for 18FDG-PET. Visvikis D, Costa DC, Crosadale I and Ell PJ. European Journal of Nuclear Medicine, 30, 344-353, 2003.

857. Strategy for the provision of PET in the UK. Ell PJ. Nuclear Medicine Communications, 24, 229-231, 2003.

858. Do we need more nuclear cardiologists in Europe? Against. Ell P J. European Journal of Nuclear Medicine, 30, 459-961, 2003.

859. Impact of technology in the utilization of positron emission tomography in lymphoma: Current and future perspectives. Visvikis D and Ell PJ. European Journal of Nuclear Medicine. 30(Suppl1), S106-S116, 2003.

860. Kinetic modelling of the novel NMDA receptor tracer [123I]CNS-1261 for SPET: a potential tracer for the NMDA receptor. Erlandsson KJ, Bressan RA, Mulligan RS, Owens J, Wyper D, Gunn RN, Cunningham VJ, Ell PJ and Pilowsky LS. Nuclear Medicine and Biology, 30(4), 441-454, 2003.

861. Treatment of Neuroendocrine tumours in adults with 131I-MIBG therapy. Bomanji JB, Wong W, Gaze MN, Cassoni A, Waddington W, Solano J and Ell PJ. Clinical Oncology, 15, 193-198, 2003.

862. Potential impact of [18F]3'-deoxy-3'-fluorothymidine versus [18F] fluoro-2-deoxy-D-glucose in Postron Emission Tomography for colorectal cancer. Francis DL, Visvikis D, Costa DC, Arulampalam THA, Townsend C, Luthra I, Taylor I and Ell PJ. European Journal of Nuclear Medicine, 30, 988-994, 2003.

863. Comparison of methodologies for the in vivo assessment of 18FLT utilisation in colorectal cancer. Visvikis D, Francis D, Mulligan R, Costa DC, Croasdale I, Luthra SK, Taylor I, and Ell PJ. European Journal of Nuclear Medicine and Molecular Imaging, 31, 169-178, 2003.

864. Education and Training in Developing Countries. Hutton BF, Nair PGG and Ell PJ. Seminars in Nuclear Medicine, 30, 988-994, 2003.

865. In vivo imaging of cellular proliferation in colorectal cancer using Positron Emission Tomography. Francis DL, Freeman A, Visvikis D, Costa DC, Luthra SK, Novelli M, Taylor I and Ell PJ. GUT, 52, 1602-1606, 2003.

866. Analysis of D2 dopamine receptor occupancy with quantitative SPET using the high-affinity ligand [123I]epidepride: resolving conflicting findings. Erlandsson KJ, Bressan RA, Mulligan RS, Ell PJ, Cunningham VJ and Pilowsky LS. NeuroImage, 19(3), 1205-1214, 2003.

867. Concentration-dependent effects of polytethylene glycol 400 on gastrointestinal transit and drug absorption. Schulze JDR, Waddington WA, Ell PJ, Parsons GE, Coffin MD and Basit AW. Pharmaceutical Research, 20, 12, 1984-1988, 2003.

868. Evaluation of NMDA receptors in vivo in schizophrenic patients with [123I]CNS 1261 and SPET: Preliminary findings. Bressan RA, Erlandsson K, Mulligan RS, Gunn RN, Cunningham VJ, Owens J, Ell PJ and Pilowsky LS. Annals of New York Academy of Sciences, 1300, 1-4, 2003.

869. A new approach to pre-treatment assessment of the NO neck in oral squamous cell carcinoma: the role of sentinel node biopsy and positron emission tomography. Hyde NC, Prvulovich E, Newman L, Waddington WA, Visvikis D and Ell PJ. Oral Oncology 29, 350-360, 2003.

870. Positron emission and computed X-ray tomography: a coming together. Costa DC, Visvikis D, Croasdale I, Pigden I, Townsend C, Bomanji J, Prvulovich E, Lonn A and Ell PJ. Nuclear Medicine Communications, 24, 351-358, 2003.

871. Is regionally selective D2/D3 dopamine occupancy sufficient for atypical antipsychotic effect? An in vivo quantitative [123I] epidepride SPET study of amisulpride-treated patients. Bressan RA, Erlandsson K, Jones HM, Mulligan R, Flanagan RJ, Ell PJ and Pilowsky LS. American Journal of Psychiatry, 160, 1413-1420, 2003.

2004

872. Myocardian perfusion scintigraphy – the evidence. Underwood SR, Anagnostopoulos C, Cerqueira M, Ell PJ, Flint J, Harbinson M, Kelion AD, Al-Mohammad A, Prvulovich EM, Shaw LJ and Tweddel AC. European Journal of Nuclear Medicine and Molecular Imaging, 31, 261-291, 2004.

873. Clinical audit in Nuclear Medicine. Peters AM, Bomanji JB, Costa DC, Ell PJ, Gordon I, Henderson BH and Hilson AJ. Nuclear Medicine Communications, 25, 97-103, 2004.

874. A bolus/infusion paradigm for the novel NMDA receptor SPET tracer [123I]CNS 1261. Bressan RA, Erlandson K, Mullingan RS, Gunn RN, Cunningham VJ, Owens J, Cullum ID, Ell PJ, and Pilowsky, LS. Nuclear Medicine and Biology, 31, 2, 155-164, 2004.

875. The use of formulation technology to assess regional gastrointestinal drug absorption in humans. Basit AW, Podczeck F, Newton JM, Waddington WA, Ell PJ and Lacey LF. European Journal of Pharmaceutical Sciences, 21, 179-189, 2004.

876. Does 18FDG-PET/CT as compared to dedicated CT alter management of pancreatobiliary tumours? Pakzad F, Syed R, Nagabushan N, Shankar A, Taylor I, and Ell PJ. Journal of Nuclear Medicine, 45, 87, 2004.

877. A comparison of FDG PET/CT and MRI versus histology for staging of primary head and neck cancers and detection of recurrent disease. Hughes SJ, Prvulovich EM, Witherow H, Kalavrezos N and Ell PJ. Journal of Nuclear Medicine, 45, 80, 2004.

878. Measuring SSRI occupancy of SERT using the novel SPET tracer [123I]ADAM. Erlandsson K, Warrington S, Sivanathan T, Lui D, Spezzi A, Townsend CE, Fry P, Lucas R, and Ell PJ. Journal of Nuclear Medicine, 45, 397, 2004.

879. Impact of 18F-FDG PET/CT in the management of pancreatobiliary tumours. Syed R, Pakzad F, Nagabhushan N, Groves A, Copland C, Taylor I, Ell PJ and Bomanji JB. Journal of Nuclear Medicine, 45, 344, 2004.

880. Samarium-153 Lexidronam Complex for the treatment of painful bone metastases in hormone-refractory prostate cancer. Sartor O, Reid RH, Hoskin PJ, Quick DP, Ell PJ, Coleman RE, Kotler JA, Freeman LM, and Olivier P; Quadramet 424Sm10/11 Study Group. Urology, 63, 940-945, 2004.

881. Issues undermining the provision of diagnostic imaging in the UK. Ell PJ, O'Doherty MJO, and Cook GJR. Lancet Oncology, 5, 467-468, 2004.

882. SPET imaging of central muscarinic receptors with (R,R) [123I]I-QNB: Methological considerations. Norbury R, Travis MJ, Erlandsson K, Owens J, Ell PJ and Murphy DG. Nuclear Medicine and Biology, 31(5), 583-590, 2004.

883. Prolactinemia is uncoupled from central D2/D3 Dopamine receptor occupancy in amisulpride treated patients. Bressan RA, Erlandsson K, Spencer EP, Ell PJ and Pilowsky LS. Psychopharmacology (Berl), 175 (3), 367-373, 2004.

884. Development of a bolus/infusion paradigm for the novel NMDA receptor tracer [123I]CNS 1261: Comparison with bolus studies. Bressan RA, Erlandsson K, Mulligan RS, Gunn RN, Cunningham VJ, Owen J, Cullum, ID, Ell PJ, Pilowsky LS. Nuclear Medicine and Biology, 31(2),155-164, 2004.

885. Myocardial perfusion scintigraphy: patients' perception of benefit and risk. Groves AM, Kayani I, Syed R, Gacinovic S, Nagabhushan N and Ell PJ. Nuclear Medicine Communications, 25(12), 1219-1222, 2004.

886. FDG-PET for the pre-operative staging of colorectal liver metastases. Arulampalam THA, Francis DL, Visvikis D, Taylor I and Ell PJ. European Journal of Surgical Oncology, 30, 286-291, 2004.

887. Assessment of recurrent colorectal cancer following 5-fluorouracil chemotherapy using both 18FDG and 18FLT PET. Francis DL, Visvikis D, Costa DC, Croasdale I, Arulampalam TH, Luthra SK, Taylor I, and Ell PJ. European Journal of Nuclear Medicine and Molecular Imaging, 31, 928, 2004.

888. Sentinel lymph node biopsy in patients with multifocal breast cancer. Goyal A, Newcombe RG, Mansel RE, Chetty U, Ell PJ, Fallowfield L, Kissim M, Sibbering M; ALMANAC Trialists Group. European Journal of Surgical Oncology, 30, 475-479, 2004.

889. Sentinel lymph node biopsy in male breast cancer patients. Goyal A, Horgan K, Kissim M, Yiangou C, Sibbering M, Lansdown M, Newcombe RG, Mansel RE, Chetty U, Ell PJ, Fallowfield L; ALMANAC Trialists Group. European Journal of Surgical Oncology, 30, 480-483, 2004.

890. The role of PET imaging in lymphoma. Burton C. Ell PJ and Linch D. British Journal of Haematology, 126, 772-784, 2004.

891. Tumour vaccine associated lymphadenopathy and false positive positron emission tomography scan changes. Jones RL, Cunningham D, Cook G and Ell PJ. British Journal of Radiology, 77, 74-75, 2004.

892. Thyroid blocking policy – revisited. Solanki KK, Bomanji JB, Waddington WA, and Ell PJ. Nuclear Medicine Communications, 25, 1071-1076, 2004.

893. In vivo imaging of muscarinic receptors in the aging female brain with (R,R)[123I]-I-QNB and Single Photon Emission Tomography. Norbury R, Travis MJ, Erlandsson K, Waddington W, Owens J, Ell PJ, et al. Journal of Experimental Gerontology, 40, 137-145, 2004.

894. Comparison of methodologies for the in vivo assessment of [18]FLT utilisation in colorectal cancer. Visvikis D, Francis D, Mulligan R, Costa DC, Croasdale I, Luthra SK, Taylor I and Ell PJ. European Journal of Nuclear Medicine and Molecular Imaging, 31(2), 169-178, 2004.

2005

895. How often do patients undergo repeat PET or PET/CT examinations? Experience from a UK Institution. Groves AM, Cullum ID, Syed R, Nagabhushan N, Kayani I, Pakzad F and Ell PJ. Nuclear Medicine Communications, 26, 2, 137-139, 2005.

896. Highlights of the Annual Congress of the European Association of Nuclear Medicine, Helsinki 2004, and a dashof horizon scanning. Ell PJ. European Journal of Nuclear Medicine and Molecular Imaging, 32(1), 113-126, 2005.

897. A training simulator for sentinel node biopsy in breast cancer: A new standard. Keshtgar MRS, Chicken DW, Waddington WA, and Ell PJ. European Journal of Surgical Oncology, 31(2), 134-140, 2005.

898. Use of 18F-FDG positron emission tomography following allogeneic transplantation to guide adoptive immunotherapy with donor lymphocyte infusions. Hart DP, Avivi I, Thomson KJ, Peggs KS, Morris EC, Goldstone AH, Linch DC, Ell PJ, Bomanji JB and McKinnon S. British Journal of Haematology, 128(6), 824-829, 2005.

899. Imaging bronchial carcinoma in situ: possible roles for combined positron emission tomography – PET/CT. Kayan I, Groves AM, Ell PJ, George PJ and Bomanji J. Lancet Oncology, 6(3), 190, 2005.

900. Oral contrast medicine in PET/CT: should you or shouldn't you? Groves AM, Kayani I, Dickson JC, Townsend C, Croasdale I, Syed R, Nagabhushan N, Hain S and Ell PJ. European Journal of Nuclear Medicine and Molecular Imaging, 32, 1160-1166, 2005.

901. Clinical evaluation of 2D versus 3D whole body PET image quality using a dedicated BGO PET scanner. Visvikis D, Griffiths D, Costa DC, Bomanji J and Ell PJ. European Journal of Nuclear Medicine and Molecular Imaging, 32, 1050-1056, 2005.

902. Molecular imaging in animal models of disease – every detail counts. Pakzad F, Ell PJ and Carrio I. European Journal of Nuclear Medicine and Molecular Imaging, 32, 899-960, 2005.

903. Impact of combined 18F-FDG PET/CT in head and neck tumours. Syed R, Bomanji JB, Nagabhushan N, Hughes S, Kayani I, Groves AM, Gacinovic S, Hydes N, Visvikis D, Copland C and Ell PJ. British Journal of Cancer, 92(6), 1046-50, 2005.

904. Impact of schizophrenia and chronic antipsychotic treatment on [123I]CNS-1261 binding to NMDA receptors in vivo. Bressan RA, Erlandsson K, Stone JM, Mulligan RS, Krystal JH, Ell PJ and Pilowsky LS. Biological Psychiatry, 58(1), 41-46, 2005.

905. Anti-CD20 monoclonal antibody (rituximab) as an adjunct in the treatment of giant cell arteritis. Bhatia A, Ell PJ and Edwards JC. Ann Rheum Dis, 64(7), 1099-100, 2005.

906. Non-uniform blockade of intrastriatal D2/D3 receptors by risperidone and amisulpride. Stone JM, Bressan RA, Erlandsson K, Ell PJ and Pilowsky LS. Psychopharmacology, 180(4), 664-9, 2005.

907. Measuring SSRI occupancy of SERT using the novel 123I-ADAM tracer: a SPET validation study. Erlandsson K, Sivananthan T, Lui D, Spezzi A, Townsend CE, Hu S, Lucas R, Warrinton SL and Ell PJ. European Journal of Nuclear Medicine and Molecular Imaging, 32, 1329-1336, 2005.

908. 18F-FDG PET scanning and lymphoma. Bomanji JB and Ell PJ. British Journal of Cancer Management, 2, 8-11, 2005.

2006

909. The contributions of PET/CT to improved patient management. Ell PJ. British Journal of Radiology, 79, 32-36, 2006.

910. First in vivo evidence of an NMDA receptor deficit in medication-free schizophrenic patients. Pilowsky LS, Bressan RA, Stone JM, Erlandsson K, Mullingan RS, Krystal JH and Ell PJ. Molecular Psychiatry, 11, 118-119, 2006.

911. PET and SPECT in common neuropsychiatric disease. Tatsch K and Ell PJ. Clinical Medicine, 6, 259-262, 2006.

912. Randomized multicenter trial of sentinel node biopsy in breast cancer: The Almanac Trial. Mansel RE, Fallowfield L, Kissin M, Goyal A, Newcombe RG, Dixon JM, Yiangou C, Horgan K, Bundred N, Monypenny I, England D, Sibbering M, Abdullah TI, Barr L, Chetty U, Sinnett DH, Fleissig A, Clarke D and Ell PJ. Journal of the National Cancer Institute, 98, 599-609, 2006.

913. A comparison of Tl-201, Tc-99m sestamibi, and Tc-99m tetrofosmin myocardial perfusion scintigraphy in patients with mild to moderate coronary stenosis. Reyes E, Loong C Y, Harbinson M, Rahman SH, Prvulovich E, Ell PJ, Anagnostopoulos C and Underwood SR. Journal of Nuclear Cardiology, 13(4), 488-494, 2006.

914. CT Pulmonary Angiography versus Ventilation-Perfusion scintigraphy in pregnancy: Implications from a survey of Doctors' knowledge of Radiation Exposure. Groves AM, Yates SJ, Win T, Kayani I, Gallagher FA, Syed R, Bomanji J and Ell PJ. Radiology, 240, 765-770, 2006.

915. The Role of Positron Emission Tomography in the Management of Pancreatic Cancer. Pakzad F, Groves A, Ell P J. Seminars in Nuclear Medicine, 36, 248-256, 2006.

916. Implications from an international survey of imaging scaphoid trauma. Groves AM, Kayani I, Syed R, Bearcroft PW, Hutton BF, Dixon AK and Ell PJ. American Journal of Roentogenology, 187, 1260-1265, 2006.

917. 186Re-HEDP in the Treatment of Patients with Inoperable Osteosarcoma. Syed R, Bomanji J, Nagabhushan N, Kayani I, Groves AM, Waddington WA, Cassoni A and Ell PJ. The Journal of Nuclear Medicine, 47(12), 1927-1935, 2006.

918. 99mTc-MAG3 Scintigraphy with Full Bladder in Patients with Severe Bladder Dysfunction. Nagabhushan N, Syed R, Hoh I, Syed I, Ell PJ, Neild G, Woodhouse C and Bomanji J. The Journal of Urology, 176(4), 1481-1486, 2006.

919. Ketamine displacement of [123I]CNS-1261 – a novel NMDA receptor SPET probe. Stone JM, Erlandsson K, Arstad E, Bressan RA, Squassante L, Teneggi V, Ell PJ, Pilowsky L. Nuclear Medicine and Biology, 33(2), 239-243, 2006.

920. An international survey of hospital practice in the imaging of acute scaphoid trauma. Groves A, Kayani I, Syed R, Hutton BF, Bearcroft PP, Dixon AK, Ell PJ. Am J Roentgenology 187, 1453-1456, 2006

921. Dose escalation study of Rhenium-186-HEDP in the treatment of patients with inoperable osteosarcoma. Syed R, Waddington W, Cassoni A, Kayani I, Groves AM, Ell PJ, Bomanji J. Journal of Nuclear Medicine, 47, 1927-1935, 2006.

922. [(123)I]TPCNE-A novel SPET tracer for the sigma-1 receptor: First human studies and in vivo haloperidol challenge. Stone JM, Arstad E, Erlandsson K, Waterhouse RN, Ell PJ, Pilowsky LS. Synapse, 60(2), 109-117, 2006.

923. Cortical serotonin 5-HT2A receptor binding and social communications in adults with Asperger's syndrome: an in vivo SPECT study. Murphy DG, Daly E, Schmitz N, Toal F, Murphy K, Curran S, Erlandsson K, Eersels J, Kerwin R, Ell P, Travis M. Am J Psychiatry, 163(5), 934-936, 2006.

2007

924. Safety and Efficacy of Repeat Administration of Samarium Sm-153 Lexidronam to Patients With Metastatic Bone Pain. Sartor O, Reid RH, Bushnell DL, Quick DP, Ell PJ. Cancer, 109, 637-643, 2007.

925. Detection of tumour thrombus by 18F-FDG-PET/CT imaging. Lai P, Bomanji JB, Mahmood S, Nagabhushan N, Syed R, Gacinovic S, Lee SM, Ell PJ. Eur J Cancer Prev., 16(1), 90-94, 2007.

926. Estrogen Therapy and brain muscarininc receptor density in healthy females: A SPET study. Norbury R, Travis MJ, Erlandsson K, Waddington W, Ell PJ, Murphy DG. Horm Behav., 51(2), 249-257, 2007.

927. Does PET imaging have a role in renal cancers after all? Powles T and Ell PJ. The Lancet Oncology, (8), 279-281, 2007.

928. Allergy to technetium-labelled nanocolloidal albumin for sentinel node identification. Chicken DW, Mansouri R, Ell PJ, Keshtgar MR. Ann R Coll Surg Engl., 89(2), 12-3, 2007.

929. Fusion of metabolic function and morphology: sequential [18F]fluorodeoxyglucose positron emission tomography/computed tomography studies yield new insights into the natural history of bone metastases in breast cancer. Du Y, Cullum I, Illidge T and Ell PJ. Journal of Clinical Oncology, 10, 3440-3447, 2007.

930. Non F18 FDG in Clinical Oncology. Groves A, Win T, Ben Haim S and Ell PJ. The Lancet Oncology 8, 822-830, 2007.

931. The impact of 18F-FDG PET/CT in patients with liver metastases. Chua SC, Groves AM, Kayani I, Menezes L, Gacinovic S, Yong Du, Bomanji J and Ell PJ. European Journal of Nuclear Medicine, 34, 34, 1906-1914, 2007.

932. Cardiac 82Rubidium PET/CT: Initial European Experience. Groves AM, Speechly-Dick ME, Dickson JC, Kayani I, Blanchard P, Endozo R, Shastry M, Menezes LJ, Prvulovich E, Townsend C, Waddington WA, Ben-Haim S, Bomanji JB, Hutton BF, McEwan JR and Ell PJ. European Journal of Nuclear Medicine, 34, 1965-1972, 2007.

933. Effect of the Abnormal Bladder When Full on Upper Tract Drainage Using a Combined Cystometrogram – 99 mTc-MAG 3 Renogram: a prospective study. Hoh IMY, Bomanji JB, Nagabhushan N, Chu A, Ell PJ, Neild GH, and Woodhouse CRJ. British Journal of Urology Int., 100(5), 1131-1136, 2007.

934. 'Click Labeling' with [18F]fluoroethylazide for Positron Emission tomography (PET) Arstad, E. Bioconjugate chem., 18(3), 989, 2007.

935. Multi-modality imaging on track. Beekman F, Hutton BF Eur J Nucl Med Mol I, 34, 1410-1414, 2007.

936. Giant cervical parathyroid adenoma mimicking a sternocleidomastoid mass and presenting as a brown tumor of the mandible. Desigan S, Syed R, Conway GS, Kurzawinski TR, Bomanji JB. Clinical Nuclear medicine, 32(4), 306-308, 2007.

937. Misregistration of emission and CT attenuation correction data in 82Rb cardiac PET/CT. Dickson JC, Groves AM, Kayani I, Hutton BF, Ell PJ, Waddington WA, Cullum I. Eur J Nucl Med Mol I, 34, S145, 2007.

938. Perfusion scintigraphy still has important role in evaluation of majority of pregnant patients with suspicion of pulmonary embolism. Groves AM, Yates SJ, Win T, Kayani I, Bomanji JB, Ell PJ. Radiology, 244, 623-625, 2007.

939. Combined 82Rb cardiac PET/64 slice CT angiography: initial experience. Groves AM, Kayani I, Endozo R, Menezes LJ, Habib SB, Prvulovich E, Shastry M, Rajasekharan S, Prakash V, Goh V, Ben-Haim S, Bomanji JB, Ell PJ. Eur J Nucl Med Mol, 34, S171, 2007.

940. Optimal parallel hole collimator for cardiac imaging with iterative reconstruction and resolution recovery. Kacperski K, Hutton BF. Proc 3D Image Reconstruction in Radiology and Nuclear medicine, 174-177, 2007.

941. Potential to Normalise Myocardial Perfusion SPECT Using CT: Technical Considerations. Rajasekharan S, Hutton B, Groves AM, Goh V, Dickson J, Endozo R, Menezes L, Shastry M, Ell P.J. Eur J Nucl Med Mol, 34, 262, 2007.

942. The effect of lung resection on pulmonary function and excercise capacity in lung cancer patients. Win T, Groves AM, Ritchie AJ, Wells FC, Cafferty F, Laroche CM. Respiratory Care, 52(6), 720-726, 2007.

943. Functional recovery after lung resection for bronchogenic carcinoma. Win T, Groves AM, Momday H, Nathan J, Oscroft N, Laroche CM. Respiratory Care, 52, 720-726, 2007.

2008

944. Functional imaging of Neuroendocrine tumors with combined PET/CT using 68Ga-DOTATATE (DOTA-dPhe1,Tyr3-octreotate) and 18F-FDG. Kayani I, Bomanji JB, Groves AM, Conway G, Gacinovic S, Win T, Dickson J, Caplin M, Ell PJ. Cancer, 112(11), 2447-55, 2008.

945. Relationship between ketamine-induced psychotic symptoms and NMDA receptor occupancy—a [123I]CNS-1261 SPET study. Stone JM, Erlandsson K, Arstad E, Squassante L, Teneggi V, Bressan R, Krystal J, Ell PJ, Pilowsky L. Psychopharmacology (Berl), 197(3), 401-408, 2008.

946. Sugar rush: the early days of molecular imaging. Ell PJ Lancet Oncol., 9(4), 400, 2008.

947. How do patients perceive the benefits and risks of peripheral angioplasty? Implications for informed consent. Habib SB, Sonoda L, See TC, Ell PJ, Groves AM. J Vasc Interv Radiol., 19(2 Pt 1), 177-81, 2008.

948. Stage migration and pilot studies of reduced chemotherapy supported by positron-emission tomography findings suggest new combined strategies for stage 2 non-seminoma germ cell tumour. Haba Y, Williams MV, Neal DE, Ong JY, Ostrowski MJ, Ell PJ, Nargund V, Shamash J, Oliver RT. British Journal of Urology Int., 101(5), 570-574, 2008.

949. Long-term estrogen therapy and 5-HT(2A) receptor binding in postmenopausal women; a single photon emission tomography (SPET) study. Compton J, Travis MJ, Norbury R, Erlandsson K, van Amelsvoort T, Daly E, Waddington W, Matthiasson P, Eersels JL, Whitehead M, Kerwin RW, Ell PJ, Murphy DG. Horm Behav., 53(1), 61-68, 2008.

950. CT coronary angiography: Quantitative assessment of myocardial perfusion using test bolus data-initial experience. Groves AM, Goh V, Rajasekharan S, Kayani I, Endozo R, Dickson JC, Menezes LJ, Shastry M, Habib SB, Ell PJ, Hutton BF. Eur Radiol., 18(10), 2155-2163, 2008.

951. Clinical governance improves de quality of nuclear medicine reporting. Peter AM, Bomanji, J, Ell, PJ, Gordon I, Hilson, JW, Murrain, C. Nuclear Medicine Communications, 29, 999-1001, 2008.

952. High-grade mucoepidermoid carcinoma of the accessory parotid gland with distant metastases identified by 18F-FDG PET-CT Marcelo Gomes, Giovanna Pepe, Jamshed Bomanji, Omar Al-Salihi, Yong Du, Svetislav Gacinovic, Peter Ell. Pediatric blood & cancer, 50(2), 395-397, 2008.

953. Guidelines for the use of PET-CT in children. Barrington SF, Begent J, Lynch T, Schleyer P, Biassoni L, Ramsden W, Kane T, Stoneham S, Brooks M, Hain SF. Nuclear Medicine Communications, 29(5), 418-424, 2008.

954. Initial experience with fast dynamic single photon emission computed tomography for myocardial perfusion imaging. Ben-Haim S, Hutton B, Van Gramberg D, Prakash V, Waddington WA, Bomanji JB, Prvulovich E, Groves A, Kacperski K, Ell PJ. Nucl Med Commun., 29, 468, 2008.

955. Is low blood pool clearance due to low LVEF a contraindication to Rb PET/CT? Dickson JC, Groves AM, Kayani I, Endozo R, Waddington W, Hutton B, Ell PJ. Journal of Nuclear Medicine, 49, 193-194, 2008.

956. Reduction of CT artifacts due to respiratory motion in a slowly rotating SPECT/CT. Erlandsson K, Núñez M, Hutton BF. IEEE Nuclear Science Symposium and Medical Imaging Conference, 3775-3778, 2008.

957. HICAM: development of a high-resolution Anger Camera for nuclear medicine. Fiorini C, Gola A, Peloso R, Longoni A, Lechner P, Strüder L, Hutton BF, Erlandsson K, Mahmood S, Van Mullekom P, Pedretti A, Moretti R, Poli GL, LucignaniG. IEEE Nuclear Science Symposium and Medical Imaging Conference, 3961-3964, 2008.

958. Methods for 18F-labeling of RGDpeptides: comparison of aminooxy [18F]fluorobenzaldehyde condensation with 'click labeling' using 2-[18F]fluoroethylazide, and S-alkylation with [18F]fluoropropanethiol. Glaser M, Solbakken M, Turton DR, Pettitt R, Barnett J, Arukwe J, Karlsen H, Cuthbertson A, Luthra SK, Årstad E. Amino Acids, DOI 10, 2008.

959. Imaging HOCM on combined Rb PET/CTA: Initial Experience. Groves AM, Elliott PR, Kayani I, Endozo R, Menenzes L, Moon JC, Habib S, Woldman S, McKenna W, Ell PJ. Journal of Nuclear Medicine, 49, 195-196, 2008.

960. Vascular uptake of 18F-FDG Uptake: data from the latest PET/CT machine. Groves AM, Endozo R, Menezes LJ, Kayani I, Bomanji J, Hutton BF, Ell PJ. Journal of Nuclear Medicine, 49, 184-185, 2008.

961. How do patients perceive benefits and risks of peripheral angiography? Implications for obtaining informed consent. Habib SH, See TC, Sonoda L, Ell PJ, Groves AM. Journal of Vascular and Interventional Radiology, 19, 177-181, 2008.

962. Evaluation of a low-dose/slow-rotating SPECT-CT system. Hamann M, Aldridge M, Dickson J, Endozo R, Lozhkin K, Hutton B. Phys Med Biol., 53, 2495-2508, 2008.

963. Iterative Deconvolution of Simultaneous Dual Radionuclide Projections for CdZnTe Based Cardiac SPECT. Kacperski K, Erlandsson K, Ben-Haim S, Van Gramberg D, Hutton BF. IEEE Nuclear Science Symposium and Medical Imaging Conference, 5260-5263.

964. Functional imaging of neuroendocrine tumors with combined PET/CT using 68Ga-DOTATATE (DOTA-DPhe1,Tyr3-octreotate) and 18F-FDG. Kayani I, Bomanji JB, Groves A, Conway G, Gacinovic S, Win T, Dickson J, Caplin M, Ell PJ. Cancer 112(11), 2447-2455, 2008.

965. Thymic 18F-fluorodeoxyglucose uptake on positron emission tomography scanning after doxorubicin, bleomycin, vincristin and dacarbazine chemotherapy and highly-active antiretroviral therapy in HIV-associated Hodgkin's disease in an adult. Lee S, Buchler T, Bomanji J, Ramsay A, Edwards S. GAIDS, 22(1), 159-160, 2008.

966. Proceedings of the IASLC International Workshop on Advances in Pulmonary Neuroendocrine Tumors 2007. Lim E, Goldstraw P, Nicholson A, Travis W, Jett J, Ferolla P, Bomanji J, Rusch V, Asamura H, Skogseid B, Baudin E, Caplin M, Kwekkeboom D, Brambilla E, Crowley J. J Thorac Oncol., 3(10), 1194-120, 2008.

967. Improved Reconstructed Image Quality in a SPECT System with Slit-Slat Collimation by Combination of Multiplexed and Non-Multiplexed Data. Mahmood S, Erlandsson K, Hutton B. IEEE Nuclear Science Symposium and Medical Imaging Conference, 4598-4603, 2008.

968. A comparison between respiratory-induced attenuation-correction artefacts in PET/CT and SPECT/CT. McQuaid S, Hutton B. (2008). Eur J Nucl Med Mol Imaging 35, 1117-1123, 2008.

969. Statistical shape modeling of the diaphragm for application to 82-Rb cardiac PET-CT studies. McQuaid, S., Lambrou, T, Hutton, B. (2008). IEEE Nuclear Science Symposium and Medical Imaging Conference, 3651-3655, 2008.

970. Assessment of left ventricular function at rest using Rb myocardial perfusion PET; Comparison of 4 different software algorithms with simultaneous 64 detector coronary CT. Menezes LJ, Groves AM, Kayani I, Bomanji J, Hutton BF, Ell PJ. Journal of Nuclear Medicine, 49, 73-74, 2008.

971. Clinical governance improves the quality of nuclear medicine reporting. Peters AM, Bomanji J, Ell PJ, Gordon I, Hilson AJ, Murrain C. Nucl Med Commun., 29(11), 999-1001, 2008.

972. New Method for Radiosynthesis of 11C-Labeled Carbamate Groups and its Application for a Highly Efficient Synthesis of the Kappa-Opioid Receptor Tracer [11C]GR103545. Schoultz BW, Årstad E, Marton J, Willoch F, Drzezga A, Wester HJ, Henriksen GA. The Open Medicinal Chemistry Journal, 2(3), 72-74., 2008.

973. High-speed myocardial perfusion imaging: Initial clinical comparison with conventional dual detector Anger camera imaging. Sharir T, Ben-Haim S, Merzon K, Prochorov V, Dickman D, Ben-Haim S, Berman DS. J Am Coll Cardiol., 1(2), 156-163, 2008.

974. Design, synthesis, and biological characterization of a caspase 3/7 selective isatin labeled with 2-[18F]fluoroethylazide. Smith G, Glaser M, Perumal M, Nguyen QD, Shan B, Årstad E, Aboagye EO. J Med Chem, 51(24), 8057-8067, 2008.

975. Guidelines for 18F-FDG PET and PET-CT imaging in paediatric oncology. Stauss J, Franzius C, Pfluger T, Juergens KU, Biassoni L, Begent J, Kluge R, Amthauer H, Voelker T, Højgaard L, Barrington S, Hain S, Lynch T, Hahn K. European Journal of Nuclear Medicine and Molecular Imaging, 35(8), 1581-1588, 2008.

976. Relationship between ketamine-induced psychotic symptoms and NMDA receptor occupancy: a [(123)I]CNS-1261 SPET study. Stone JM, Erlandsson K, Arstad E, Squassante L, Teneggi V, Bressan RA, Krystal JH, Ell PJ, Pilowsky LS. Psychopharmacology (Berl), 197(3), 401-408, 2008.

977. Dynamic single photon emission computed tomography - novel technology for fast myocardial perfusion imaging: a technologist's perspective. Van Gramberg D, Ben-Haim S, Hutton B, Prakash V, Waddington W, Townsend C, Ell P. Nucl Med Commun. 29, 480-480, 2008.

978. CT Screening for cerebral metastases in patients with potentially resectable non small cell lung cancer: Experience from a UK Cardiothoracic Centre. Win, T, Laroche CM, Groves AM, Nathan J, Clements L, Screaton NJ. Clinical Radiology, 59, 936-939, 2008.

979. Predicting survival in potentially curable lung cancer patients. Win T, Sharples L, Groves A, Jackson A, Wells F, Ritchie A, Laroche C. Lung, 186, 97-102, 2008.

2009

980. 18F-FDG PET and PET/CT in the evaluation of cancer treatment response. Ben-Haim S, Ell P. Journal of Nuclear Medicine, 50(1), 88-99, 2009.

981. EANM-EORTC general recommendations for sentinel node diagnostics in melanoma. Chakera AH, Hesse B, Burak Z, Ballinger JR, Britten A, Caracò C, Cochran AJ, Cook MG, Drzewiecki KT, Essner R, Even-Sapir E, Eggermont AM, Stopar TG, Ingvar C, Mihm MC Jr, McCarthy SW, Mozzillo N, Nieweg OE, Scolyer RA, Starz H, Thompson JF, Trifirò G, Viale G, Vidal-Sicart S, Uren R, Waddington W, Chiti A, Spatz A, Testori A. Eur J Nucl Med Mol Imaging, 36(10), 1713-42, 2009.

982. Partial volume correction in SPECT using anatomical information and iterative FBP. Erlandsson K, Hutton BF. Proc 10th International Meeting on Fully Three-dimensional Reconstruction in Radiology and Nuclear Medicine 287-290, 2009.

983. Performance evaluation of D-SPECT: a novel SPECT system for nuclear cardiology. Erlandsson K, Kacperski K, van Gramberg D, Hutton BF. Physics in Medicine and Biology, 54(9), 2635-2649, 2009.

984. A novel high sensitivity rapid acquisition single photon molecular imaging camera. Gambhir SS, Berman DS, Ziffer J, Nagler M, Dickman D, Rousso B, Sandler M, Patton J, Hutton B, Dichterman E, Ziv O, Melman H, Zilberstein Y, Ben-Haim S, and Ben-Haim S. Journal of Nuclear Medicine, 50, 635-643, 2009.

985. First experience of combined cardiac PET/64-detector CT angiography with invasive angiographic validation. Groves AM, Speechly-Dick ME, Kayani I, Pugliese F, Endozo R, McEwan J, Menezes LJ, Habib SB, Prvulovich E, Ell PJ. European Journal of Nuclear Medicine and Molecular Imaging, 36(12), 2027-33, 2009.

986. Idiopathic Pulmonary Fibrosis and Diffuse Parenchymal Lung Disease: Implications from Initial Experience with 18F-FDG-PET/CT. Groves AM, Win T, Screaton NJ, Berovic M, Endozo R, Booth H, Kayani I, Menezes LJ, Dickson JC, Ell PJ. Journal of Nuclear Medicine, 50(4), 538-545, 2009.

987. Metabolic-flow relationships in primary breast cancer: feasibility with combined PET/dynamic contrast-enhanced CT. Groves AM, Wishart GC, Shastry M, Moyle P, Britten P, Iddles S, Brtton P, Gaskarth M, Warren RM, Ell PJ, Miles KA. European Journal of Nuclear Medicine and Molecular Imaging, 36(3), 416-421, 2009.

988. Evidence for pre and postsynaptic nigrostriatal dysfunction in the fragile X tremor-Ataxia syndrome. Healy DG, Bressman S, Dickson J, Silveira-Moriyama L, Schneider SA, O'Sullivan SS, Massey L, Bhatia KP, Shaw K, Bomanji J, Wood NW, Lees AJ. Movement Disorders, 24(8), 1245-1247, 2009.

989. Increased Metabolic Activity in Abdominal Aortic Aneurysm Detected by 18F-Fluorodeoxyglucose ((18)F-FDG) Positron Emission Tomography/Computed Tomography (PET/CT). Kotze CW, Menezes LJ, Endozo R, Groves AM, Ell PJ, Yusuf SW. European Journal of Vascular and Endovascular Surgery, 38(1), 93-99, 2009.

990. Design of a novel slit-slat collimator system for SPECT imaging of the human brain. Mahmood ST, Erlandsson K, Cullum I, Hutton BF. Physics in Medicine and Biology, 54(11), 3433-3449, 2009.

991. The application of a statistically shape model to diaphragm tracking in respiratory gated PET images. McQuaid S, Lambrou T, Cunningham VJ, Bettinardi V, Gilardi MC, Hutton BF. Proceedings IEEE 97, 2039-2052, 2009.

992. Vascular inflammation imaging with 18F-FDG PET/CT: when to image? Menezes LJ, Kotze CW, Hutton BF, Endozo R, Dickson JC, Cullum I, Yusuf SW, Ell PJ, Groves AM. Journal of Nuclear Medicine, 50(6), 854-857, 2009.

993. Procedure guideline for planar radionuclide cardiac ventriculogram for the assessment of left ventricular systolic function. Nicol A, Avison M, Harbinson M, Jeans S, Waddington W, Woldman S. BNCS/BNMS/IPEM Nucl Med Commun., 30(3), 245-52, 2009.

994. Attenuation correction for lung SPECT: evidence of need and validation of an attenuation map derived from the emission data. Nunez M, Prakash V, Vila R, Mut F, Alonso O, Hutton BF. European Journal of Nuclear Medicine and Molecular Imaging, 36(7), 1076-1089, 2009.

995. Hybrid Imaging Technology: from dreams and vision to clinical devices. Patton JA, Townsend DW, Hutton BF. Seminars in Nuclear Medicine, 39, 247-263, 2009.

996. Sentinel node imaging in breast cancer using superficial injections: Technical details and observations. Somasundaram S, Chicken D, Waddington W, Bomanji J, Ell P, Keshtgar M. European Journal of Surgical Oncology, 35, 1250-1256, 2009.

2010

997. Why do clinicians request DaT scans ? An analysis of requesting practice and outcome in 455 consecutive scans. Aguirregomozcorta M, Edwards MJ, Prvulovich E, Schneider SA, Quinn NP, Lees AJ, Dickson JC, Bhatia KP. Mov Disord 25 (suppl 2), S368-369, 2010.

998. Scans with ipsilateral dopaminergic deficit (SWIDDs) – a new entity? Aguirregomozocorta M, Edwards MJ, Schwingenschuh P, Prvulovich E, Quinn NP, Dickson J, Bhatia KP. Mov Disord 25, (Suppl 2) S368-36, 2010.

999. Comparison of (68)Ga-DOTATATE and (18)F-fluorodeoxyglucose PET/CT in the detection of recurrent medullary thyroid carcinoma. Conry B, Papathanasiou N, Prakash V, Kayani I, Caplin M, Mahmood S, Bomanji J. European Journal of Nuclear Medicine and Molecular Imaging, 37(1), 49-57, 2010.

1000. The impact of reconstruction method on the quantification of DaTSCAN images. Dickson J, Tossici-Bolt L, Sera T, Erlandsson K, Varrone A, Tatsch K, Hutton BF. European Journal of Nuclear Medicine and Molecular Imaging, 37(1), 23-35, 2010.

1001. Simultaneous dual-radionuclide myocardial perfusion imaging with a solid-state dedicated cardiac camera. Ben-Haim S, Kacperski K., Hain S, Van Gramberg D, Hutton BF, Erlandsson K, Sharir T, Roth N, Waddington WA, Berman DS, Ell PJ Eur J Nucl med Mol Imaging, 37, 1710-1721, 2010.

1002. The effect of reconstruction method on DaTSCAN quantification. Dickson JC, Tossici-Bolt L, Sera T, Erlandsson K, Varrone A, Tatsch K, Hutton BF. Eur J Nucl Med Mol Imaging, 37, 23-35, 2010.

1003. Changes in the initial slope of the QRS in ischemic patients and normal subjects undergoing scintigraphy with dipyridamole. Dori G, Gershinsky M, Ben-Haim S, Lewis BS, Bitterman H. Computers Biol Med, 40, 869-875, 2010.

1004. "Partial volume correction in SPECT using anatomical information and iterative FBP" Erlandsson K, Hutton BF. Tsinghua Science and Technology, 15(1), 50-55, 2010.

1005. "Tracer Kinetic Modeling: Basics and Concepts", Erlandsson K, in M Kahlil (Ed) "Basic Sciences of Nuclear Medicine", Springer-Verlag, 2010.

1006. Automated synthesis of [11C]-(+)-PHNO from [11C]methyl iodide. Conference Information: 8th International Symposium on Functional Neuroreceptor Mapping of the Living Brain, JUL 22-24, 2010 Glasgow, SCOTLAND. Garcia-Arguello SF, Arstad E, Brickute D, Luthra SK, Turton DR, Glaser M, Fortt R, Robins EG. Neuroimage, 52 (Supplement), S218-S218, 2010.

1007. New SPECT technology: potential and challenges. Hutton BF. Eur J Nucl Med Mol Imaging, 37, 1883-1886, 2010.

1008. Prognostic role of PET scanning before and after reduced intensity allogeneic stem cell transplant for lymphoma Lambert JR, Bomanji JB, Peggs K S, Thomson K J, Chakraverty R K, Fielding A K, Kottaridis P D, Roughton M, Morris E C, Goldstone A H, Linch D C, Ell P J, and Mackinnon S. Blood, 115, 2763-2768, 2010

1009. Potential for mixed multiplexed and non-multiplexed data to significantly improve reconstruction quality of a Multi-Slit-Slat collimator SPECT System. Mahmood S, Erlandsson K, Cullum I, Hutton BF. Phys Med Biol, 55, 2247-2268, 2010.

1010. What is the Natural History of 18F-FDG Uptake in Arterial Atheroma on PET/CT. Menezes LJ, Kayani I, Bomanji J, Hutton BF, Ell PJ, Groves AM. Atherosclerosis, 211, 136-140, 2010.

1011. Pediatric and adolescent lymphoma: Comparison of whole-body STIR half-Fourier RARE MR imaging with an enhanced PET/CT reference for initial staging. Punwani S, Taylor SA, Bainbridge A, Prakash V, Bandula S, De Vita E, Olsen OE, Hain SF, Stevens N, Daw S, Shankar A, Bomanji JB, Humphries PD. Radiology, 255(1), 182-90, 2010.

1012. Synthesis and in vitro evaluation of F-18-labelled S-fluoroalkyl diarylguanidines: Novel high-affinity NMDA receptor antagonists for imaging with PET. Robins EG, Zhao YJ, Khan I, Wilson A, Luthra SK, Årstad E. Bioorg Med Chem Lett., 20(5), 1749-1751, 2010.

1013. Evaluation of the kappa-opioid receptor-selective tracer [(11)C]GR103545 in awake rhesus macaques. Schoultz BW, Hjornevik T, Willoch F, Marton J, Noda A, Murakami Y, Miyoshi S, Nishimura S, Årstad E, Drzezga A, Matsunari I, Henriksen G. Eur J Nucl Med Mol Imaging, 37(6), 1174-1180, 2010.

1014. Distinguishing SWEDDs patients with asymmetric resting tremor from Parkinson's disease: a clinical and electrophysiological Study. Schwingenschuh P, Ruge D, Edwards MJ, Terranova C, Katschnig P, Carrillo F, Silveira-Moriyama L, Schneider SA, Kägi G, Palomar FJ, Talelli P, Dickson J, Lees AJ, Quinn N, Mir P, Rothwell JC, Bhatia Kp. Mov Disord., 25(5), 560-9, 2010.

1015. Multicenter trial of high-speed versus conventional SPECT imaging: results of myocardial perfusion and left ventricular function. Sharir T, Slomka PJ, Hayes SW, Di Carli MF, Ziffer JA, Martin WH, Dickman D, Ben-Haim S, Berman DS J Am Coll Cardiol., 55, 1965-74, 2010.

1016. Distribution pattern of 68Ga-DOTATATE in disease-free patients. Shastry M, Kayani I, Wild D, Caplin M, Visvikis D, Gacinovic S, Reubi JC, Bomanji JB. Nucl Med Commun., 31(12), 1025-32, 2010.

1017. The role of 68Ga-DOTATATE PET in patients with neuroendocrine tumors and negative or equivocal findings on 111In-DTPA-octreotide scintigraphy. Srirajaskanthan R, Kayani I, Quigley AM, Soh J, Caplin ME, Bomanji J. J Nucl Med., 51(6), 875-82, 2010.

1018. PET/CT Colonography. J Nucl Med. Taylor SA, Bomanji JB. [Epub ahead of print] August 18, 2010, doi: 10.2967/jnumed.110.080374

1019. Nonlaxative PET/CT colonography: feasibility, acceptability, and pilot performance in patients at higher risk of colonic neoplasia. Taylor SA, Bomanji JB, Manpanzure L, Robinson C, Groves AM, Dickson J, Papathanasiou ND, Greenhalgh R, Ell PJ, Halligan S. J Nucl Med. 51(6), 854-61, 2010.

1020. Procedure guidelines for PET/CT tumour imaging with 68Ga-DOTA-conjugated peptides: 68Ga-DOTA-TOC, 68Ga-DOTA-NOC, 68Ga-DOTA-TATE. Virgolini I, Ambrosini V, Bomanji JB, Baum RP, Fanti S, Gabriel M, Papathanasiou ND, Pepe G, Oyen W, De Cristoforo C, Chiti A. Eur J Nucl Med Mol Imaging, 37(10),2004-10, 2010.

1021. 'Running on empty'. Wild D, Theodoraki A, Kurzawinski TR, Bomanji J, Reubi JC, Khan R, Bouloux P, Khoo B. Eur J Nucl Med Mol Imaging, 37(7), 1439-1440, 2010.

1022. Exendin-4-based radiopharmaceuticals for Glucagon-like-peptide-1 (GLP-1) Receptor PET/CT and SPECT/CT imaging. Wild D, Wicki A, Mansi R, Baumann A, Storch D, Béhé M, Bernhardt P, Christofori G, Ell P, and Mäcke H. European Journal of Nuclear Medicine and Molecular Imaging, 51(7), 1059-1067, 2010.

1023. Distribution pattern of 68Ga-DOTATATE in disease-free patients. Shastry M, Kayani I, Wild D, Caplin M, Visvikis D, Gacinovic S, Reubi JC, Bomanji JB. Nucl Med Commun., 31(12), 1025-32, 2010.

1024. Procedure guidelines for PET/CT tumour imaging with 68Ga-DOTA-conjugated peptides: 68Ga-DOTA-TOC, 68Ga-DOTA-NOC, 68Ga-DOTA-TATE. Virgolini I, Ambrosini V, Bomanji JB, Baum RP, Fanti S, Gabriel M, Papathanasiou ND, Pepe G, Oyen W, De Cristoforo C, Chiti A. Eur J Nucl Med Mol Imaging, 37(10), 2004-10, 2010.

1025. The role of 68Ga-DOTATATE PET in patients with neuroendocrine tumors and negative or equivocal findings on 111In-DTPA-octreotide scintigraphy. Srirajaskanthan R, Kayani I, Quigley AM, Soh J, Caplin ME, Bomanji J. J Nucl Med, 51(6),875-82, 2010

1026. Pediatric and adolescent lymphoma: Comparison of whole-body STIR half-Fourier RARE MR imaging with an enhanced PET/CT reference for initial staging. Punwani S, Taylor SA, Bainbridge A, Prakash V, Bandula S, De Vita E, Olsen OE, Hain SF, Stevens N, Daw S, Shankar A, Bomanji JB, Humphries PD. Radiology, 255(1), 182-90, 2010

1027. ^{18}F-FDG PET and biomarkers for tumour angiogenesis in early breast cancer. Groves AM, Shastry M, Rodriguez-Justo M, Malhotra A, Endozo R, Davidson T, Kelleher T, Miles KA, Ell PJ, Keshtgar MR. Eur J Nucl Med Mol Imaging, 38(1), 46-52, 2010.

2011

1028. Glucagon-like Peptide-1 versus somatostatin receptor targeting reveals 2 distinct forms of malignant insulinomas. Wild D, Christ E, Caplin ME, Kurzawinski TR, Forrer F, Brändle M, Seufert J, Weber WA, Bomanji J, Perren A, Ell PJ, Reubi JC. J Nucl Med, 52(7), 1073-1078, 2011.

1029. What is the relationship between (18)F-FDG aortic aneurysm uptake on PET/CT and future growth rate? Kotze CW, Groves AM, Menezes LJ, Harvey R, Endozo R, Kayani IA, Ell PJ, Yusuf SW. Eur J Nucl Med Mol Imaging, 38(8), 1493-1499, 2011.

1030. The role of ^{18}fluoro-deoxy glucose combined position emission and computed tomography in the clinical management of anal squamous cell carcinoma. Engledow AH, Skipworth JR, Blackman G, Groves A, Bomanji J, Warren SJ, Ell PJ, Boulos PB. Colorectal Dis., 13(5), 532-537, 2011.

1031. The importance of appropriate partial volume correction for PET quantification in Alzheimer's disease. Thomas BA, Erlandsson K, Modat M, Thurfjell L, Vandenberghe R, Ourselin S, Hutton BF. Eur J Nucl Med Mol Imaging, 38(6), 1104-1119, 2011.

1032. Iterative deconvolution of simultaneous 99mTc and 201Tl projection data measured on a CdZnTe-based cardiac SPECT scanner. Kacperski K, Erlandsson K, Ben-Haim S, Hutton BF. Phys Med Biol., 56(5), 1397-1414, 2011.

1033. PET imaging for prediction of response to therapy and outcome in oesophageal carcinoma. Chua S, Dickson J, Groves AM. Eur J Nucl Med Mol Imaging, 38(9), 1591-1594, 2011.

1034. What is the relationship between (18)F-FDG aortic aneurysm uptake on PET/CT and future growth rate? Kotze CW, Groves AM, Menezes LJ, Harvey R, Endozo R, Kayani IA, Ell PJ, Yusuf SW. Eur J Nucl Med Mol Imaging, 38(8), 1493-1499, 2011.

1035. Commercial software upgrades may significantly alter Perfusion CT parameter values in colorectal cancer. Goh V, Shastry M, Engledow A, Reston J, Wellsted DM, Peck J, Endozo R, Rodriguez-Justo M, Taylor SA, Halligan S, Groves AM. Eur Radiol., 21(4), 744-749, 2011.

1036. 18F-FDG PET/CT and 123I-metaiodobenzylguanidine imaging in high-risk neuroblastoma: diagnostic comparison and survival analysis. Papathanasiou ND, Gaze MN, Sullivan K, Aldridge M, Waddington W, Almuhaideb A, Bomanji JB. J Nucl Med, 52(4), 519-25, 2011.

1037. 177Lu-DOTATATE Molecular Radiotherapy for Childhood Neuroblastoma. Gains JE, Bomanji J, Fersht NL, Sullivan T, D'Souza D, Sullivan KP, Aldridge M, Waddington W, Gaze MN. J Nucl Med., 52(7), 1041-1047, 2011.

1038. 18F-Fluorodeoxyglucose PET/CT in the evaluation of large-vessel vasculitis: diagnostic performance and correlation with clinical and laboratory parameters. Papathanasiou ND, Du Y, Menezes LJ, Al-Muhaideb A, Shastry M, Beynon H, Bomanji JB. Br J Radiol. 2011 Mar 8. Epub DOI: 10.1259/bjr/16422950

1039. Combined PET and X-ray computed tomography imaging in pulmonary infections and inflammation. Bomanji J, Almuhaideb A, Zumla A. Curr Opin Pulm Med., 17(3), 197-205, 2011.

1040. "Partial volume correction in SPECT reconstruction with OSEM", Erlandsson K, Thomas B, Dickson J, Hutton BF. Nucl Instr Methods Phys Res A, 648, S85-88, 2011.

1041. Investigating Vulnerable Atheroma Using Combined 18F-FDG-PET/CT Angiography of Carotid Plaque with Immunohistochemical Validation. Menenzes L, Kotze CW, Endozo R, Rodriguez-Justo M, Yusuf SW, Groves AM. J Nucl Med., In Press, 2011.

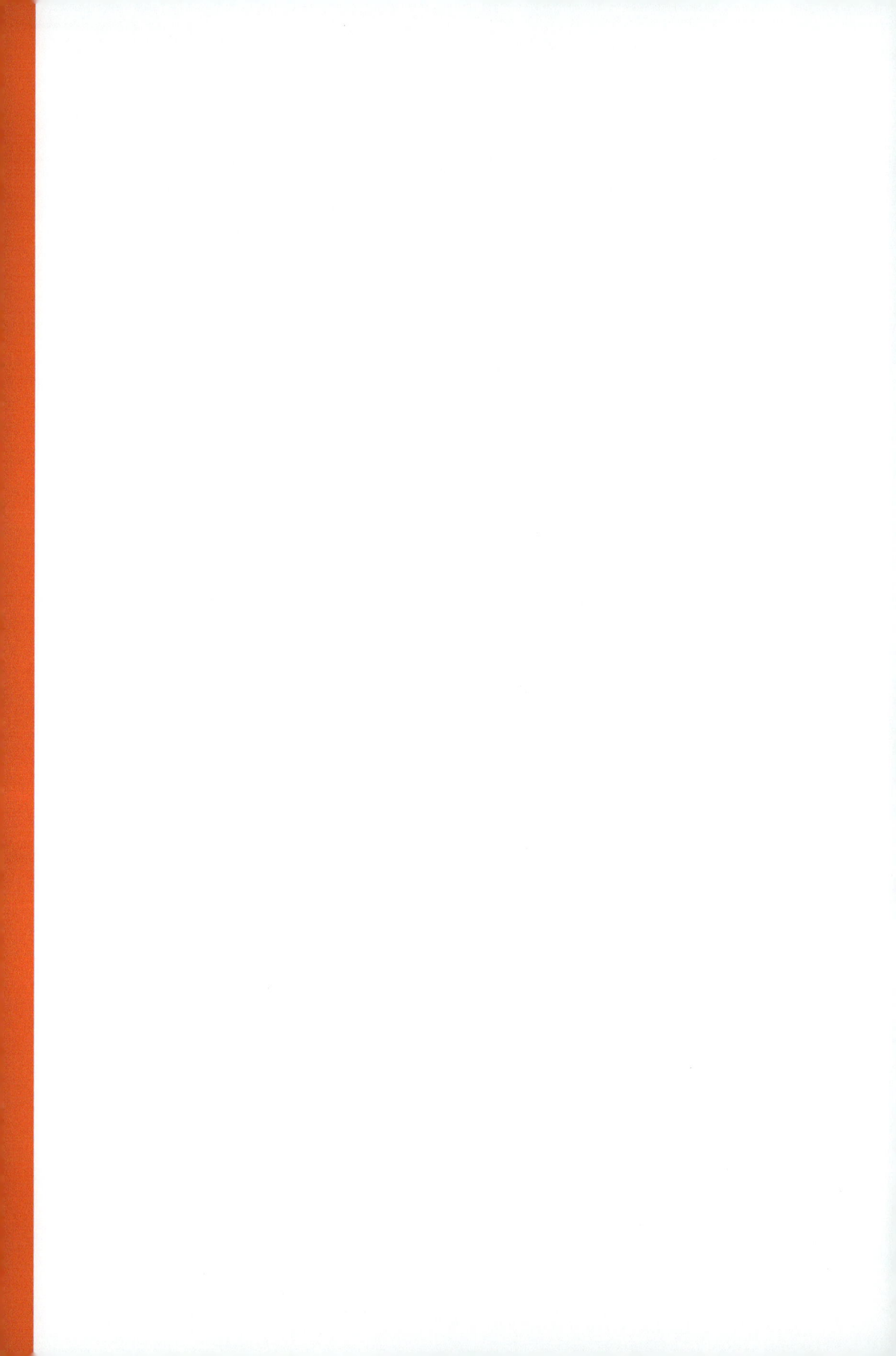

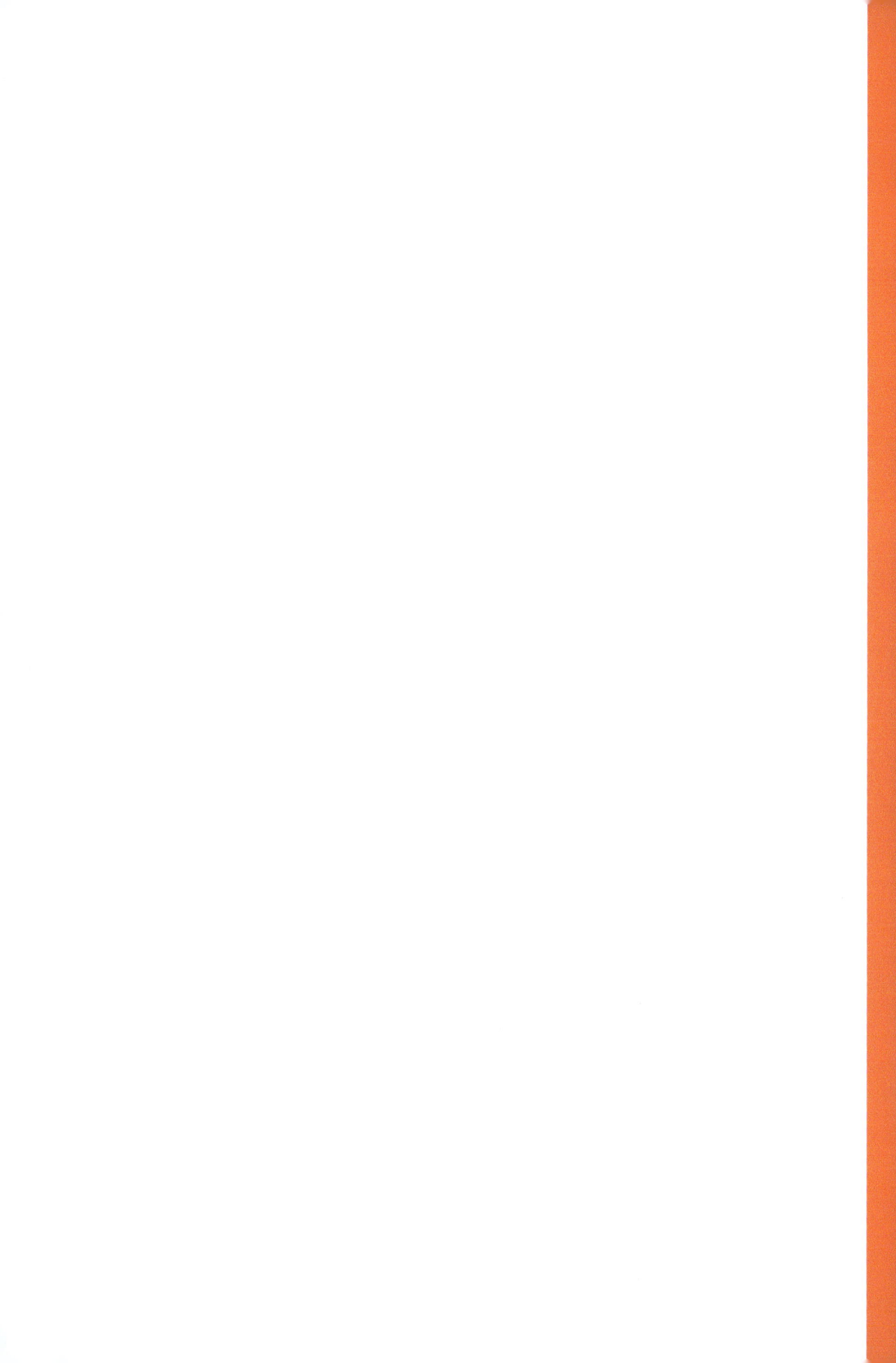

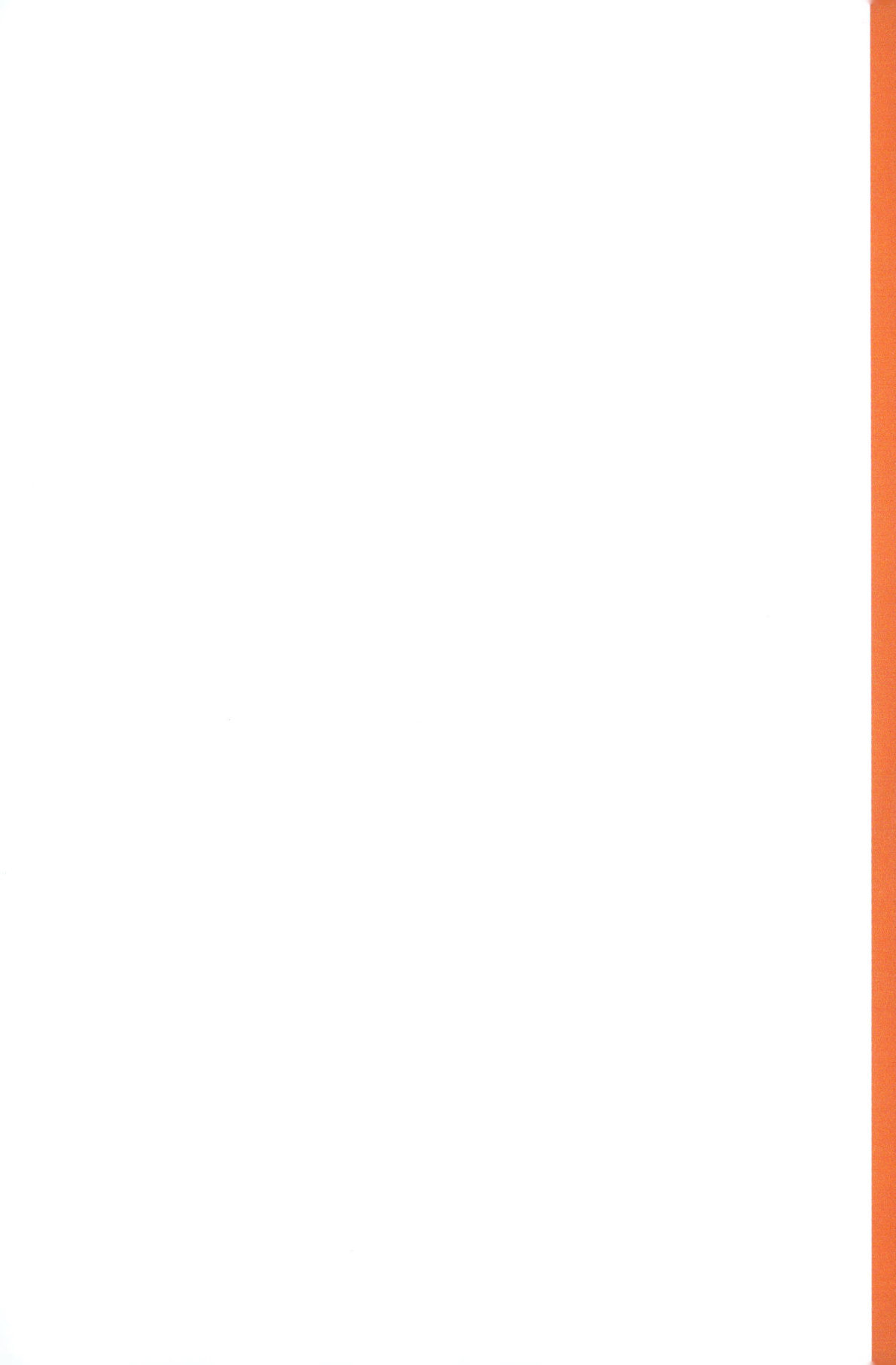

Printing: Ten Brink, Meppel, The Netherlands
Binding: Stürtz, Würzburg, Germany

GPSR Compliance

The European Union's (EU) General Product Safety Regulation (GPSR) is a set of rules that requires consumer products to be safe and our obligations to ensure this.

If you have any concerns about our products, you can contact us on ProductSafety@springernature.com

In case Publisher is established outside the EU, the EU authorized representative is:

Springer Nature Customer Service Center GmbH
Europaplatz 3
69115 Heidelberg, Germany

Batch number: 09635259

Printed by Printforce, the Netherlands